Workbook for Egan's Fundamentals of Respiratory Care

Tenth Edition

Stephen F. Wehrman, RRT, RPFT, AE-C
Professor/Program Director
Respiratory Care Program
Kapi'olani Community College
University of Hawaii
Honolulu, Hawaii

with 44 illustrations

3251 Riverport Lane
St. Louis, Missouri 63043

WORKBOOK FOR EGAN'S FUNDAMENTALS OF RESPIRATORY CARE, TENTH EDITION

ISBN: 978-0-323-08202-0

Notice

Knowledge and best practice in this field are constantly changing. As new research and experience broaden our understanding, changes in research methods, professional practices, or medical treatment may become necessary.

Practitioners and researchers must always rely on their own experience and knowledge in evaluating and using any information, methods, compounds, or experiments described herein. In using such information or methods they should be mindful of their own safety and the safety of others, including parties for whom they have a professional responsibility.

With respect to any drug or pharmaceutical products identified, readers are advised to check the most current information provided (i) on procedures featured or (ii) by the manufacturer of each product to be administered, to verify the recommended dose or formula, the method and duration of administration, and contraindications. It is the responsibility of practitioners, relying on their own experience and knowledge of their patients, to make diagnoses, to determine dosages and the best treatment for each individual patient, and to take all appropriate safety precautions.

To the fullest extent of the law, neither the Publisher nor the authors, contributors, or editors, assume any liability for any injury and/or damage to persons or property as a matter of products liability, negligence or otherwise, or from any use or operation of any methods, products, instructions, or ideas contained in the material herein.

Content Manager: Billie Sharp
Senior Content Development Specialist: Kathleen Sartori
Content Coordinator: Andrea Hunolt
Publishing Services Managers: Catherine Jackson/Hemamalini Rajendrababu
Senior Project Managers: Rachel E. McMullen/Srividhya Vidhyashankar
Design Direction: Amy Buxton

Printed in the United States

Last digit is the print number: 9 8 7 6 5 4 3 2 1

This book is dedicated to Jessica Michiko Chow Wehrman
She is my inspiration to write and the best daughter
any dad could hope to love.

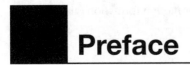

Preface

EAGER FOR EGAN's!
"Anyone who keeps learning stays young."
Henry Ford

Dear Student:

The year was 1977. I had just started school to become a respiratory technician. My first textbook was *Egan's Fundamentals of Respiratory Therapy*. I have to confess that I had to read everything three times to understand it. Egan's really bent my brain out of shape! I was really glad to graduate and be done with the difficult task of understanding that book. When I began teaching, there was Egan's waiting for me. A new edition and a new challenge to help students make the most of a book that is full of everything you need to know to prepare for this exciting career.

The problem for all health students is information overload. This is just as true for teachers as it is for anyone else. It is just as true for you today as it was for me 35 years ago. This workbook will help you learn and help you sort out the important information you will need to succeed in practice and to pass your credentialing exams.

If you want to get the most out of this book and the textbook, here's what you should do. First, read the assigned chapter in *Egan's*. I read lightly and quickly using a highlighter to touch on key points. Next, open the workbook and *Egan's* and go through the chapter answering the questions. I suggest you get in the habit of noting the page numbers where you find answers. The Answer Key can be found on the Evolve site.

At the end of the chapters you will find questions written in the same style as your NBRC examinations. You'll also find cases, exercises, and internet tools. When you graduate and prepare for your credentialing examinations, you'll find *Egan's Fundamentals* and this workbook waiting to help you succeed.

Learning how to be a Respiratory Therapist is a challenging, fun, difficult, and sometimes painful experience. Don't ever give up along the way. Your instructors, textbooks, and clinical faculty are all there to help you succeed. You've chosen a dynamic and exciting field that will always keep you on your toes and give you a feeling of pride and satisfaction in helping people breathe better.

I want to add that no book is merely the invention of the author. A lot of people are involved in creating a text. I especially want to thank my editor Ms. Kathleen Sartori for her work on this edition. Her insight, encouragement, and skill have brought you a powerful learning tool.

Aloha,
Stephen

P.S. Want to talk? Your feedback, questions, or comments are always welcome at wehrman@hawaii.edu. I am always glad to help you if you get stuck!

ADDITIONAL LEARNING AIDS

Mosby's Respiratory Care Online

This web-delivered course supplement, available as a separate purchase, has been carefully designed to reinforce the learning and synthesis of the concepts presented in the text through a range of visual, auditory, and interactive elements.

This unique program offers additional learning opportunities while accommodating different learning styles and environments. The online course features:

- Animations, slideshows, videos—with audio narration!
- Image enlarge function
    - Interactive learning activities: labelling, fill-in, sequencing, short answer, matching, image association, and more!
- Mini Clini Challenges with representative patient photos and simulated patient data records
- Special Features: **Formulas** that are organized by content area and printable, and a comprehensive **Glossary** that includes audio pronunciations
- Breath sounds are included in some activities
- Ventilator graphics accompany many modules
- Module exam are written in NBRC exam format; automatically scored and reported to the instructor grade book
- And much more!

This online course supplement is only accessible with purchase of an access code. For more information, visit http://evolve.elsevier.com/Egans/

Evolve Resources—http://evolve.elsevier.com/Egans/

Evolve is an interactive learning environment designed to work in coordination with *Egan's Fundamentals of Respiratory Care*. It contains the following for students:

- A detailed cross-reference of the content in *Egan's* to the National Board for Respiratory Care (NBRC) matrices for the certified respiratory therapist (CRT) and registered respiratory therapist (RRT) credentialing examinations: This handy reference will help you use Egan's to prepare for the credentialing exams.
- Student lecture notes. Students can choose to print these and can make notations when following along with our Instructor-only PowerPoint chapter presentation.

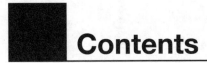

Contents

History of Respiratory Care

It is history that teaches us to hope.
General Robert E. Lee

Respiratory therapists today have a lot more evidence to help guide them toward effective and efficient practice. The rapid shallow breathing index, for example, makes it easier to identify which patients are ready to breathe again on their own. In Chapter 1, we take a look at the past with an eye toward the future. Pay special attention to the descriptions of the profession, basic areas of care, and milestones that mark the path to respiratory therapists' expanded role in disease management and acute cardiopulmonary care.

WORD WIZARD

Getting to know the terminology of medicine can be a challenge. Each chapter in this workbook starts off with some word work to help you learn to "talk the talk" of a professional respiratory therapist.

Match the following terms to their definitions.

Definitions	Terms
_____ 1. caregiver who acts as a physician extender after receiving additional education	A. AARC
_____ 2. national professional association for respiratory care	B. CoARC
_____ 3. health care discipline that specializes in the promotion of optimum cardiopulmonary health	C. NBRC
_____ 4. name suggesting increased involvement in disease prevention and management and promotion of health and wellness	D. cardiopulmonary system E. respiratory care F. respiratory therapy G. respiratory therapist(s)
_____ 5. one of the primary treatments for asthma uses this method of delivery	H. oxygen therapy I. aerosol medications
_____ 6. widely prescribed in hospitals by the 1940s and still a mainstay of respiratory care	J. mechanical ventilation K. airway management
_____ 7. organization responsible for the respiratory credentialing examinations	L. pulmonary function testing M. physician assistant
_____ 8. iron lung is an example of this therapy that helps patients who cannot breathe	N. respiratory care practitioner(s)
_____ 9. professional organization that accredits respiratory care schools and programs	
_____ 10. heart and lungs working together is the "bread and butter" of our profession	
_____ 11. method to test the ways that height, age, obesity, and disease alter lung function	

_____ 12. another name for the RT is this more formal term

_____ 13. individual trained to deliver care to patients with heart and lung disease

_____ 14. relieving obstruction is the key to this respiratory procedure

MEET THE OBJECTIVES

Chapter 1 presented four main objectives for learning. Test how well you understand these mysteries of history by providing short answers.

15. Define the respiratory care profession in your own words. Include at least three main concepts. How did the profession get started? Why are we here?

16. Respiratory care has three main professional associations. Describe the role and write out the full name for:
    A. CoARC

    Full name _____

    Role _____
    B. NBRC

    Full name _____

    Role _____
    C. AARC

    Full name _____

    Role _____

17. Describe how RT schools got started. What kinds of programs do they have now? How is this different from the early days?

18. Name three major events in the history of science and medicine that were foundations for respiratory physics or physiology.

A.

B.

C.

SUMMARY CHECKLIST

19. Respiratory therapists apply scientific principles to _____, identify,

and _____ dysfunction of the cardiopulmonary system.

20. The _____ is the professional organization for the field. It was started in _____

and was called _____ .

21. The iron lung was used extensively during the _____ epidemics of the 1940s and 1950s.

22. In the future, there will be a(n) _____ in demand for respiratory care due to advances in

_____ and increases in _____ of the population.

FOOD FOR THOUGHT

The associate degree is the entry point into the respiratory care profession, as the authors make clear. These days, if you want to advance your career and be competitive with similar medical professionals, you will need more education.

23. Describe at least four careers that would open up for you as a result of baccalaureate or graduate education.

A. _____

B. _____

C. _____

D. _____

24. Heroes are found in history. Name three important historical figures in respiratory care. Pick one, and briefly explain how this person might inspire you in your career!

2 Quality and Evidence-Based Respiratory Care

Mediocrity killed the cat.
Forrest Gump

Everyone expects quality, from the goods we buy to the services we receive. Health care is no different. You want to work for a quality-oriented organization. You try to deliver quality care to your patients. Patients expect to be treated by qualified providers and to receive the best care at all times. In Chapter 2 we look at what quality means in the health care setting and at specific ways we can monitor and achieve quality in the respiratory care profession. We also look at the trend toward using evidence-based methods for determining best practices in our profession.

WORD WIZARD

The Key terms in Chapter 2 are more complicated because they describe organizations, methods for disease management, and outcome monitoring.

Increase your understanding by matching the terms below to the Big Ideas.

Word

Big Idea

1. CoARC   _____ Responsible for quality of credentialing exams

2. The Joint Commission   _____ Responsible for quality of schools

3. Evidence-based medicine   _____ Uses meta-analyses to find best care

4. NBRC   _____ Uses site visits to check quality of care

MEET THE OBJECTIVES

Chapter 2 presented five main objectives for learning. How well do you understand these important ideas about delivering the best care? Fill in your answers in the space provided.

5. Providing quality care to the patient involves many dimensions. Name at least three elements that are part of quality respiratory care.

    A. _____

    B. _____

    C. _____

6. Quality must be monitored to ensure it is being obtained. Give an example of each main monitoring strategy.

    A. _____

    B. _____

7. How can protocols enhance the quality of respiratory care services? Support your answer with evidence from the text.

8. What are the four essential components of a disease management programs?

   A. _____

   B. _____

   C. _____

   D. _____

9. Evidence-based medicine specifies precise methods for analyzing data and making decisions. Explain how this method was used to treat ARDS. Be sure to include the ARDSNet study.

SUMMARY CHECKLIST

Identify eight key points from Chapter 2. Complete the following statements by writing the correct term(s) in the blank(s) provided.

10. Educated _____ respiratory care personnel are crucial elements for providing quality care.

11. Ordering too many respiratory care services is called _____ and hinders delivery of quality care.

12. Specific guidelines for delivering appropriate respiratory care services are called _____.

13. The _____ respiratory therapist is the highest credential in the profession.

14. Respiratory care credentialing examinations are administered by the _____.

15. Maintaining and improving quality require ongoing _____ and repeated _____ testing of the RTs.

16. Evidence suggests that the use of _____ can improve allocation of services.

17. An approach to determining optimal patient management based on research _____- _____ medicine.

Case 1

A 25-year-old woman has returned to a medical/surgical nursing unit following an appendectomy. She has no history of lung disease and is wearing a nasal cannula delivering oxygen at 3 L/min. She is alert and oriented, with a respiratory rate of 18 breaths/min and a heart rate of 82 beats/min. Her SpO$_2$ (pulse oximeter reading) is 99% on the nasal cannula. Her physician orders "respiratory therapy protocol," and you are asked to assess this patient.

Use the protocol found in Figure 2-2 in the text to help you answer the following questions.

18. What are the clinical signs of hypoxia/hypoxemia? Name at least three.

    A. _____

    B. _____

    C. _____

19. Using the oxygen therapy protocol, determine if the oxygen therapy is appropriate for this patient. Support your answer with information from the textbook.

20. What action would you recommend at this time?

Case 2

A 54-year-old man with a history of asthma and cigarette smoking was admitted to the hospital for a hernia repair. Following the procedure, his chest radiograph shows elevated diaphragms with bilateral atelectasis. Vital capacity is acceptable, but the patient is unable to hold his breath. The pulse oximetry reading is 95% on room air. His heart rate is 84 beats/min, blood pressure 110/78 mm Hg, respiratory rate 17 breaths/min, and temperature 36.8° C. Breath sounds are decreased bilaterally with apical wheezes. He has a weak nonproductive cough. The patient is alert and oriented.

21. Use the algorithm in Figure 2-1 to determine how to give this patient his medications. If you've never used an algorithm before, it may be useful to write out the steps in your path. Start with "Is the patient alert?" and put your answer in Step 1.

    Step 1 _____

    Step 2 _____

    Step 3 _____

    Step 4 _____

Respiratory therapists routinely plan, deliver, and assess the effects of care!

The National Board for Respiratory Care (NBRC) expects you to be able to participate in the development of care plans. You might expect to see five questions on this area in the Entry-Level Examination. Following are questions that are similar in style to the ones on the boards for practice. If you are a beginner, you will need to look up the therapeutic interventions and disease management options in other parts of your text.

Circle the best answer for the following multiple choice questions.

22. A patient with chronic obstructive pulmonary disease complains of difficulty breathing when he is ambulating. His SpO_2 is 88% at rest. Which of the following would you recommend?
    A. oxygen therapy
    B. PEEP therapy
    C. antibiotic therapy
    D. aerosolized bronchodilator therapy

23. An alert 18-year-old patient is admitted with difficulty breathing. A diagnosis of asthma is determined, and you are asked to instruct the patient in the use of an MDI. An MDI is a device used for
    A. oxygen therapy
    B. PEEP therapy
    C. antibiotic therapy
    D. aerosolized bronchodilator therapy

24. A patient with pneumonia is receiving oxygen via nasal cannula at 2 L/min. The SpO_2 is 89%, heart rate is 110 beats/min, and respiratory rate is 24 breaths/min. Which of the following would you recommend?
    A. Increase the liter-per-minute flow to the cannula.
    B. Intubate and begin mechanical ventilation.
    C. Initiate aerosolized bronchodilator therapy.
    D. Initiate postural drainage.

FOOD FOR THOUGHT

25. Protocol-based therapy and quality assurance efforts do not always work! Discuss some of the reasons you think these two strategies might fail.

26. Evidence-based medicine (EBM) uses meta-analysis. What does this term mean? Why is meta-analysis different than standard reviews of literature? Is it better?

3 Patient Safety, Communication, and Recordkeeping

So, our prime purpose in this life is to help others. And if you can't help them, at least don't hurt them.

Dalai Lama

Chapter 3 combines a huge amount of information that can be hard to swallow all at once. Let's break this down into bite-sized pieces, and you see if you can digest the material.

WORD WIZARD

Read Chapter 3 in your textbook, and see if you can fill in the missing words.

You'll Get a Charge out of This

The medical center is filled with electrical equipment. The flow of electricity is called _____. Everything

has a three-prong plug. The third prong is the neutral wire, or _____, which helps prevent electrocution. For this reason, no outside electrical devices are allowed in the hospital unless they are checked by the biomedical

staff. Electrocution can occur in the form of a(n) _____ shock. This might happen if you are standing on a wet floor and a power cord fell onto the floor. Many of the power cords are detachable, so this is a potential hazard. Always clean up spills.

A small shock, or _____ shock, is a hazard to patients who have pacemakers, ECG leads, and indwelling

heart catheters. This may result in ventricular fibrillation and death! This could happen if the _____ wire gets broken, so don't ever roll beds or other equipment over the electrical power cords. Report frayed cords, and take suspect equipment out of use.

Burn, Baby, Burn

Because high oxygen concentrations are used in respiratory care, fire is a real hazard.

Even though oxygen is _____ and does not burn, it greatly speeds up an existing fire. In fact, oxygen is

necessary for fires to exist. For a fire to start, you also need _____ material, and heat. Remove any of these

three, and the fire will go out. You must make sure that ignition sources such as _____ are not allowed when oxygen is in use. Most hospitals will call a "Code Red" if a fire exists, and you must respond. One of the respiratory therapist's responsibilities in a fire is to shut off the zone valve to the affected area if the fire is near a patient using oxygen. (See Chapter 37: Storage and Delivery of Medical Gases.)

KEEP IT MOVING!

Anyone who stays immobile in a bed for too long will suffer consequences. You need to ambulate the patient as soon as he or she is stable.

Here are some guidelines for safe ambulation. Number them 1 through 7 in the right order.

_____ Dangle the patient.

_____ Sit them up.

_____ Assist to a standing position.

_____ Encourage slow, easy breathing.

_____ Lower the bed, and lock the wheels.

_____ Move the IV pole close to the patient.

_____ Provide support while walking.

9

I CAN'T HEAR YOU

Communication plays a big part in your ability to gain patient cooperation, evaluate progress, and make recommendations for care. What you do (nonverbal) is just as important as what you say (verbal). Communication will also play a role in your satisfaction on the job. Exchanging information and working out problems with other members of the health care team are an everyday part of hospital life.

MEET THE OBJECTIVES

Chapter 3 presents 16 objectives for learning. We've already covered some of them. How well do you understand safety and communication? Fill in your answers in the spaces provided.

1. Name at least three risks that are common among patients receiving respiratory care.

   A. _____

   B. _____

   C. _____

2. Describe two problems of bed rest and two benefits of ambulation.

   A. _____

   B. _____

3. What is the main reason you should use good body mechanics?

   _____

4. State at least two factors you should monitor during patient ambulation. (There are a total of five!)

   A. _____

   B. _____

5. Name at least four of the many factors that influence the communication process.

   A. _____

   B. _____

   C. _____

   D. _____

6. The text lists five ways to improve your effectiveness as a sender of messages. Describe two of these that apply to you. Give examples of situations where you communicated well (or not!).

   I need to improve in...

   A. _____

   B. _____

Give an example of good communication.

Give an example of unsuccessful communication.

7. Name four sources of conflict in health care organizations. Give an example of each.

   A. _____

   B. _____

   C. _____

   D. _____

8. What is a medical record? Who owns the record? Who is allowed to read it?

9. State one legal and one practical essential of recordkeeping.

   A. _____

   B. _____

10. One of the most common formats that respiratory therapists (and others) use in charting is the SOAP format. What does SOAP mean? Give examples of information you would chart for each category.

	MEANING	EXAMPLE
S		
O		
A		
P		

SUMMARY CHECKLIST

Identify eight key points from Chapter 3. Complete the following statements by writing the correct term(s) in the blank(s) provided.

11. You should begin _____ as soon as a patient is stable.

12. A(n) _____ is a small current that enters the body through external catheters and may cause ventricular fibrillation.

Chapter **3** **Patient Safety, Communication,and Recordkeeping**

13. Prevent electrical shocks by always _____ your equipment.

14. You can minimize fire hazards by removing flammable materials and ignition sources from areas where

_____ is in use.

15. _____ skills play a key role in your ability to achieve desired patient outcomes.

16. Accommodating, avoiding, collaborating, competing, and compromising are basic strategies for handling

_____.

17. A medical record is a _____ document.

18. You must _____ each treatment, medication, or procedure you provide.

CASE STUDIES

Case 1

The physician orders ambulation for a patient who is receiving oxygen. The nurse asks you to assist. The patient is in bed wearing a nasal cannula running at 2 L/min.

19. What equipment will you need *before* you try to walk with this patient?

_____

_____

After 5 minutes of walking, you notice that the patient is breathing at a rate of 24 breaths/min and using his accessory muscles of ventilation. His skin appears sweaty, and he is exhaling through pursed lips.

20. What observations are important to note in this situation? What action would you take?

Case 2

You are caring for a patient who is on a mechanical ventilator. You need to transport the patient to radiology for a CT scan. The nurse unplugs the IV pump and pulse oximeter from the *back* of each unit. The pumps and the pulse oximeter are now running on their battery systems. As you prepare to leave, you notice that the power cords are still plugged into the wall outlets. The physician and the nurse are anxious to get the transport under way.

21. Describe the actions you would take if you encountered this situation.

22. What potential conflict/communication problems exist? How will you deal with them?

WHAT DOES THE NBRC SAY?

By now you should be asking the question, "Does any of this apply to my board examinations?" The answer is yes and no. Fire and electrical safety do not appear on the exam, they are just practical things a respiratory therapist should know. However, the content outline for the board exams in Section III, Therapeutic Procedures, with "Maintain Records and Communicate Information" includes:

- **Explain** therapy to patients in terms they can understand.
- **Document** a treatment correctly.
- **Note responses** to therapy—includes vital signs, adverse reactions, and so on; but it also includes interpreting subjective and attitudinal response to therapy!
- **Verify computations** and correct errors.
- **Communicate clinical information** to other health care practitioners.
- **Communicate to avoid conflicts**, maintain scheduling and sequencing of treatments.
- **Communicate results of therapy** and alter therapy per protocols.
- **Counsel patient and family** about smoking cessation/disease management.

You should expect seven questions on this specific material on the certified respiratory therapist (CRT) examination and five harder ones about the same material on the written registry examination (WRE).

Try a few problems in board exam style. Circle the best answer for the following multiple choice questions.

23. A respiratory therapist has completed SOAP charting in the progress notes following a bronchodilator treatment. While signing the chart form, she notices that the wrong amount for the medication has been entered. Which of the following actions should be done at this time?
    1. Draw one line through the error.
    2. Notify the physician of the error.
    3. Write "Error" and initial.
    4. Recopy the progress notes.
       A. 1 and 2
       B. 1 and 3
       C. 2 and 4
       D. 3 and 4

24. An asthmatic patient has orders for albuterol by medication nebulizer every 2 hours. During the shift, the patient improves, and the order is changed to every 4 hours. In regard to the new frequency, what action should you take?
    1. Note the change in your charting.
    2. Inform the registered nurse of the order.
    3. Frequency will change on the next shift.
       A. 1 and 2
       B. 1 and 3
       C. 2 and 3
       D. 1, 2, and 3

25. A patient's heart rate increases from 88 to 134 beats/min following a breathing treatment. After reassuring the patient, the respiratory therapist should
    A. discontinue the therapy
    B. reduce the dosage of the medication
    C. place the patient on oxygen
    D. notify the physician

Chapter **3** **Patient Safety, Communication, and Recordkeeping**

FOOD FOR THOUGHT

Every year people die in work-related fires and electrocutions. The hospital can be a busy, stressful environment, and it is easy to skip some of the steps in the safety process. That is one of the reasons the Occupational Safety and Health Administration (OSHA) requires health care institutions to train workers in fire, electrical, blood-borne pathogen, back injury, and other safety areas *every year!*

26. What do you think is the most common type of injury in health care? _____

_____

27. On what shift do most injuries, accidents, and patient incidents occur? _____

_____

4 Principles of Infection Prevention and Control

The doctor is to be feared more than the disease.
Latin proverb

Nobody comes to the hospital to get sick! But let's face it, 5% to 10% of all the patients who enter a hospital get an infection while they are there. To make matters worse, up to 40% of these infections involve the respiratory system. It costs billions of dollars to treat patients with hospital-acquired illnesses, and even more to pay for lost work time. Patients are not the only ones who get sick. Each year, thousands of health care practitioners are exposed to "bugs" like hepatitis, HIV, and TB (or, worse, SARS), and some of them will be infected. Fortunately, there are plenty of simple, easy ways you can protect yourself and the patients.

WORD WIZARD

Chapter 4 introduces a lot of new terms that you should know if you want to be able to beat bacteria and viruses. After you read about this timely topic, you will be able to make these key definitions match up.

Definitions	Terms
_____ infections that are acquired in the hospital	A. fomites
_____ inanimate objects that help transfer pathogens	B. nosocomial
_____ death of all microorganisms	C. sterilization
_____ universal method of protection for health workers	D. disinfection
_____ death of pathogenic microorganisms	E. standard precautions

MEET THE OBJECTIVES

Chapter 4 presented 10 objectives for learning. How well do you understand these important ideas about infection control? Fill in your answers in the spaces provided.

1. What is a health care–associated infection (HAI)? How many people get sick?

   A. HAI = _____

   B. How many get sick? _____ What percent of patients? _____

2. Why are HAIs important to our profession?

3. Name the three elements that are required for these infections to take place.

   A. _____

   B. _____

   C. _____

4. A susceptible host may be elderly, have HIV, or have chemotherapy, but we can still reduce host susceptibility by focusing on employees and chemoprophylaxis. Name five vaccinations that might help you decrease the risk.

   A. _____

   B. _____

   C. _____

   D. _____

   E. _____

5. Respiratory therapists must know about the routes of transmission of disease so we can avoid infection. What are the three **major** routes? Give an example of each.

	ROUTE	EXAMPLE
A		
B		
C		

6. Interrupting the route of transmission involves special equipment processing. What is the first step in cleaning equipment that is going to be resterilized after a critical procedure like bronchoscopy?

7. State the six methods of sterilization. For each method, give an example of applicable equipment to be sterilized. Refer to Table 4-5 in your text if you get lost.

	METHOD	EQUIPMENT
A.		
B.		
C.		
D.		
E.		
F.		

8. You will need to decide how to clean the RT equipment. Use the Mini-Clini on "Selection of Equipment Processing Methods" of your text to help decide how to clean and sterilize these items:

ITEM	DISINFECT	STERILIZE
A. Laryngoscope blade		
B. Humidifier		
C. Mechanical ventilator		

9. List the three general barrier methods used to prevent exposure to organisms. Describe a situation or an organism where you need this type of protection as a respiratory therapist.

A. _____

B. _____

C. _____

SUMMARY CHECKLIST

Identify the key points from Chapter 4. Complete the following statements by writing the correct term(s) in the blank(s) provided.

10. _____ is the best choice for high-level disinfection of semicritical respiratory care equipment.

11. Among respiratory care equipment, _____ have the greatest potential to spread infection.

12. Always use _____ fluids for tracheal suctioning and to fill nebulizers and humidifiers.

13. Thoroughly _____ your _____ after any patient contact, even when gloves are used.

14. Use standard (universal) precautions in caring for _____ patients, regardless of their diagnosis or infection status.

15. Wear _____ and _____ during any procedure that can generate splashes or sprays of body fluids.

16. The use of _____ is part of routine care when there is skin contact.

17. Ventilator circuits may be used up to _____ days before they need to be changed.

Chapter **4** **Principles of Infection Prevention and Control**

Case 1

You work in the surgical intensive care unit (ICU) of a large urban hospital. Over the past 2 days, a number of patients in the unit have developed serious *Staphylococcus aureus* infections.

18. Why do postoperative patients have an increased risk of infection?

19. What is the most common source of *S. aureus* organisms? _____

_____

20. Identify three ways to disrupt the route of transmission in this situation.

  A. _____

  B. _____

  C. _____

Case 2

During your third day of clinical, you are assigned to go with a therapist who has an extremely heavy workload on a medical floor of the hospital. The therapist puts on gloves for each patient contact, and asks you to do so also. When you go to wash your hands after the first treatment, the therapist tells you, "We don't have time for that, and besides the gloves will keep our hands clean."

21. Explain the role of gloves in protecting practitioners and preventing the spread of infection.

22. What does the CDC say about cleaning your hands in regard to washing? Are there any alternatives?

Chapter **4** **Principles of Infection Prevention and Control**

A serious tuberculosis outbreak occurs in a local prison facility. You are called to the emergency department as four of the sickest patients are being admitted together to your hospital for treatment.

23. By what route does tuberculosis spread?

24. When transporting these patients out of the emergency department, what action should you take?

25. What kind of precautions should be taken to prevent the spread of infection once these patients are admitted?

26. What special guidelines exist in regard to cough-inducing and aerosol-generating procedures for patients with active tuberculosis?

27. What other concerns do you have in working with these patients?

28. What should you do if enough private rooms are not available with airborne precautions for this group of patients?

Chapter **4** **Principles of Infection Prevention and Control**

Your board exams will place an emphasis on infection control. The Entry-Level Examination Matrix says:
"Will assure selected equipment cleanliness" and
1. Choose the right method or agent for disinfection and sterilization.
2. Perform disinfection and sterilization procedures.
3. Monitor sterilization effectiveness.
4. Protect the patient from nosocomial infection.
5. Follow infection control policies and procedures.

Following are some questions like the ones you might see on the test. Here they are in the form of a single case, but they will normally be spread throughout the exam. In general, students learn about this early in their training and tend to forget for the boards, so be sure to review this topic!

Circle the best answer for the following multiple-choice questions.

The following questions refer to this situation:
A 72-year-old female patient with COPD has a tracheostomy tube in place following prolonged intubation and mechanical ventilation. She is currently in the medical intensive care unit. After you take her off the ventilator, you will need to set up a heated aerosol system with an FiO_2 of 40%.

29. What type of water should be placed in the nebulizer?
    A. distilled water
    B. tap water
    C. normal saline solution
    D. sterile distilled water

30. To help lower the risk of a nosocomial infection when using heated aerosol systems, the respiratory therapist should do which of the following?
    1. Label the equipment with the date and time it is started.
    2. Avoid draining the tubing to prevent contamination.
    3. Use aseptic technique during the initial setup.
    4. Use a filter or heat and moisture exchanger (HME) to reduce airborne bacteria.
        A. 1 and 3
        B. 1 and 2
        C. 2 and 4
        D. 3 and 4

31. The best way to prevent the spread of infection in the ICU is to
    A. ensure that sterilized equipment is used
    B. wash your hands after every patient contact
    C. wear gloves when you come in contact with body fluids
    D. isolate infected patients

FOOD FOR THOUGHT

Because many hospitalized patients acquire respiratory infections, the respiratory therapist is really under a microscope at work. We have to maintain the highest standards of behavior to protect ourselves, our patients, and our loved ones.

32. One of your fellow students comes to clinical with a cold. He asks you not to tell your clinical instructor, because missed clinical days are hard to make up. What is your reaction to this situation? What are the potential problems with this scenario?

33. The college recommends that you get immunized against hepatitis B before attending clinical. The consent form lists a number of possible side effects of the vaccine, and the vaccination is expensive. What are the pros and cons of vaccines? What will you choose?

34. What is respiratory etiquette? Can you name the five elements?

5 Ethical and Legal Implications of Practice

Ignorance of the law excuses no one from practicing it.
A. Mizner

Malpractice is a word that strikes fear into the hearts of physicians. We live in a society where lawsuits are commonplace; you hear about them every day. Do respiratory therapists ever get sued? You bet they do. To make matters worse, the ethical issues that are always present in health care are crossing into the legal arena more and more. Should we terminate life support? How can health services be rationed? What if the patient cannot afford the care? Your two safeguards are knowledge and good defensive recordkeeping. Chapter 5 gives you the tools you need to provide care with confidence.

WORD WIZARD

Law, like medicine, has a language of its own that most people do not understand. (Shakespeare said, "It was Greek to me.") You will need clear comprehension of some basic legal terminology to avoid ending up in court. For these words, let's skip the ethics and go directly to legal issues in your text. Complete the following paragraphs by writing in the correct terms in the blanks provided.

The two basic types of law in the United States are public and civil law. Public law is further divided into adminis-

trative law and _____ law. Health care facilities operate under a mountain of regulations set by

government agencies. Private, or _____, law protects citizens who feel they have been harmed.

The individual who brings a complaint is called the _____, and those accused of wrongdoing are

known as _____. A(n) _____ is a civil wrong. These cases could easily

involve a health care practitioner. There are three types. _____ is the failure to perform your duties competently. Cases in which the patient falls, is given the wrong medication, or is harmed by equipment revolve around a provider's duty to anticipate harm and prevent it from happening.

Expert testimony, professional guidelines, or even circumstantial evidence can determine what a reasonable and pru-

dent respiratory therapist would have done in a given situation. The Latin term _____ ("the thing speaks for itself") is sometimes invoked to show that harm occurred because of inappropriate care. When a professional

fails to act skillfully, breaches ethics, or falls below a reasonable standard, it is called _____.

Wrongdoing may be considered intentional or unintentional. Intentional acts include _____, or

placing another person in fear of bodily harm, _____, or physical contact without consent. Other

common intentional harm occurs through _____, which is verbal defamation of character, and

_____, which is written defamation of character. Finally, information about patients is considered

private, or _____, and cannot be shared with anyone who is not involved in their care.
There are two good defenses against all of these problems. The first is to show that actions were not intentional. For example, fainting during a procedure is not a voluntary act. The second defense is to obtain consent from the patient. Consent, whether verbal or written, should be obtained from the patient for most procedures. Of course you have to explain the risks and the procedure in clear language the patient can understand.

Chapter 5 is packed with solid objectives. Meet them and you will have a strong ethical and legal foundation for practice.

1. The basis of ethics is found in philosophy and is a science in itself. What is the fundamental question of ethics?

2. What is the one primary purpose of a professional code of ethics?

3. Describe some of the information you might gather or consider before making a decision that involves ethics. For example, before discontinuing life support for a patient who is "brain dead," what might you consider?

4. Health care is constantly changing and evolving in ways that affect ethical and legal decision making. Please discuss one example, such as managed care, and briefly explain how this new kind of medicine might shape our choices.

CASE STUDIES

Be sure to look at the Mini-Clinis in this chapter.

Case 1

You get a chance to meet with your fellow students for lunch in the hospital cafeteria during a busy clinical day. One of your classmates is bursting with excitement as you sit down to eat. "You won't believe what I got to do today! I was taking care of Mr. Brainola, a patient in the intensive care unit (ICU), and he started to go bad, and we had to intubate. Then he coded, and I got to do CPR! It was so cool!"

5. What's the problem with this picture? What violation has your classmate committed?

6. What are the possible consequences of this scenario?

7. What action should you take?

8. Is this situation simply a breach of ethics or a violation of law?

Case 2

You receive an order to administer a bronchodilator to a 27-year-old asthmatic. The patient refuses the therapy, stating, "I just can't take any more of this today!" He appears alert and oriented.

9. Does the patient have a legal right to refuse in this case? Cite evidence from the text to justify your answer.

10. How would you respond to this situation?

11. What other action should you take at this time?

Chapter **5** **Ethical and Legal Implications of Practice**

After finishing with the previous patient, you receive a stat call to the orthopedic floor. The registered nurse informs you they are having problems with a 76-year-old woman who recently had surgical repair of a broken hip. As you enter the room, you notice that she has removed her oxygen mask. She is breathing rapidly, and her color is not good. The pulse oximeter shows a saturation of 84%. When you try to get the patient to wear the oxygen mask, she screams at you to get out of the room.

12. Does the patient have a legal right to refuse in this case? Cite evidence from the text to justify your answer.

13. How would you respond to this situation?

14. Would physical restraints be an option or a possible case of battery?

WHAT ABOUT ETHICS?

No, we haven't forgotten about ethics (although this subject *is* less clear-cut than the legal issues). The law sets minimum standards that we all must try to follow. Ethics, on the other hand, are a set of guidelines for doing your job in a way that is morally defensible. The problem is not that there are a lot of immoral people working in health care, but rather that ethical dilemmas cannot be avoided.

Start at the Beginning

The most famous ethical code in medicine is the Hippocratic Oath. Respiratory therapist's have a code of ethics that was developed by the AARC. You can find it on page 85 in *Egan's*.

Do No Harm versus Save Lives

When two or more "right" choices are in direct conflict, an ethical dilemma exists. A hot topic in medicine and government right now involves how we end our lives, or "assisted suicide." On one hand, we don't want people to suffer needlessly. Watching a terminally ill patient suffer is a sad and demoralizing experience for respiratory therapists. On the other hand, taking someone's life is an equally difficult decision with far-ranging consequences (some of which could be legal). Reducing these issues to simple rules and formulas is not easy, perhaps not even possible. Every ethical principle involves two parts: professional duty and patient rights.

Case 1

A 17-year-old male is admitted for pneumonia. This young man is depressed and has expressed thoughts of ending his life if "my worst fears are true about this illness." Laboratory studies reveal that the patient is HIV positive. His physician expresses concern to the other caregivers about revealing the patient's diagnosis to him.

15. Under what circumstances can you lie (or not tell the truth) to patients?

16. What are your feelings about telling the truth to patients?

17. What would you do if the patient asks you if he has AIDS?

Ethical Decision-Making Model

Let's apply the ethical decision-making model to Case 1 (see Box 5-2, in your text). Write your answer in the spaces provided.

18. What is the problem or issue in this case?

19. Who are the individuals involved?

20. What ethical principle(s) apply here?

21. Who should make the decision to tell the patient?

22. What is your role as a respiratory therapist who is giving treatments to this patient?

23. Are there short-term consequences to either decision? Long-term consequences?

24. Make the decision! (What would you do?)

25. How would you proceed after you made your choice?

A respiratory therapist who is a deeply religious individual has strong feelings about homosexuality. When he is assigned to provide therapy for an openly homosexual patient, he objects to the supervisor, saying, "I do not want to take care of him. It is against my religious principles. Assign someone else."

26. What are some of the possible problems for the respiratory department that could arise out of this situation?

27. Patients are allowed to refuse even life-sustaining treatment for religious reasons. What about professional caregivers?

28. What would you do if you were the supervisor?

I would rather be the man who bought the Brooklyn Bridge than the man who sold it.

Will Rogers

SUMMARY CHECKLIST

Identify seven key points from Chapter 5. Complete the following statements by writing the correct term(s) in the blank(s) provided.

29. Ethical _____ occur when there are two equally desirable or undesirable outcomes.

30. Professional codes of ethics are general guidelines to identify _____ behavior.

31. The two basic ethical theories are _____ and _____.

32. _____ law deals with the relationships of private parties and the government.

33. Professional _____ is negligence in which a professional has failed to provide the

    _____ expected, resulting in _____ to someone.

34. Practitioners must carry out their duties with an eye toward _____ themselves in the case

    of _____ action.

35. A(n) _____ act defines who can perform specified duties in health care. The purpose of

    _____ is to provide for the public's safety.

FOOD FOR THOUGHT

A law that affects all health care workers is called HIPAA. The Health Insurance Portability and Accountability Act of 1996 was not actually ready for enforcement until 2002. HIPAA provides for both civil and criminal penalties for violations. Respiratory therapist students can get into trouble in many ways besides simply breaching confidentiality, which is now a part of HIPAA.

Chapter **5** **Ethical and Legal Implications of Practice**

36. You are asked to do a clinical case study by your instructor. What is PHI? What things do you think you should take out of the case to avoid identifying the patient to others?

Patients are asked about their living will when admitted. Do you have a living will or advanced directive? Try asking around and see if your instructors or the respiratory therapists at clinic have one. You might be surprised....

37. What is the difference between advanced directives and a living will?

HIPAA may seem complicated, but the bottom line has never changed: Keep your lips zipped about the patients. Period.

6 Physical Principles of Respiratory Care

Mrs. Peter's Law:
Today if you're not confused you're just not thinking clearly.
Irene Peter

Physics is a subject that many struggle to understand. The purpose of this chapter is to help you figure out what is important and how to apply the information. You don't have to be a rocket scientist to understand the physical principles of respiratory care. We are applied scientists, after all, so the secret to physics is to find examples, analogies, and experiments that help you understand the rules and how to use them in the Respiratory World.

WORD WIZARD

Words are the keys that open up your mind so you can start to learn a difficult subject. After you read *Egan's*, you will be able to put the right words into the blanks. There's a lot to this chapter, so material you may need to know for work and your examinations will be emphasized.

Complete the following paragraph by writing the correct terms in the blanks provided.

Yes, but It's a Dry Heat

Without humidity, our airways get irritated and mucus gets thick and nasty. The actual amount, or weight, of water

vapor in a gas is called _____ humidity. As respiratory therapists, we compare the weight of water vapor to the amount it could hold if the gas was fully saturated. This ratio of content to capacity is known as

_____ humidity. You hear about this on the weather report every day. I'm more interested in how much vapor gas can hold inside the airways. This amount is called percent _____

humidity. When inspired gas has less than 100% of its capacity, a humidity _____ exists. Humidifiers are used to make up the difference. When you get a can of icy soda on a hot day, water droplets begin to form on the outside of the can. That's because the air around the can is cooling (everyone knows cold air does not hold as much water vapor as warm air). When air cools, and gaseous water returns to a liquid form, we say that

_____ has occurred. The opposite effect occurs when the drink sits out. Water molecules

escape from the liquid into the air. This process is called _____ and adds to the humidity in the air.

Some Like It Hot

Heat moves in mysterious ways—four of them, to be precise. Newborn babies are especially sensitive to heat loss. Keeping a preemie warm can make the difference between life and death! When babies are born, we dry them off to

prevent loss through _____.

Then the little one is wrapped in cloth to prevent _____, or loss that occurs when you are touching a cooler object. Finally, we put the tyke in an incubator. The incubator provides warmth in two ways. First,

a special light _____ heat toward the baby. Second, warm air blows into the incubator.

Transfer of heat through movement of fluids (or gas) is called _____.

1. Oxygen normally exists as a gas at sea level. What has to happen to turn gaseous oxygen into liquid oxygen for medical use?

2. What happens to the temperature when liquid oxygen is converted into gaseous oxygen?

3. Which temperature scale would a respiratory therapist be *least* likely to use clinically?

4. At sea level, what is the primary factor that determines the state of matter? Maybe you should use water as an example.

5. Liquid water can easily turn into its gaseous or vapor form. Water vapor content of gas is important for comfort and airway health. What factors affect the amount and rate of vaporization of water?

6. Explain why visible moisture, a mist, comes out when you exhale on a cold day. If you get stuck, look at Figure 6-13.

7. What is the general name of the laws that RTs have to know to predict how oxygen and nitrogen will behave when you heat them, cool them, or pressurize them in a cylinder?

8. Gases and liquids belong to the family called fluids. Just like plumbers need to know how liquids flow through pipes, we need to know how gases flow through tubes and airways. What is the name of the primary law that governs resistance, or opposition, to flow through the airway and the amount of pressure, or work, you have to perform to overcome resistance and move air in and out?

OBEY THE LAWS

Remember the bumper sticker: "Gravity: it's not just a good idea, it's the law!"? Gases have to follow the laws of physics, too. Because respiratory therapists work with different gases, like oxygen, nitrogen, carbon dioxide, and helium, it's important that you know the laws and how gases behave. This section provides some real examples of gas laws in action.

In the space provided, identify which law is being demonstrated. If you get stuck, go to Table 6-4 for the scoop on Boyle, Charles, and Gay-Lussac.

Example 1

A registered pulmonary function technologist (RPFT) is performing lung testing on a patient. The patient inhales 1.5 L from the spirometer.

9. What will happen to the volume of gas inside the patient's lungs? _____

_____

10. What is the gas law? _____

Example 2

A home care respiratory therapist places an oxygen cylinder in the van so that she can take it to a client's house. The sun is shining through the window on the cylinder.

11. What will happen to the pressure inside the cylinder as it gets warmer? _____

_____

12. What is the gas law? _____

Example 3

When you start to inhale, your diaphragm drops and your chest expands. In other words, you increase the size, or volume, of your chest.

13. What happens to the pressure inside your chest? _____

_____

14. What is the gas law? _____

TRY IT, YOU'LL LIKE IT!

Here are some safe, easy experiments you can perform in the lab at school or at home.

Experiment 1

Place a dry, empty *glass* soda bottle in the freezer for at least 15 minutes. Take the bottle out and *immediately* cover the mouth of the bottle with a balloon. Wait a few minutes and watch!

15. What happened to the balloon? _____

16. What gas law is responsible for the result? _____

Experiment 2

Cut a 1-inch strip of notebook paper. Hold one end of the paper to your chin, just below your lip. Blow steadily across the top of the paper.

17. What happened to the paper? _____

18. What principle is responsible for this action? _____

Another experiment that shows this same principle can be accomplished with balloons. Blow up two round balloons and tie them off. Attach about 1 foot of string to each balloon. Tape the string to a stick (like a ruler, or yardstick) so the balloons are about 6 to 8 inches apart. Blow between the balloons.

19. What happened to the balloons? _____

Experiment 3

Get a coffee stirrer, an ordinary straw, and a big straw (like the kind you use for a milkshake). Now get two cups. Put some water in one cup. Put some honey in another. Suck the water up through each straw. Now try the honey. To make this more interesting, get a 6-foot length of oxygen-connecting tubing. Try the two fluids again!

20. Which tube is easiest to suck through? _____

21. Which fluid is easiest to suck up? _____

22. What hard-to-pronounce, French-sounding law explains all this? _____

Experiment 4 (A virtual experiment)

If you had a teacher to supervise the situation, you could take an oxygen cylinder and put a regulator on it with a gauge to show pressure. You could measure the room temperature and record the pressure in the cylinder. *If* you put that cylinder out into the sun, it would get warm (don't do this, of course) and matter would be affected.

23. What do you predict would happen to the pressure in the cylinder?

24. What gas law explains the change? _____

25. Why don't we put cylinders out in the sun?

Experiment 5

Surface tension can be hard to grasp when you think of physics, but it is easy to see. Take a cup or glass and fill it with water up to the top. Slowly add more water until the cup is about to overflow. Observe the water surface as it sits slightly above the rim of the cup.

26. What law explains your ability to fill a cup above the rim without it overflowing?

_____

27. What is the name of the curved surface of the water?

_____

Experiment 6

Blow up one balloon with air. Fill the next one with water. Keep them small, about the size of your fist. Now try to squeeze the air-filled balloon. Next, try to squeeze the water-filled balloon.

28. Could you compress the water balloon in the same way as the air balloon?

_____

29. What physical difference between water and air explains this phenomenon?

_____

30. What law governs this phenomenon?

_____

Because gases and liquids are both fluids, the same rules apply to the inhaling!

CASE STUDIES

Case 1

A respiratory therapist decides to attend the AARC International Congress. To get there, the therapist must travel by air. Before taking off, the flight attendant explains about the oxygen system. The therapist pays attention (unlike everyone else) when he sees the partial rebreathing mask. He also knows that something interesting happens to oxygenation at 30,000 feet.

31. What is the barometric pressure (P_B) and inspired (PiO_2) partial pressure of oxygen at this altitude?

P_B _____

PiO_2 _____

32. A properly fitting oxygen mask can deliver about 70% oxygen to passengers. What would the PiO_2 be while wearing the mask?

_____

33. What gas law did you use to make these conclusions?

_____

Case 2

Respiratory therapists frequently draw arterial blood samples to measure the partial pressures of oxygen and carbon dioxide in the blood. Many patients have elevated or decreased body temperatures.

34. What effect does a fever have on these partial pressure readings?

_____

35. A normal arterial carbon dioxide pressure (PaCO$_2$) is 40 mm Hg (torr) at a body temperature of 37° C. Estimate the new PaCO$_2$ if body temperature was 40° C.

36. Why is temperature correction of arterial blood gas readings controversial?

MATHEMATICS

You must be able to perform calculations in the clinical setting and on board examinations. Chapter 6 gave several examples of problems found in both settings. Write the formula, and then solve the following problems **without using a calculator.** (Because your board examinations do not allow use of electronic calculators, only use a calculator to check your work.) You can write out the formula first, and then plug in the numbers to avoid mistakes.

37. Convert 30° C to degrees Kelvin.

Formula _____

Solution _____

Answer _____

38. Convert 68° F to degrees Celsius.

Formula _____

Solution _____

Answer _____

39. Convert 40° C to degrees Fahrenheit.

Formula _____

Solution _____

Answer _____

40. At body temperature, gas has a saturated capacity of about 44 mg of water vapor per liter. If a gas has an absolute humidity of 22 mg/L, what is the relative humidity?

Formula _____

Solution _____

Answer _____

41. What is the humidity deficit in Question 40?

Formula _____

Solution _____

Answer _____

42. Convert a pressure reading of 10 millimeters of mercury (mm Hg) to centimeters of water (cm H_2O).

Formula _____

Solution _____

Answer _____

43. Convert a pressure reading of 10 centimeters of water (cm H_2O) to kilopascals (kPa). Hint: It's okay to round off.

Formula _____

Solution _____

Answer _____

44. Air is normally about 21% oxygen. Calculate the partial pressure of oxygen in air (PiO_2) when the barometric pressure is 760 mm Hg.

Formula _____

Solution _____

Answer _____

45. Now calculate the new PiO_2 that would result if the barometric pressure is 500 mm Hg.

Formula _____

Solution _____

Answer _____

Did we forget anything? Let's check on the end of the chapter summary and highlight a few important ideas.

46. Two temperature scales are used in hospitals in the United States. The _____ scale is used universally in health care around the world.

47. Transfer of heat energy can occur through _____, convection, radiation, and _____.

48. The total _____ pressure of a mixture of gases must equal to the sum of

    the _____ pressures of the constituent gases.

49. A gas's _____ and pressure vary directly with _____.

50. When temperature is constant, a gas's volume and pressure vary _____.

WHAT DOES THE NBRC SAY?

Math may be hard for some of us. Getting good at it can make the difference between success and failure on the board exams! Pay special attention to the sections "Obey the Laws" and "Mathematics" and the two case studies, because these are the areas you'll need to focus on for credentialing. Dalton's law, temperature conversions, and Poiseuille's law are among the concepts you might see on the tests.

51. A blood gas analyzer is being calibrated with a 5% mixture of carbon dioxide and balance nitrogen. If the barometric pressure is 747 mm Hg, what reading would be most correct for the CO_2 electrode of the analyzer?
    A. 35 mm Hg
    B. 37 mm Hg
    C. 7.47 mm Hg
    D. 74.7 mm Hg

52. What is the most significant factor affecting airway resistance?
    A. Airway length
    B. Airway radius
    C. Gas viscosity
    D. Gas flow rate

FOOD FOR THOUGHT

Your knowledge of physics could be pretty useful in the real world. You know your garden hose needs a rubber washer to make a leak-proof connection where the metal of the hose joins the metal of the faucet. Same thing is true for an oxygen cylinder. A washer, or gasket, is needed where the metal of the cylinder joins the metal of the regulator.

53. What property of liquid oxygen makes it especially difficult and potentially harmful to work with at home?

7 Computer Applications in Respiratory Care

The real danger is not that computers will begin to think like humans, but that humans will begin to think like computers.

Sydney Harris

We are living in the "Information Age." Microprocessor technology is part of everyday life in the intensive care unit (ICU), respiratory therapists use computers to chart at most clinical sites, and you can download medical podcasts to keep up-to-date. If you can learn to use these tools effectively, you will be a more proficient respiratory therapist.

WORD WIZARD

Many of the words that describe computers are not yet in the dictionary. If you want to travel the information highway, you will need to be able to talk the talk. Let's get started with a few key terms.

Complete the following paragraphs by writing the correct term in the blank provided.

Computerese

The most common computers in use today are personal computers. Desktop, laptop, and handheld computers are all commonly used. In each case you need software applications. We write a paper or a memorandum using

_____ processing programs. My students learn to make presentations using a popular

presentation software called _____. When a manager wants to make a budget, a(n)

_____ program like Microsoft Excel is useful. Your state respiratory society might keep member

records in a _____-base program for easier retrieval of information in organized chunks.

Talk to Me!

Computers can talk to each other through local networks inside the hospital, or they can go outside the institution. The

global network of computer networks is called _____. Inside the hospital, a similar network

called the _____ serves as a conduit for information. If you want to go surfing, you've got to go

to Hawaii or you can navigate using the _____.

COMPUTERS IN HEALTH CARE

Clinicians use computers to help interpret data, reach a diagnosis, and automate certain aspects of patient care. Now you need to open your textbook and look up some information about this subject. Fill in your answers in the space provided.

1. Give five examples of clinical and diagnostic computer applications useful to the respiratory therapist.

   A. _____

   B. _____

   C. _____

   D. _____

   E. _____

39

2. In addition to staffing and billing, how do respiratory therapists use Respiratory Care Management Information Systems (RCMIS)?

3. What are the advantages of wireless handheld systems? List three.

   A. _____

   B. _____

   C. _____

4. What does the term "benchmarking" mean? How does a manager use benchmarking to assess performance?

5. Health care providers are using computers in several emerging areas. Tell us a little more about these three emerging applications of information technology. How will respiratory therapists use technology to better care for patients?

   A. Tobacco cessation: _____

   _____

   _____

   B. Telemedicine: _____

   _____

   _____

   C. Disease management: _____

   _____

   _____

GARBAGE IN, GARBAGE OUT

The ability to find information and sort out the good from the bad is one thing that identifies the best medical practitioners in our modern age. Evidence-based medicine is our best tool to improve practice, and we find the evidence using information technology.

Fill in your answers in the spaces provided.

6. What is Cochrane, and what do they collect? _____

   _____

7. Google may be lovely for routine stuff, but you can get more from Google Scholar. Give one pro and one con for this site.

A. Pro _____

B. Con _____

8. What happens to a search engine like Google when you:

A. Use the term "AND"? _____

B. Use the term "OR"? _____

9. The National Library of Medicine provides a free search engine for health information.

A. What is the name of this powerful engine?

_____

B. Why would you want to use this tool and not a commercial site?

CASE STUDIES

Case 1

A respiratory student is about to go to the ICU to learn how to care for patients on mechanical ventilation. Unfortunately for the student, the Charge Therapist corners him in the department and decides to test his knowledge. See if you can answer these questions as well.

10. The first question the Charge Therapist asks is,

"What is the common control mechanism of conventional mechanical ventilators?"

_____

11. Next, the therapist wants to know,

"Why are software driven systems less expensive for the Respiratory Department?"

_____

12. As the Charge Therapist gets warmed up, he asks,

"Can you name the four reasons why computerized charting is better on the ventilator than manual charting?"

A. _____

B. _____

C. _____

D. _____

13. When the student finally gets to the ICU, the preceptor smiles and says,

"What is this computer's proportional assist mode designed to enhance?"

_____

A respiratory care student is asked by her instructor to explain how you can tell if information from a Web site is likely to be trustworthy. In reading Chapter 7, the student knew there was a code of conduct for medical and health Web sites that would provide the information she needed. You can look at Table 7-3 if you need some help.

14. What term indicates that a Web site shows clearly where they got their information and the date when the page was modified?

_____

15. Justifiability is a critical concept in evaluating claims that a product, device, or drug will benefit patients. Explain this concept and why it is important.

16. Explain the phrase "transparency of sponsorship."

17. What difference do ads make?

_____

PRACTICE MAKES PERFECT!

You will need a computer with access to the World Wide Web so you can practice some of the skills discussed in the text. Most colleges will provide a free e-mail account for students and have wireless hot spots and computers with Web access. If your college does not, you can try your bookstore, coffee shop, or supermarket and get onto a free hot spot. I recommend getting an additional free e-mail account from a provider like Microsoft or Google for your personal mail. It's a good idea to practice separating your personal and work (or school) emails to avoid big headaches!

Activity 1: Information Search

Start up your browser and go to your search engine of choice. Now you can enter a keyword or phrase to look for information on a specific topic. Initially, it is alright to use natural language such as "asthma causes" or "what causes asthma" as keywords. You may find too much information and need to narrow your search. Box 7-1 of your text contains examples of Boolean operators, or special ways to refine searches. For example, try "asthma AND causes." When you find a site or an article that looks worthwhile, bookmark the URL for future reference.

Google (www.google.com) is now considered the top search engine, for ordinary searches. But watch out because Internet-savvy librarians estimate that between 80% and 90% of all the information on the Web is NONSCIENTIFIC and NONEDUCATIONAL! The first few sites that pop up are usually provided by paying sponsors, so move on and refine your search.

42

Activity 2: Evaluate!

Not all the information on the Internet is reliable. There is a lot of "junk science," amateur material, and sales and marketing you will have to sort through to get worthwhile information. Once you have found a Web site that contains the information you want, you can test it!

Find a Web site now, and answer these simple questions:

Site: _____

- Is it clear who is sponsoring the page? Look at the URL. Does the address end in ".edu" or ".gov"? These sites tend to be more reliable than the ".com" URL sites. In any case, it should be very clear who is sponsoring the page.
- Can you verify the legitimacy of the sponsor? Look for a telephone number or address for more information, not just an e-mail address.
- Is it clear who wrote the material (and the author's qualifications)?
- Is the information free of spelling, grammatical, and typographical errors?
- Is the information free of advertising?
- Are there dates on the page to indicate when the material was written or revised?
- Is it clearly stated when data or statistical information was collected?

The more "YES" answers you got, the more reliable is the information! Refer to Table 7-3 for more information on evaluating Web sites.

Activity 3: Respiratory Care!

In this exercise, you will locate a specific document from the AARC's Web site.

- Open the AARC home page (www.aarc.org).
- Click on "Resources" and find the section on Clinical Practice Guidelines (CPGs).
- Open the guideline on pulse oximetry.
- Print this guideline, and use it as a study reference. Why? One reason is the reliability of this material. Another good reason is that the National Board for Respiratory Care says in its newsletter: "CPGs are a valuable tool for preparing for board examinations."

How about that! The AARC Web site is the single most useful resource for respiratory therapy students and practitioners on the World Wide Web.

Portions of the AARC Web site are only accessible to members of the association. You can gain full access by joining. All respiratory students are eligible for free AARC memberships if their faculty belong and sign you up. If you do not have a free membership, you can join for about $0.20 per day.

FOOD FOR THOUGHT

It is easy to learn how to use the computer for more than just games. Besides the activities listed earlier, you may want to try the following:

- Locate the home page for your college.
- If your program has a Web site, locate it and print the home page or find some specific information from the page. If you do not have a page, find one from another program. These sites are easily accessed from the AARC Web site.
- If you do not have a program Web site, design one as a class project. Ask your media or learning center to provide skills and access to the campus server. With the new software available, anyone can learn to make a Web site.
- If your college offers e-mail accounts for students, get the entire class to sign up. Create an address list for the class, and send messages via e-mail. Ask your instructors to e-mail assignments, the class syllabus, and so on. Search any of the Web sites in Table 7-2 in the textbook. Find a specific article, protocol, practice guideline, or other information that can be linked to a class activity or a personal need. For example, GOLD has diagnostic criteria and treatment plans for COPD. You could use this to help write a report or complete a journal assignment. The NBRC (www.nbrc.org) has your examination blueprint and practice board exams! For free!
- Visit the Evolve site available with *Egan's:* http://evolve.elsevier.com/Egans. Evolve is an interactive learning environment designed to work in coordination with your text. Your instructors may use Evolve to provide an Internet-based course component that reinforces and expands the concepts presented in class. Even if your instructor hasn't incorporated Evolve into your course, you may access a list of helpful Web links to sites of interest. You can also access an NBRC exam cross-reference of the content in *Egan's* to the exam matrices for the CRT and RRT exams.

A FINAL THOUGHT

Smartphones, iPods, and other handheld devices can be invaluable. There are many VERY USEFUL medical applications, and many are free to download. For example, there is a program that allows users to look up almost any drug and check doses, costs, side effects, and so on. Also available is a blood gas calculator, Henderson-Hasselbalch calculator, peak flow and PFT norms, cylinder duration—you name it. Many students buy handheld devices because there is no better digital tool. You can shoot video of procedures in the lab or take photos of equipment to use for study purposes. Plus they fit in your lab coat pocket! (But remember, don't take pictures in the hospital and use "airplane" mode or turn off your Wi-Fi and alarms.)

8 The Respiratory System

Anatomy is destiny.
Sigmund Freud

Remember anatomy? It was one of those required courses, the one where you memorized a lot of body parts. It turns out that structure and function have a lot to do with each other. Anatomy even has clinical applications! In this chapter, we'll be trying to bring anatomy back to life. Before we go there, let's check and see if you still remember some important terms that relate to the anatomy of the respiratory system.

WORD WIZARD

Egan really puts the key in "key terms" in this chapter. It's like learning a new language. Perhaps you can help translate some of the more important words. The first one is done for you.

	MEDICAL TERMINOLOGY	IN PLAIN LANGUAGE, PLEASE
A.	Alveoli	Tiny air sacs for gas exchange
B.		Place where trachea splits into R+L
C.	Cilia	
D.		Primary muscle of breathing
E.	Epiglottis	
F.		Hole that opens into your windpipe
G.	Hilum	
H.		Voice box
I.	Pharynx	
J.		Wrapping that lines the lungs
K.	Sternum	
L.		Windpipe

JUST LIKE DEAR OLD DAD

Several very important pulmonary conditions find their origins in our genetics. Cystic fibrosis is the most famous example but even emphysema and lung cancer have genetic components. Lung cancer therapies are being tailored to individual genetics. It is important for the respiratory therapist to find out about family health when making assessments or taking the pulmonary history. The board exams (NBRC) agree.

Respiratory therapists take care of a wide range of patients from the tiniest preemie to elderly adults. That means you need to know about the ways in which lungs grow and develop.

1. During what stage and week of development is alveolar capillary surface area considered sufficient to support extrauterine life?

   Stage: _____

   Week: _____

2. What is the primary organ of gas exchange for the fetus? _____

   _____

3. Describe the umbilical cord blood vessels.

4. The fetus lives in a relatively hypoxic environment. What is considered to be a major factor that enables the fetus

   to survive under these conditions? _____

   _____

5. About half of the blood entering the right atrium is shunted to the left atrium via what structure?

   _____

6. Why is fetal pulmonary vascular resistance so high?

7. What percentage of blood entering the pulmonary artery actually flows through the lungs? Where does the rest of the blood go?

   _____

   _____

8. Describe the events that occur in the first few breaths after birth in terms of transpulmonary pressure, blood gases, and circulatory changes.

9. Compare the development of lung structures in newborns and adults.

    A. Number of alveoli

    B. Surface area of the lung

THEY AREN'T JUST LITTLE ADULTS...

10. Let's compare the head and upper airway of adults and babies.

	ANATOMY	BABY	ADULT
A.	Head		
B.	Tongue		
C.	Nasal passages		
D.	Larynx		
E.	Narrow point		
F.	Dead space		
G.	Airways		

11. Most infants breathe exclusively through what part of the airway? _____

12. Why are infant lung volumes relatively lower than those of adults?

13. Grunting is a type of maneuver used by infants that is now known by what more modern term? What does it mean when an infant is grunting?

    A. _____

    B. _____

14. Why do infants experience severe hypoxemia more readily than adults?

47

Identify the structures labeled in these figures.

15. What's in a chest?

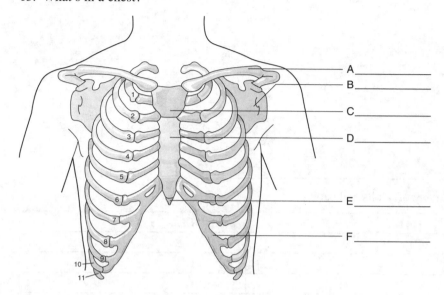

A_____
B_____
C_____
D_____

E_____

F_____

Anterior view of the bones of the thorax.
(From Hicks GH: *Cardiopulmonary Anatomy and Physiology*, Philadelphia, 2000, WB Saunders.)

Pneumopnuggets

When you put your stethoscope just below the clavicle you are listening over the upper lobes. You can also see that the lower lobes aren't really on the front of the chest at all! There's a little on the side, but mostly in the back. If you know your locations, your auscultation improves. If you look at the location of the apices, you will see they are **above** the clavicle! So if someone inserts a subclavian line, the lung could get punctured in the process!

16. Imagination 1

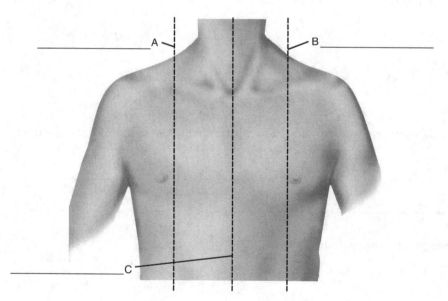

Imaginary lines on the anterior chest wall.

17. Imagination 2

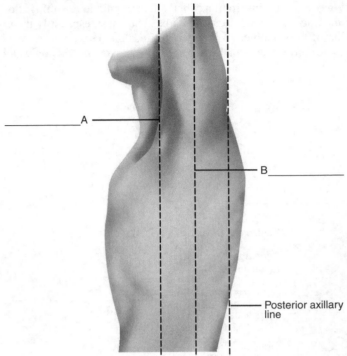

A _____

B _____

Posterior axillary
line

Imaginary lines of the lateral chest wall.

Pneumopnuggets

You can use these imaginary lines for a couple of things. First, when you perform a 12-lead ECG on a patient, you use the lines to guide placement of the electrodes (plus counting the ribs). The lines are also good if you notice something unusual (like a scar or a lesion) and want to document where it is located.

18. Pump me up

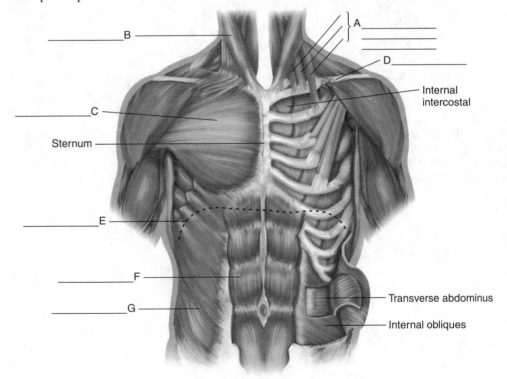

B _____

A _____

D _____

Internal
intercostal

C _____

Sternum _____

E _____

F _____

Transverse abdominus

G _____

Internal obliques

The muscles of ventilation.

49

Pneumopnuggets

Watch closely when someone breathes. See the belly move out on inspiration. That's diaphragmatic breathing. See the relaxed exhalation. That's normal. Many people use their accessory muscles to breathe. The chest, especially the upper chest, moves on inspiration, but no outward excursion of the abdomen! When we get into distress, or exercise really hard, you will see the abdominal group come into play to force exhalation. Sharpen your assessment skills by watching the *anatomy* of breathing!

19. What's up, doc?

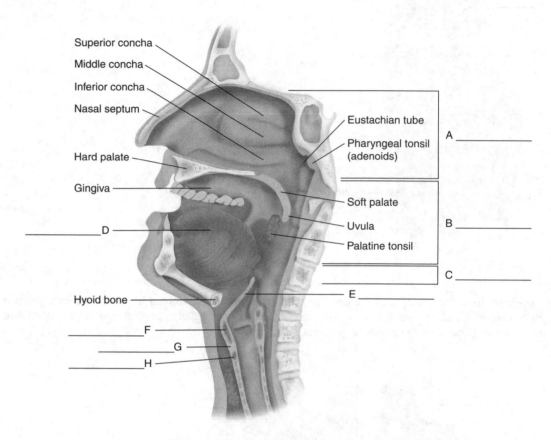

Structures of the upper airway and oral cavity.

Pneumopnuggets

Look at the nasopharynx. You'll be sticking tubes in there. It's fun if you know your anatomy. Notice that it goes straight back (a short distance) then drops down into the oropharynx. When you insert a catheter or airway, don't go straight back (very far), aim downward. Stay midline along the septum or you'll ram the turbinates (ouch!). In this cross-sectional view, it's easy to see how the tongue could block the airway if it falls back.

20. "Adam's apple"

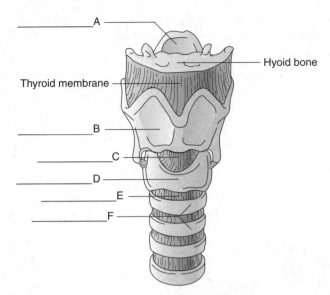

Thyroid membrane

Hyoid bone

A

B

C

D

E

F

Anterior view of the larynx.

Pneumopnuggets

The thyroid cartilage sticks out on males. Find a willing male example. Palpate the thyroid cartilage. Feel the front and the sides. Now move your finger down (just a little) from the big bump on the front. Feel the soft spot? That's the cricothyroid membrane. (You might learn how to do a cricothyrotomy in school.) The cartilage just below that is the cricoid, the trachea's only complete ring. Keep going and feel the rings of the trachea. Gently (!) grasp the whole box in your fingers and wiggle back and forth. It's supposed to be mobile! Now ask your friend to swallow while you keep your fingers on the thryoid cartilage. What happened?

21. See cilia

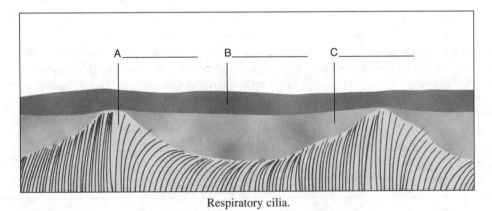

A _____   B _____   C _____

Respiratory cilia.

Pneumopnuggets

Your airway makes more than 100 ml of mucus every day. Where does it all go? Without good ciliary function where would it go? Drugs (like smoking tobacco for instance) can impair ciliary function. Hot or toxic gases (like smoking for instance!) can destroy cilia. There are diseases that involve the cilia, too!

22. You can call me Al

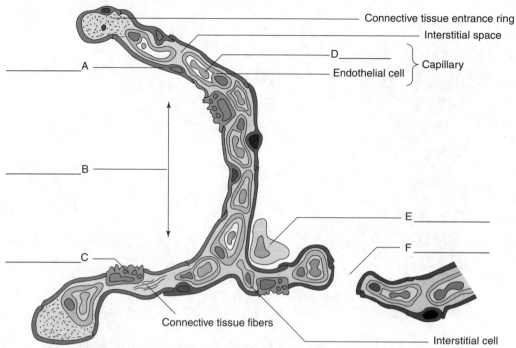

Cross-sectional sketch of the cells and organization of the alveolar septa. (From Hicks GH: *Cardiopulmonary Anatomy and Physiology*, Philadelphia, 2000, WB Saunders.)

Pneumopnuggets

The distance from alveoli to blood is only about 0.2 microns. (Remember, there are 1000 microns in a millimeter!) Oxygen has less than 1 second to cross this distance and combine with the RBC. So anything, like the fluid from pulmonary edema, that increases this distance will impair gas exchange. There are about 300 million alveoli in an adult lung. If you flatten them out, the area would be the size of a tennis court!

LOBES AND SEGMENTS

Students are always dismayed when they have to learn postural drainage and find out that the lungs have 5 different lobes and 18 individual segments. It's not so hard when you know there are some duplicates and break the whole thing down into little pieces. Fill in the following chart. You can make your own version of this and fill it in until you get them memorized. This will really help you with postural drainage. Notice that the left lung only has 8 segments, even though they are numbered 1-10! Refer to Table 8-8 for help.

	RIGHT LUNG		**LEFT LUNG**
	Right Upper Lobe		Left Upper Lobe
1			Upper Division
2		1 and 2	
3		3	
	Right Middle Lobe		Lower Division (Lingula)
4		4	
5		5	
	Right Lower Lobe		Left Lower Lobe
6		6	
7		7 and 8	
8		9	
9		10	
10			

We've covered most of the material in Chapter 8. Here are a few more ideas that are important to know about the respiratory system. Fill in your answers in the space provided.

23. Name the nerves that innervate the diaphragm, intercostal muscles, and larynx. State the origin of these nerves and describe what will happen if they are damaged.

24. Describe the pathway gas follows as it is conducted through the lower airway. Use Table 8-7 as a guide.

SUMMARY CHECKLIST

Fill in the blanks to identify eight key points from the Summary Checklist at the end of Chapter 8.

25. The _____ houses and protects the lungs.

26. The _____ is the primary muscle of ventilation.

27. The upper respiratory tract _____ and _____ inspired air and protects

    the lungs against _____ substances.

28. The lower respiratory tract _____ gases from the upper airway to the respiratory

    _____ of the lung.

29. The airways branch into _____ which are in turn made up of _____
    in both the left and right lungs.

30. The respiratory bronchioles and _____ provide a large _____ for
    exchange of gases between air and blood.

31. Fetal _____ and _____ differ markedly from those functions in the
    postnatal period.

32. Closure of the _____ and ductus _____ are important events in the
    transition from intrauterine to extrauterine life.

A cruel respiratory instructor forces the students to learn the anatomy of the lung. Completely by coincidence, the instructor slips while running with scissors, and the sharp shears puncture his right chest. The students gather around their fallen facilitator to discuss the anatomic consequences of this tragedy.

33. What would happen to the lung on the affected side?

34. What would happen to the pleural space on the affected side?

35. What is this condition called? _____

_____

36. What is the treatment for this condition?

_____

Case 2

A respiratory care practitioner (RCP) is working the night shift at a large urban medical center. As he makes his rounds, he hears loud snoring coming from a patient's room. Even though snoring is a commonly heard sound at night, the RCP stops to investigate.

37. What anatomic change results in snoring?

38. What is OSA, and how is it treated?

39. What is the similarity between snorers and unconscious victims who require resuscitation?

40. How would you approach management of the airway of an unconscious person?

WHAT DOES THE NBRC SAY?

Respiratory anatomy is not on the boards, but the kinds of applications we've been using in this chapter are part of the test. For example, you'll probably see several questions about pneumothorax. Airway management, assessment, and ECG are all areas on the boards that incorporate anatomy into questions. An endotracheal tube may be seen at the level of the aortic knob on an x-ray, lead IV is placed on the midclavicular line, and the leaf-shaped cartilage seen on intubation is the epiglottis.

FOOD FOR THOUGHT

What happens to these structures when disease is present?

41. What happens to the airways and alveoli when a patient is having an acute episode of asthma?

42. What changes to the airways and alveoli occur in emphysema?

9 The Cardiovascular System

What the heart knows today, the head will understand tomorrow.

James Stephens

Your heart beats, on average, about 38 million times in 1 year! No matter how well the respiratory system works to exchange gas with the blood, it would be meaningless without the heart pushing that blood out to the organs via the vascular system. Those blood vessels are the best transportation network in the world, constantly reacting to the need for more or less flow of nutrients to the tissues.

WORD WIZARD

Because the cardiovascular function is closely connected to the respiratory system, you will meet up with it again and again in the course of your training. The words you learn today will help you throughout your career. Match the following terms to their definitions as they apply to respiratory care.

Terms	Definitions
_____ 1. afterload	A. membranous sac that surrounds the heart
_____ 2. automaticity	B. stroke volume multiplied by heart rate
_____ 3. baroreceptors	C. ventricular stretch provided by end-diastolic volume
_____ 4. cardiac output	D. biologic sensors that monitor arterial blood pressure
_____ 5. chemoreceptors	E. pathologic narrowing or constriction
_____ 6. pericardium	F. force against which the ventricle pumps
_____ 7. preload	G. biologic sensors that monitor arterial blood oxygen
_____ 8. stenosis	H. ability to initiate a spontaneous electrical impulse

MEET THE OBJECTIVES

Chapter 9 presented eight objectives for learning. We'll cover five here and do the math problems at the end. How well do you know your cardiovascular system?

9. We all know there are four valves in the heart. Patients commonly have disorders of the mitral valve. Where is it? What is the effect of mitral stenosis on the lung?

10. Explain how specialized tissue allows the muscle cells in the ventricle to contract in a coordinated and efficient manner.

11. Compare and contrast local control of blood vessels with central control mechanisms.

12. Describe how the cardiovascular system responds to exercise and blood loss by balancing blood volume and vascular resistance.

13. Match the mechanical events to their corresponding electrical events in the normal cardiac cycle. Hint: Take a look at Figure 9-14 on page 222 of your text.

	ELECTRICAL EVENT	CARDIAC EVENT (MECHANICAL)
A.		
B.		
C.		

SUMMARY CHECKLIST

Identify six key points from Chapter 9. Complete the following questions by writing the correct term(s) in the blank(s) provided.

14. The _____ system consists of the heart and vascular network, which maintain

_____ by regulating the distribution of blood flow in the body.

15. Cardiac _____ is primarily determined by preload, _____,

contractility, and _____.

16. Under conditions of increased _____, special _____ mechanisms are called on to maintain stable flow.

17. The heart and vascular systems ensure that tissues receive sufficient blood to meet their _____ needs.

18. Blood pressure is regulated by changing the _____ of the blood, changing the

_____ of the vascular system, or changing _____.

19. _____ heart rate will _____ cardiac output.

Case 1

A 57-year-old patient is admitted to the coronary care unit with a diagnosis of mitral stenosis. The patient is breathing rapidly and complains of shortness of breath. Her pulse oximetry readings reveal hypoxemia. Auscultation reveals inspiratory crackles in the posterior lower lobes.

20. What is mitral stenosis? _____

21. What mechanical events are occurring to cause pulmonary edema and stiffening of the lung tissue?

22. What action should the respiratory therapist take at this time? _____

_____

Case 2

A respiratory care student is giving an aerosolized bronchodilator to a 27-year-old patient with asthma. Breath sounds reveal bilateral wheezing. The pulse oximeter shows 98% saturation on room air. The student notices the heart rate rising from 82 to 98 beats/min during the therapy.

23. What are the effects of sympathetic and parasympathetic stimulation on the sinus node in the heart?

    A. _____

    B. _____

24. Describe the two ways that drugs produce bronchodilation.

    A. _____

    B. _____

25. Based on this information, why would you expect increased heart rate to be a common side effect of drugs that cause bronchodilation?

Cardiac anatomy, like respiratory anatomy, does not have a particular place on the national exams. That doesn't mean it's not important; we just use this material as a foundation for clinical applications like hemodynamics and electrocardiography. Advanced cardiac life support certification course instructors expect you to know cardiac concepts before you try to understand emergency cardiovascular pharmacology. Having said that, hemodynamics is on the test. Expect to need to know normals and some mathematics. More on this topic later...of course!

Circle the best answer for the following questions.

26. A patient has a heart rate of 70 beats/min and a stroke volume of 60 ml with each ejection of the ventricle. What is the approximate cardiac output in liters per minute?
    A. 3.6 L/min
    B. 4.2 L/min
    C. 5.0 L/min
    D. 6.0 L/min

27. Calculate systemic vascular resistance if mean arterial pressure is 90 mm Hg, central venous pressure (CVP) is 10 mm Hg, and cardiac output is 4 L/min.
    A. 2.5 mm Hg/L/min
    B. 8.6 mm Hg/L/min
    C. 20 mm Hg/L/min
    D. 22.5 mm Hg/L/min

28. What is the ejection fraction if stroke volume is 50 ml and end-diastolic volume is 75 ml?
    A. 50%
    B. 66%
    C. 75%
    D. 150%

FOOD FOR THOUGHT

29. What four mechanisms combine to promote venous return to the heart?

    A. _____

    B. _____

    C. _____

    D. _____

30. What is meant by the "thoracic pump"? What effect does positive pressure ventilation, like IPPB, have on venous return to the chest?

10 Ventilation

Keep breathing.
Sophie Tucker

Chapter 10 is loaded with heavy-duty information. Your challenge is to sort out what is important to remember, learn the basic principles, and connect the knowledge to what is clinically important. You may want to read this chapter two or three times to get the big picture!

WORD WIZARD

Let's start off by emphasizing the difference between *ventilation* and *respiration*. Complete the following paragraph by filling in the correct term(s) in the blank(s) provided.

Remember that the primary purpose of the lungs is to supply the body with oxygen and remove wastes in the form of

carbon dioxide. _____ is the process of moving air in and out of the lungs. Some of that ventilation

is _____ space, or wasted ventilation. When CO_2 builds up in the body, the pH of blood decreases, resulting in a state of acidosis. We can measure the amount of air that moves in and out with a device called a spirometer.

The pressure changes in the chest are measured using a body box, or _____. Finally, the actual

rate of air flow is measured using a(n) _____. Airway _____ is a measure-

ment of how much pressure it takes to push the gas through the conducting air passages. _____, or the distensibility (a fancy way to say stretchiness), is the change in lung volume divided by the pressure needed to take that breath. Stiff lungs increase the work of breathing.

Much of respiratory care is aimed at reducing the work of breathing and restoring adequate ventilation. The process of respiration, on the other hand, is the exchange of gas between blood and other tissues.

PICTURE THIS

1. Trans what? Air moves in and out of the chest because of pressure gradients. Label the following diagram to help improve your understanding of these pressure changes.

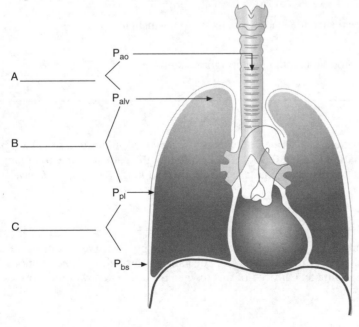

A _____

B _____

C _____

P_{ao}

P_{alv}

P_{pl}

P_{bs}

Pressures, volumes, and flows involved in ventilation. (Modified from Martin L: *Pulmonary Physiology in Clinical Practice: The Essentials for Patient Care and Evaluation*, St. Louis, 1987, Mosby.)

61

Write out the definition of each gradient.

A. _____

B. _____

C. _____

Pneumopnuggets

Our ability to generate the necessary pressure changes requires muscle power. Muscles need glucose, oxygen, and innervation (among other things) to work properly. Any clinical condition that requires bigger pressure gradients to move air (like asthma) makes the muscles work harder. Just like when you work out, a pulmonary patient can get muscle fatigue from increased work of breathing.

2. Where has all the ventilation gone? Fill in the missing pressures for the apex and base of the lung.

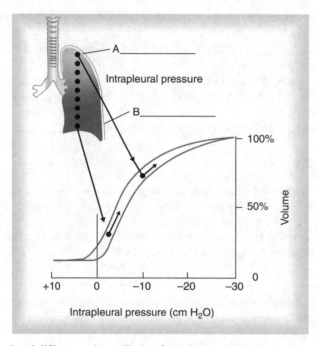

Causes of regional differences in ventilation from the apex to the base of an upright lung.

3. Where does the bulk of ventilation go during a normal breath in an upright person?

_____

Pneumopnuggets

You can use this information clinically. When a patient has serious unilateral, or one-sided, lung disease (like a bad case of pneumonia), he or she will have poor ventilation in the affected side. Positioning the patient so the good lung is dependent will preferentially increase the ventilation in that lung and away from the bad lung. Remember: *Down with the good lung!*

WORK OF BREATHING

It's time to talk about the bottom line. Work of breathing, or WOB, has a definite energy cost. We can measure the metabolic cost in terms of oxygen consumed, and we can reduce the work for patients through our interventions. A healthy person consumes about 250 ml of oxygen per minute. Only 5% of this oxygen is needed to power the muscles of

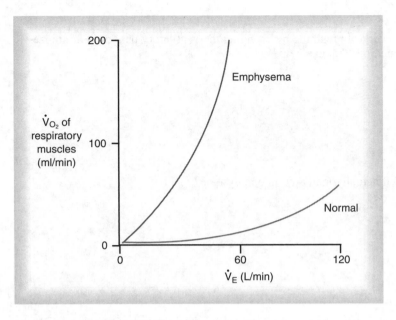

Relationship of oxygen cost of breathing to minute ventilation for a healthy subject and for a patient with emphysema.

ventilation. The cost goes up about 1 ml for each liter of additional ventilation. Look at what happens to this cost when a patient has emphysema.

There are four factors that contribute to WOB: compliance, resistance, active exhalation, and ventilatory pattern. Let's look at each of these separately and talk about strategies for improvement.

Compliance

Compliance is a measure of lung elasticity, or stretchability. It is defined as:

$$\text{Change in volume (L)} \div \text{Change in pressure (cm } H_2O)$$

A healthy lung is pretty stretchy, and compliance is 0.2 L for every cm H_2O of pressure generated.

However, the lungs sit inside the thorax, which has its own compliance. Coincidentally, the compliance of the chest wall is also 0.2 L/cm H_2O! You have to remember that the lung wants to recoil in and the chest wants to spring out, so they are pulling in opposite directions. Mathematically this is like a cancellation, so the net result is a compliance of 0.1 L/cm H_2O for health lungs in a healthy chest. However, if the lungs are overinflated or underinflated, the whole thing changes. You can understand this by trying a simple experiment.

Experiment

- Get an ordinary balloon.
- Blow it up a just a tiny bit. This is your underinflated lung.
- Blow it up some more. Hard to do, right?
- Now blow it up some more. Pretty easy.
- Now inflate the balloon until it is almost full.
- Blow in some more! Hard to do!

Lungs are a little like this balloon. A patient who has a very low lung volume has to work harder to take a breath than does a person with a normal amount of functional residual capacity. A person with air-trapping (like emphysema) is like the balloon that is overinflated.

Try this for yourself: Take a deep breath. Don't exhale. Now try to breathe in. You get the idea.

Bottom Line

You can move 500 ml of air with a pressure of 5 cm H_2O. Pretty good!

4. The text states that you can reduce frictional work of breathing by changing the ventilatory pattern to minimize airway resistance. What are the two simple methods that can help?

5. Why is the compliance of the lung tissue itself actually increased in emphysema?

Resistance

Resistance comes in two kinds: tissue and frictional. Tissues have to move when the chest expands. Obesity (outside the lung) and fibrosis (inside the lung) are examples of increased tissue resistance. The really big problem is the frictional resistance created when you move air through your pipes (80% of all resistance). Airway resistance (Raw) is defined as the driving pressure it takes to create a flow of gas. Or to put it mathematically:

$$\text{Raw} = \text{Change in pressure (cm } H_2O) \div \text{Change in flow rate (L/min).}$$

Your upper airway causes most of this resistance. The normal value is 0.5 to 2.5 cm H_2O per liter per second of flow. Conditions like asthma narrow the airways and significantly increase resistance. You can understand this with another simple experiment.

Experiment

- Get a straw and a coffee stirrer (the hollow kind).
- Breathe in and out slowly through the stirrer. Now the straw. Which one is easier?
- Now try putting your lips together and sucking in the air really fast. Feel the work?

Bottom Line

The inner diameter of the airway determines the amount of resistance. (Remember old what's-his-name's law? The French one that is so hard to pronounce. Starts with a *P*.) If the bronchi decrease from 2 mm to 1 mm in diameter, the resistance increases *16 times!* Your muscles will have to generate a much higher pressure to achieve ventilation if the airway is narrow.

Questions

6. What important change occurs in the airway of patients with COPD and asthma to increase the resistance? What airways are usually involved?

7. What class of medications can respiratory therapists use to reduce airway resistance in asthma?

Active Exhalation

Normal exhalation is passive. The power comes from energy you stored by stretching the lung and chest during inspiration. When you actively exhale, you have to use your abdominal muscles (and internal intercostals). Remember that additional muscle work takes additional energy. You can actually observe patients using their abdominal muscles when they are in distress and trying to get the air out quicker, or through narrowed airways. You can try this yourself.

Experiment

- Place your hands on your belly.
- Breathe in.
- Exhale normally.
- Breathe in again. This time, push firmly in with your hands as you exhale. Air moves faster, right?
- Release your hands, and breathe in again. This time, bear down with your abs and blow out hard and fast until your lungs are empty. Feels like work!

Bottom Line

Actively exhaling has a price. When you see a patient doing this, they are either exercising or in distress.

Questions

8. What does it mean when you see active exhalation in your patient?

9. What happens to a person with a spinal cord injury who cannot use their abdominal muscles? Hint: What other important respiratory activity uses these muscles?

Ventilatory Pattern

The way you breathe can change the amount of work. In healthy people, a big deep breath increases the elastic part of WOB. Fast breathing increases the frictional work. Healthy people adjust their tidal volume and respiratory rate to minimize the work of breathing during exercise. Our patients exhibit altered patterns, too. Patients with fibrosis (loss of elasticity) breathe with a rapid shallow pattern to reduce the mechanical work of distending the lung. Patients with obstructive diseases like asthma and emphysema need to reduce their rate to reduce work, because they have increased frictional resistance.

Experiment

- Tie something tightly around your upper chest. I use a bathrobe tie. This will restrict chest movement.
- Try breathing faster with shallow breaths.
- Now try to breathe slowly and deeply. Which way feels better?
- Now, untie yourself.
- Get out your straw or coffee stirrer. Breathe rapidly and shallowly through the tube.
- Now take slow, deep breaths. Which way feels better?

Bottom Line

You can learn a lot by observing someone's breathing pattern.

10. Describe what happens to alveolar ventilation in healthy individuals when they increase respiratory rate or decrease tidal volume?

11. What is the optimal pattern of breathing for patients with obstructive airway diseases?

DEAD SPACE

Dead space is, plainly put, wasted ventilation—gas that does not participate in exchange with the blood. You normally waste the first third of each breath, or about 1 ml per pound of ideal body weight. Alveolar dead space occurs when gas enters the alveoli but no blood comes to pick up the oxygen. A pulmonary embolus (blood clot, fat clot, air bubble, etc.) blocks blood flow to alveoli and causes increased dead space. Too much (50% to 60% of each breath) dead space will result in the inability to maintain adequate ventilation through spontaneous breathing. The patient will need mechanical ventilation until the problem improves.

12. Label the types of dead space in this diagram.

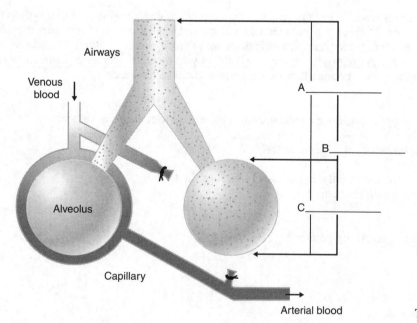

Three types of dead space.

13. What is the normal percentage of anatomic dead space for each breath? What is the value used to calculate average anatomic dead space? Why is this method a problem for us now? What would be better?
    A. Percentage
    B. Value for calculation
    C. Problem? Better method?

14. What type of ventilatory pattern will be seen with significantly increased dead space?

_____

15. What is the difference between *hyperventilation* and *hyperpnea?*

MATHEMATICS

Chapter 6 mentioned that math is part of our board examination process and a clinical reality. Don't use a calculator to solve these problems! Use your calculator to check your work.

16. Calculate exhaled minute ventilation for a patient who has a tidal volume of 800 ml and a frequency of 8 breaths/min.

    Formula _____

    Calculation _____

    Answer _____

17. Calculate anatomic dead space for a patient who is 6 feet tall and weighs 180 lb.

    Formula _____

    Calculation _____

    Answer _____

18. Calculate alveolar minute ventilation using the data from Problems 1 and 2.

    Formula _____

    Calculation _____

    Answer _____

19. Calculate the physiologic dead space using the Bohr equation if $PaCO_2$ is 60 mm Hg and $PECO_2$ is 30 mm Hg.

    Formula _____

    Calculation _____

    Answer _____

The NBRC (and everyone else) will expect you to be able to calculate exhaled minute volume and alveolar minute volume and apply the information. SERIOUSLY, this is always on your boards. Here's a sample.

Circle the best answer for the following multiple-choice questions.

20. The minute volume for a 68-kg (150-lb) patient who has a respiratory rate of 12 breaths/min and a tidal volume of 600 ml would be
    A. 4800 ml
    B. 5400 ml
    C. 6000 ml
    D. 7200 ml

21. The estimated alveolar minute ventilation for an 82-kg (180-lb) patient who has a respiratory rate of 10 breaths/min and a tidal volume of 500 ml would be
    A. 3200 ml

    B. 3500 ml

    C. 4800 ml

    D. 5000 ml

22. Which of the following ventilator settings would provide the optimal alveolar ventilation?

	Rate	Volume
A.	10	600
B.	12	500
C.	15	400
D.	20	300

23. Determine the physiologic dead space percentage for a patient with an arterial CO_2 of 40 mm Hg and an exhaled CO_2 of 30 mm Hg
    A. 0.25
    B. 0.33
    C. 0.50
    D. 0.75

11 Gas Exchange and Transport

To Air is human, to Respire divine.
Paul Thackara, RRT

In Chapter 11, we go for it and jump in the deep end (of physiology that is). It may be challenging at first, but when you have mastered the basics of gas transport, you're going to feel exhilarated! It's going to feel great to get a grasp of how gas exchange works and how respiratory therapists apply physiology to patient care.

WORD WIZARD

Let's get on the hemoglobin-oxygen train and take a little ride. First you're going to learn the different names for all those forms that hemoglobin (Hb) takes when it combines. Complete the following paragraphs by filling in the correct term(s) in the blank(s) provided.

All Aboard

It's natural for this complex molecule to want to be in a relationship. Hemoglobin meets oxygen. When they get

together, the new name is _____. Their newfound affinity is likely to end when they meet up

with the _____ effect at the tissue level. So hemoglobin takes up with carbon dioxide and we get
carbaminohemoglobin. The fickle heme will drop CO_2 off at the lung when they run into the _____

effect. Life could go on like this unless our conjugated protein meets up with a really unusual gas like carbon monoxide.

This combination is called _____, and it really lasts because hemoglobin's affinity for CO is

_____ times greater than its affinity for oxygen.

Why Be Normal?

Not all hemoglobins are created equal. Some are downright unnatural. Abnormal hemoglobins are given letter designations. Complete the following paragraph by filling in the correct term(s) in the blank(s) provided.

HbS, whose common name is _____ _____ hemoglobin, not only car-
ries on poorly with O_2 but also causes red blood cells to deform and clump together into thrombi. Babies are born with

_____ hemoglobin, which causes a(n) _____ shift of the curve and makes
babies more prone to cyanosis. Sometimes heme is altered in other ways. When the iron compound is oxidized, we get

_____, which causes the blood to turn a brownish color. Poisoning from nitric oxide is one thing
that can cause this transformation of our gas-loving protein.

OXYGEN TRANSPORT

Before oxygen can go to the tissues, it has to get into the alveoli. There is a useful formula for calculating the partial pressure of O_2 (PAO_2) in those little grapelike clusters. True, this equation has never won any popularity contests with students, but it is clinically useful (and can show up on those board exams). So put on your thinking caps, and we'll show them who's in charge here! The fancy formula looks like this:

$$PAO_2 = F_iO_2(P_B - PH_2O) - PaCO_2(F_iO_2 + 1 - F_iO_2/R)$$

We usually simplify this to read:

$$PAO_2 = F_iO_2(P_B - 47) - PaCO_2/0.8$$

Or you can go one step farther (especially if the F_iO_2 is ≥60%) and use this one:

$$PAO_2 = F_iO_2(P_B - 47) - PaCO_2$$

Or in English...

The partial pressure of O_2 in the alveoli is equal to the inspired O_2 percent multiplied by the barometric pressure minus water vapor pressure.

Why?

Dalton's law gives us the first part (partial pressure = concentration × total pressure). Because water vapor in the lung acts like a gas, it takes up space. That's space that oxygen can't occupy.

Next: Subtract arterial CO_2 × a factor.

Why?

What we want to know is how much CO_2 is in the alveoli. (CO_2 takes up space, too.) It's hard to measure; solution: Use a converted arterial value in its place. You don't really need to do this when the patient is breathing a high F_iO_2, like 60% or more.

Who Cares?

All of this sounds like pulmonary laboratory stuff, except for the fact that we can use this baby to find out how *efficiently* the lungs are at transferring oxygen into the blood by comparing *alveolar PO_2* with *arterial PO_2!* This relationship is called the A–a gradient. A normal A–a gradient is about 5 to 10 mm Hg on room air, or about 10%.

MATHEMATICS

1. Calculate alveolar oxygen tension for a person breathing room air. Assume that barometric pressure is 760 mm Hg, F_iO_2 is 21%, and $PaCO_2$ is 40 mm Hg.

    Formula _____

    Solution _____

    Answer _____

2. If the patient in problem 1 has an arterial PO_2 of 90 mm Hg, what is the A–a gradient?

    Formula _____

    Solution _____

    Answer _____

3. Calculate alveolar O_2 tension for a person breathing 60% O_2 (P_B = 760 mm Hg, CO_2 = 40 mm Hg).

    Formula _____

    Solution _____

    Answer _____

4. If the patient in Problem 3 has an arterial PO_2 of 90 mm Hg, what is the A–a gradient?

    Formula _____

    Solution _____

    Answer _____

Both patients have identical PaO_2 values of 90 mm Hg. If you only look at PO_2, or only look at oxygen saturation, they appear to be the same.

However, the A–a gradients are very different. The second patient is having serious problems getting O_2 from the lung into the blood. In fact, the patient breathing 60% oxygen should have a PaO_2 of about 340 mm Hg (PAO_2 – 10%).

"By the Pricking of My Thumbs..."

Everyone loves a good rule of thumb. If you're in a big hurry and don't have a calculator at the bedside, you can try this shortcut. To estimate alveolar PO_2 for a patient breathing room air, multiply F_iO_2 by 5 ($5 \times 20 = 100$). For 40% or more, multiply by 6 ($40 \times 6 = 240$). *Remember,* this only works when the CO_2 is normal. Besides, what respiratory therapist doesn't have a calculator at the bedside?

BARRIERS TO DIFFUSION

5. Do not pass "go" until you pass through the three barriers to diffusion. List them here.

   A. _____

   B. _____

   C. _____

Pneumopnuggets

The partial pressure of a gas is the main driving force across the aveolar-capillary (A-C) membrane. Respiratory therapists routinely increase the driving pressure of oxygen by increasing the PAO_2. CO_2 has a much lower driving pressure, but is about 20 times more soluble than O_2, so it has little difficulty in making the journey. In some cases, time can limit diffusion due to increased blood flow. Fever and septic shock are clinical examples.

LET'S GET MOVING!

Once it gets into the blood, O_2 is only transported two ways. First, it dissolves in the plasma. To calculate dissolved O_2, multiply PaO_2 by 0.003.

$$\text{Dissolved } O_2 = PaO_2 \times 0.003$$

The second way that O_2 is transported is as oxyhemoglobin; 1.34 ml of O_2 binds to each gram of hemoglobin (per 100 ml of blood). If all the hemoglobin carried O_2, this would be simple, but it doesn't. Remember the anatomic shunt? Hemoglobin saturation is usually less than 100%.

$$\text{Combined } O_2 = 1.34 \times Hb \times \text{\% saturation}$$

Put them together and what have you got?

$$O_2 \text{ content} = PaO_2 \times 0.003 + 1.34 \times Hb \times \text{\% saturation}$$

MATHEMATICS

Although computers in the hospital will usually calculate content for you, the National Board for Respiratory Care (NBRC) thinks you should be able to do this yourself (and without a calculator)!

6. Calculate O_2 content for Patient 1 with an Hb of 15 g/dL, SaO_2 of 97%, and PaO_2 of 100 mm Hg.

   Formula _____

   Solution _____

   Answer _____

7. Calculate O_2 content for Patient 2 with an Hb of 15 g, SaO_2 of 80%, and PaO_2 of 50 mm Hg.

   Formula _____

   Solution _____

   Answer _____

Chapter **11** **Gas Exchange and Transport**

8. Calculate O_2 content for Patient 3 with an Hb of 10 g, SaO_2 of 97%, and PaO_2 of 100 mm Hg.

Formula _____

Solution _____

Answer _____

Now compare the results. Patient 2 has pretty crummy values but a good hemoglobin level. Patient 3 has good values but a crummy hemoglobin level. Who has better oxygenation?

The Moral of the Story

Looking at pulse oximetry values, or any other simple indices of oxygenation like PaO_2, doesn't tell the whole story. You *always* have to consider hemoglobin. A patient may need blood as a treatment for poor O_2 content. Remember that there may be enough hemoglobin, but it may not be able to combine with oxygen, like in CO poisoning.

THROW ME A CURVE

The last piece of the oxygenation puzzle (for now at least) is to look at the relationship of O_2 and hemoglobin. This relationship is described by the oxyhemoglobin dissociation curve. Look at the curve shown in Figure 11-9 of your text. The flat upper part of the curve means that you can have a large drop in PaO_2 and only get a small drop in saturation. In fact, PaO_2 can drop from 600 mm Hg to 60 mm Hg, and the saturation will only drop from 100% to 90%! The steep part of the curve is equally cool, physiologically speaking. A small increase in PaO_2 will give you a large increase in saturation. If you raise the PaO_2 from 27 mm Hg to 60 mm Hg, the saturation will rise from 50% all the way to 90%. Normally, a given PaO_2 will produce a predictable hemoglobin saturation.

Fill in the correct values for partial pressure of O_2 and saturation (with a normal pH) on the chart below. Use the Mini-Clini on hemoglobin saturation (Page 260) if you need help.

	PaO_2	SaO_2
9.	40 mm Hg	
10.		80%
11.	60 mm Hg	
12.		97%

But the curve doesn't always stay in the same place! Fill in the correct answers for how the curve will shift in the following chart:

	Factor	Shift
13.	Acidosis	
14.	Hypothermia	
15.	High 2,3-diphosphoglycerate (2,3-DPG)	
16.	Fever	
17.	Hypercapnia	
18.	Carboxyhemoglobin	

The shift of the curve to the right facilitates O_2 unloading to the tissues, but a given PaO_2 will have a lower hemoglobin saturation. A left shift does the opposite.

FICK IT

Fick was a physiologist who figured out something pretty cool—how to calculate cardiac output using O_2 content data and tissue O_2 consumption. Your instructors may want you to learn this now, or later in Chapter 46. Because this can show up on your NBRC exams, you may want to take a look at this old formula that keeps on working. Basically you divide the amount of O_2 the tissues are using (average of 250 for the normal adult) and divide by the difference between arterial and venous O_2 content, and you get the cardiac output. We measure output more directly these days, but Fick's formula is a good way to explain the relationships. More in Chapter 46!

CARBON DIOXIDE TRANSPORT

Carbon dioxide is transported three ways in the blood. Just like O_2, it dissolves right into the plasma. This factor is more important than dissolved O_2, because it transports a fair amount of CO_2. Just like oxygen, CO_2 is carried by hemoglobin. Unlike oxygen, this is a relatively small amount. The majority of the CO_2, about 80%, is transported in the form of bicarbonate. Sorry, there are no math problems for you to do right now. But do remember this equation:

$$CO_2 + H_2O = H_2CO_3 = HCO_3^- + H^+$$

This reaction is called hydrolysis, because it involves combining CO_2 with water. First, carbonic acid is formed, but this quickly ionizes into bicarbonate and hydrogen ions. Remember, the reaction can move in both directions. Most of the hydrolysis occurs inside the red blood cell because of the presence of an enzyme (carbonic anhydrase) that speeds up the reaction rate.

Carbon dioxide levels are inversely proportional to alveolar ventilation. If you increase alveolar ventilation, the CO_2 will decrease. A normal $PaCO_2$ is 35 to 45 mm Hg. A high CO_2 level means that the patient is not ventilating adequately. We draw arterial blood gases when we want to accurately assess ventilation. A high CO_2 in the blood indicates hypoventilation. Because CO_2 has an acidifying effect on the blood, the pH of the blood will decrease when the CO_2 rises. The normal lower limit of pH is 7.35. The normal upper limit is 7.45. Low values reflect acidosis, whereas increased pH represents an alkaline state.

BAD GAS EXCHANGE

Oxygen delivery and CO_2 removal are where it's at, physiologically speaking. The following questions will test your knowledge of the causes of poor gas exchange.

Fill in the correct term(s) in the blank(s) provided.

19. Inadequate delivery of O_2 to the tissues is known as _____.

20. _____ is the medical name for a low level of O_2 in the blood.

21. Physiologic _____ occurs when blood passes through areas of the lung that have no ventilation.

22. Ventilation-_____ imbalances are the most common cause of low blood O_2 in patients with lung disease.

23. Patients with pulmonary fibrosis have a(n) _____ defect that results in low blood O_2 levels.

24. A low blood pressure results in _____ and poor tissue CO_2 delivery.

25. Myocardial infarction is an example of _____, a localized reduction in blood flow to tissues that can result in tissue death.

26. Increased _____ space ventilation may result in increased levels of CO_2 in the blood.

27. Drug overdose may result in an inadequate _____ ventilation due to central nervous system depression.

28. Patients with severe COPD are unable to maintain adequate ventilation due to ventilation-_____ imbalances.

The NBRC thinks you should be good at assessing gas exchange and treating abnormalities. Circle the best answer for each of the following multiple-choice questions.

29. A room air blood gas reveals the following results:
pH	7.50
$PaCO_2$	30 mm Hg
PaO_2	110 mm Hg

    In regard to these data, the respiratory therapist should
    A. report the results to the physician
    B. redraw the sample because of air contamination
    C. report that the patient is on O_2
    D. place the patient on O_2

30. Calculate O_2 content for a patient with the following data:
Hb	10 g
PaO_2	80 mm Hg
SaO_2	95%

    A. 12.73 ml O_2/dL
    B. 12.97 ml O_2/dL
    C. 13.40 ml O_2/dL
    D. 13.64 ml O_2/dL

31. Calculate PAO_2 for a patient with the following data:
P_B	747 mm Hg
FiO_2	0.21
PaO_2	95 mm Hg
$PaCO_2$	40 mm Hg
SaO_2	97%

    A. 97 mm Hg
    B. 103 mm Hg
    C. 107 mm Hg
    D. 117 mm Hg

32. A man is brought to the emergency department from a house fire. He is conscious and in obvious distress on 6 L of O_2 via nasal cannula. His heart rate is 135 beats/min, respiration is 26 breaths/min, blood pressure 160/100 mm Hg. The pulse oximeter is reading SpO_2 99% and a heart rate of 136 beats/min. He has no cyanosis but complains of dyspnea. What abnormality of hemoglobin is most likely to be the source of the clinical problem?

    A. HbCO
    B. HbS
    C. anemia
    D. HbF

CASE STUDIES

Case 1

A 29-year-old housewife is brought to the emergency department following exposure to smoke during a house fire. She is breathing at a rate of 30 breaths/min. Her heart rate is 110 beats/min. Blood pressure is 160/110 mm Hg. The patient complains of headache and nausea. The pulse oximeter is reading a saturation of 99%.

33. Why are pulse oximetry readings unreliable in this setting? _____

_____

34. What is wrong with this patient?

35. What action would you take at this time?

A patient is brought back to the unit following major surgery after a motorcycle accident. He was given a massive transfusion of blood to replace loss from both the trauma and the surgical procedure. The pulse oximeter is reading 96% on room air, but the nurse has requested you to evaluate because of the patient's clinical condition. You find him sitting up and breathing 32 times per minute. He has tachycardia and tachypnea and complains of difficulty breathing. Breath sounds are clear on auscultation.

36. The patient's clinical signs are consistent with what gas exchange abnormality?

_____

37. What is one of the potential problems with banked blood?

_____

38. Name some of the other possible causes of the patient's distress.

39. What diagnostic procedure could you recommend? _____

_____

A woman is admitted with a diagnosis of pneumonia. Arterial blood gases reveal a pH of 7.55, $PaCO_2$ of 25 mm Hg (acute respiratory alkalosis), PaO_2 of 75 mm Hg, and an SaO_2 of 94%. She complains of feeling short of breath. Lab data reveal a hemoglobin level of 8 g/dL.

40. Interpret this blood gas in terms of gas exchange.

41. What other laboratory information plays a key role in helping to determine O_2 content?

_____

42. What is absolute anemia, and how is it treated?

Case 4

A young man has been brought by paramedics to the emergency department after an accidental overdose of narcotics at a party. The patient is unconscious and has a respiratory rate of 8 breaths/min. The pulse oximeter shows a saturation of 85%.

43. Why would CO_2 be elevated in this patient?

44. Why is the patient's O_2 saturation so low?

SUMMARY CHECKLIST

Let's make sure you've met the objectives and key points for this vital section on how gas exchange works.

45. The movement of gas between the lungs and the tissues depends mainly on _____.

46. The alveolar PCO_2 varies inversely with _____ ventilation.

47. _____ and _____ must be in balance to be effective.

48. Blood carries a small amount of dissolved O_2 in the plasma and a large amount carried in chemical combination with

_____.

49. The five causes of a decreased PaO_2, or O_2, level in arterial blood are low ambient PO_2, _____,

impaired _____, _____-_____ imbalances,

and physiologic _____.

50. Most of the CO_2 in your blood is transported as _____.

51. Hypoxia can occur when _____ blood O_2 content is decreased or if blood

_____ is decreased.

52. Alveolar ventilation decreases when the minute ventilation is _____ or when

_____ ventilation is increased.

FOOD FOR THOUGHT

Dysoxia

Is your brain full yet? Dysoxia is a form of hypoxia where cells do not take up O_2 properly.

53. What is the classic example of dysoxia? _____

_____

54. When does tissue O_2 consumption become dependent on O_2 delivery? _____

_____

55. Why does lactic acid form when tissues are hypoxic?

FOOD FOR THOUGHT PART DEUX

A new technology has been developed that allows pulse oximeters to look beyond the usual O_2–hemoglobin relationship. Masimo is currently the only company that offers a pulse oximeter that can detect carboxyhemoglobin and tells you how much CO you have without drawing blood. A second oximeter allows you to assess methemoglobin or sulfhemoglobin or whatever you want. It is a noninvasive co-oximeter. This will become a standard of care in emergency medicine in the near future, so you'll want to check out this important new generation of pulse oximeters.

REMEMBER: When new devices come out, they may not appear in your board exams right away. Currently, the answer is "pulse oximeters can't detect carbon monoxide," and we don't know if that will change in the next revision of the boards; but we'll all be watching.

12 Solutions, Body Fluids, and Electrolytes

If you can't convince 'em, confuse 'em.
Harry S. Truman

Imagine yourself swimming in a warm ocean lagoon. The salty water is filled with life. Currents move you and waves propel you through this complex ecology. Now think about the inside of your body. Warm, wet, and filled with salts; an intricate environment where life depends on the relationships of fluids and electrolytes. Chapter 12 reviews various types of solutions, the mechanisms that control fluid movement, acid-base basics, and the role of major electrolytes in body function. We start on the second half of the chapter first. Then we'll wrap up with a look at solutions.

WORD WIZARD

You'll need to have some new vocabulary to keep you afloat in the sea of salts and solutions. See if you can match the definitions to the terms. You might have trouble with a chapter like this if you don't understand these fundamental phonemes of body chemistry.

Write your answer in the spaces provided.

Definitions	Terms
1. _____ A compound that gives off H⁺ in water. Vinegar is a good example in the kitchen.	A. acid
	B. active transport
2. _____ The opposite of inactive transport; movement across membranes.	C. normal solution
	D. solvent
3. _____ Negatively charged ion; Cl⁻ and HCO₃⁻ are common in the body.	E. solute
	F. base
4. _____ A compound that gives off OH⁻ in water. Sodium bicarbonate is an example in the kitchen.	G. cations
	H. hypertonic
5. _____ Minimizing the change in pH. Think of how pleasant it is to buffer your stomach acids after eating chili!	I. isotonic
	J. solution
6. _____ Positively charged ion. Na⁺ and K⁺ are common in the body.	K diluent
	L. colloid
7. _____ A substance with big molecules that hold water (among other things). Like milk in the kitchen or albumin in the blood. Also an evenly dispersed mixture or gel.	M. dilute solution
	N. hypotonic
	O. buffering
8. _____ Something you use to water down a medication or solution.	P. saturated solution
	Q. anions
9. _____ The medium you dissolve something into, like your coffee.	
10. _____ The stuff that gets dissolved, like sugar.	
11. _____ A stable mixture of two substances, like sugar when it is stirred (dissolved) into coffee. Heat helps make this happen.	
12. _____ A really weak solution. The soup needs more salt.	
13. _____ A solution holding as much as it can. The soup is fine.	

14. _____ The standard solution with 1 mEq/L. I was never like this, myself.

15. _____ Has the same amount of salt as your body fluids. A good solution in your nebulizer.

16. _____ Saltier than your body fluids. Good for inducing sputum.

17. _____ Low salt or no salt, and okay to nebulize, too.

WATER, WATER EVERYWHERE

The human body is mostly water. Water makes up as much as 80% of your weight. Because water is relatively heavy, the easiest way to track gain and loss is by weighing the patient! Clinicians also monitor intake and output (I and O) of water very closely.

Now you need to open your textbook (check out Table 12-3 in your text) and look up some information about this subject.

18. Rank the relative amount of water in the following individuals. Put "1" by the group with the lowest percentage of water and "5" by the people with the largest percentage of body water.

_____ males

_____ newborns

_____ children

_____ females

_____ obese individuals

19. Name the two major compartments for body distribution of water. List subdivisions, and give the relative amount (%) of water in each area.

COMPARTMENT	% H$_2$O
A.	
B.	
1.	
2.	
3.	

WHERE HAS ALL THE WATER GONE?

A lot of water leaves your body every day through sensible and insensible losses. Give examples of these water losses and an average daily amount. Look at Table 12-4 in your text to satisfy your thirst for knowledge.

	SOURCE	AMOUNT
20.	Sensible	
	A.	
	B.	
	C.	
21.	Insensible	
	A.	
	B.	

80

You can also lose water through additive losses like sweating, diarrhea, and vomiting. The insensible loss that interests us the most is water lost through breathing. A tracheostomy patient with poor humidification can lose 700 ml/day or more. This results in dried-out secretions that clog the patient's lungs. If your tracheostomy patient has a fever, the problem is worse.

22. Describe the loss of water that occurs through fever.

23. Lost water is regained by two main methods. List these sources of liquid and give amounts.

	SOURCE	AMOUNT/DAY
A. Ingestion		
1.		
2.		
B. Metabolism		

ACID-BASE BASICS

If your body was a playground, acids and bases would be the seesaw ride! You don't have to be a chemistry major to play. Acids are substances that release hydrogen ions (H^+) when placed in a watery solution. Another definition states that acids are substances that are proton donors. Bases release hydroxyl ions (OH^-) or accept protons. Pure water is the reference point for determining acidity or alkalinity. Any solution with more H^+ ions than water is considered an acid. A solution with less hydrogen ions is considered alkaline, or basic. A logarithmic scale, called the pH scale, is used to indicate the relative amount of acidity or alkalinity of a substance. Water is assigned a value of 7.0 on the pH scale. Because the scale is logarithmic, a pH of 6 is 10 times more acidic than water. The human body exists in a narrow range of pH values. Normally, our arterial blood has a pH of 7.35 to 7.45. A prolonged pH below 7.0 or above 7.60 is usually fatal! In Chapter 13, we'll get into clinical applications and interpretations of acid-base balance, so let's make sure you have the basic ideas down pat.

24. One way your body prevents wide swings in pH is through the process of buffering. Explain the important role hemoglobin and other proteins play in buffering the blood.

25. If a patient ingested bicarbonate for stomach problems and the pH went up from 7.0 to 8.0, how much more alkaline did the body become?

26. What equation is used to calculate pH? Write it out so you begin to remember.

A. Name

B. Equation

Electrolytes are chemicals that dissociate into ions when placed into solution, thus becoming capable of conducting electricity. Positively charged ions are called cations, and negative particles are called anions. There are seven major electrolytes in the body that are essential to life. Electrolytes are naturally regulated by the kidney (mostly) and can be manipulated by oral or intravenous intake in the health care setting. Let's see if you know your electrolytes. Look at the end of the chapter for this information.

27. List the seven major electrolytes and their primary purpose in the body.

	ELECTROLYTE	SYMBOL	PURPOSE
A.			
B.			
C.			
D.			
E.			
F.			
G.			

You will also need to know the average normal plasma value for these babies. Match the value to the chemical in the list below. Seriously, learn these values if you want to pass "go" with the NBRC.

28. _____ bicarbonate

29. _____ calcium

30. _____ chloride

31. _____ magnesium

32. _____ phosphorus

33. _____ potassium

34. _____ sodium

A. 140 mEq/L

B. 24 mEq/L

C. 4.0 mEq/L

D. 5.0 mEq/L

E. 100 mEq/L

F. 2.0 mEq/L

G. 1.4 mEq/L

Electrolytes are so important that a patient will exhibit some pretty interesting signs and symptoms if these powerful substances become too high or low. Complete the chart below to match up disorders, causes, and symptoms of electrolyte disturbances. Use Table 12-5 to help you get going.

	IMBALANCE	CAUSE	SYMPTOM
35.		Sweating	
36.	Hypokalemia		
37.		Starvation	Diaphragmatic weakness
38.	Hypercalcemia		
39.		Chronic renal disease	

Notice the similarities in the symptoms of many of these imbalances. When you see muscle weakness, abnormal fatigue, or ECG disturbances or metabolic acid-base disorders, take a look at the electrolytes! When you see electrolyte disorders in the lab results, take a look at the arterial blood gas to check the acid-base status!

CASE STUDIES

Case 1

A 68-year-old man with congestive heart failure (CHF) is being treated with a combination of diet and diuretics. He returns from a trip to New Orleans complaining of difficulty breathing and swollen ankles. He is admitted to the coronary care unit for observation and treatment. Auscultation reveals bilateral inspiratory crackles in the lung bases. His respiratory rate is 28 breaths/min, and his heart rate is 110 beats/min with arrhythmias. Hint: Check out the Mini-Clini in the electrolyte section (Page 288).

40. Patients with CHF are usually placed on what special type of diet? Why?

41. Diuretics commonly cause loss of what specific electrolyte that affects cardiac function? How will this electrolyte be replaced in the hospital? The home?

  A. Electrolyte: _____

  B. Hospital replacement: _____

  C. Home replacement: _____

42. As a respiratory therapist, what action will you take to further assess cardiopulmonary status? What is likely to be your initial treatment of this patient?

43. What is the cause of this patient's lung crackles?

A 68-year-old homeless alcoholic is found in respiratory distress by the paramedics and brought to your emergency department. The patient is malnourished. Auscultation reveals bilateral inspiratory crackles in the lung bases. His respiratory rate is 28 breaths/min with a heart rate of 110 beats/min. Hint: Look at the section on Starling equilibrium. We'll get back to these two cases again and again because pulmonary edema is such a common clinical problem. So common that Chapter 27 is devoted to this topic. Now is a good time to get your feet wet in the area of flooded lungs.

44. What protein accounts for the high osmotic pressure of plasma? Why is the patient lacking this substance?

_____

45. Explain why this patient has crackles.

46. As a respiratory therapist, what action will you take to further assess cardiopulmonary status? What is likely to be your initial treatment of this patient?

MATHEMATICS

Respiratory therapists frequently work with weight/volume solutions and perform dilution calculations. Dilution calculations are used in drug preparation and in the pulmonary laboratory. You will be expected to perform some of these calculations on the NBRC board examinations. *Remember, no calculators on the boards.* Here's a hint. You need to look at the weight/volume solutions and dilution calculations as well as a Mini-Clini to do this section (Page 281).

47. Albuterol is prepared in a 5% solution (weight/volume). How many grams of albuterol are dissolved in 100 ml to make this solution?

Formula _____

Solution _____

Answer _____

48. Respiratory therapists do not usually administer 100 ml of drugs to their patients. Instead, they give 1 ml or less. How many milligrams of albuterol would be found in 1 ml of the 5% solution in problem 20?

Formula _____

Solution _____

Answer _____

49. After drawing up 1 ml of a 5% solution of albuterol into a syringe, the respiratory therapist places the bronchodilator into a nebulizer along with 2 ml of saline for dilution. The total solution is now 3 ml in the nebulizer. What is the new concentration of the drug?

Formula _____

Solution _____

Answer _____

Excuse Me, Would You Like Some Help?

Formula: $C_1 \times V_1 = C_2 \times V_2$

Where C_1 = stock strength in the bottle, 5% and V_1 = the amount you need to draw up, or 1 ml. C_2 is what we want to find out. V_2 is the 1 ml of drug and the 2 mL of saline, or 3 ml.

Solution: $5\% \times 1$ ml $= C_2 \times 3$ ml

Answer: 0.16%. You can check this out in the Mini-Clini on methacholine dilution in your text where they apply this formula to make a new formula of a stronger drug that is safe to give to asthmatics.

WHAT DOES THE NBRC SAY?

The National Board for Respiratory Care (NBRC) would give this chapter an "E" for "emphasis of important test material." Here are more sample questions in the same format as your tests. Other items you'll need for the boards from Chapter 12 include electrolyte values and some of those calculations.

Circle the best answer for each of the following multiple-choice questions.

50. A patient with severe hypokalemia is receiving an intravenous infusion of potassium to correct this serious disorder. What should you monitor?
   A. SpO_2
   B. respiratory frequency
   C. mental status
   D. ECG rhythm

51. Which of the following signs and symptoms would you expect to observe in a patient with hypokalemia?
   1. metabolic acid-base disturbance
   2. muscle spasms and tetany
   3. ECG abnormality
      A. 1 only
      B. 1 and 2 only
      C. 1 and 3 only
      D. 2 and 3 only

52. All of the following would be consistent with administration of a large amount of IV fluid *except*
   A. increased pulmonary vascular markings on the chest x-ray
   B. presence of crackles on auscultation
   C. increased urine output
   D. increased hematocrit

Chapter **12** **Solutions, Body Fluids, and Electrolytes**

53. A respiratory therapist delivers isotonic saline to a patient via nebulizer. What concentration of saline is the therapist delivering?

A. 0.0%

B. 0.45%

C. 0.90%

D. 1.0%

FOOD FOR THOUGHT

Administration of fluids with varying tonicities by both intravenous and aerosol routes is common.

54. What happens to cells in the presence of a hypertonic solution? _____

_____

55. What happens to cells when a hypotonic solution is given? _____

_____

56. What name is given for the movement of water across a semipermeable membrane? _____

_____

Here's another one for you. Once upon a time a physician asked a respiratory therapist if the saline in his nebulizer treatment would hurt her patient, who was on sodium restriction for his heart. "No problem," said the RT. Use this scenario to answer the following question.

57. If you give 3 mL of normal saline by nebulizer, how much sodium chloride is being delivered to the airway in theory? Do you think the whole thing goes into the patient?

13 Acid-Base Balance

The formula for success is simple: practice and concentration, then more practice and more concentration.

Babe Didrikson Zaharias

If our bodies are factories that use oxygen and glucose to manufacture energy, then they are also producers of waste in the form of water, heat, and carbon dioxide. The CO_2 and water will produce acid that must be buffered, or neutralized. A respiratory therapist must understand the role that the lung and the kidney play in removing all this acid and keeping our pH balanced so body systems will keep working. To do this we need to know how to interpret the results of arterial blood gases. Drawing, analyzing, and, most of all, interpreting blood gas findings are hallmarks of our profession. Learning this skill will require some memorization and lots of practice!

WORD WIZARD

There's no point in building your knowledge without a foundation. Before you can learn to use acid-base information clinically, you will have to know your terminology.

Match the following terms to their definitions.

Terms	Definitions
1. _____ acidemia	A. acid that can be excreted in gaseous form
2. _____ volatile acid	B. decreased hydrogen ion concentration in the blood
3. _____ anion gap	C. ventilation that results in decreased CO_2
4. _____ hyperventilation	D. respiratory processes resulting in increased hydrogen ions
5. _____ metabolic acidosis	E. acid that is excreted by the kidney
6. _____ alkalemia	F. abnormal ventilatory pattern in response to metabolic acidosis
7. _____ Kussmaul breathing	G. nonrespiratory processes resulting in decreased hydrogen ions
8. _____ hypoventilation	H. difference between electrolyte concentrations
9. _____ fixed acid	I. respiratory processes resulting in decreased hydrogen ions
10. _____ respiratory alkalosis	J. increased hydrogen ion concentration in the blood
11. _____ metabolic alkalosis	K. nonrespiratory processes resulting in increased hydrogen ions
12. _____ standard bicarbonate (HCO_3^-)	L. chemical substance that minimizes fluctuations in pH
13. _____ base excess	M. plasma concentration of HCO_3^- corrected to a normal CO_2
14. _____ respiratory acidosis	N. difference between normal and actual buffers available
15. _____ buffer	O. ventilation that results in increased CO_2

Body acids come in two types: fixed and volatile, or water soluble. The lungs excrete more acid each day than any other organ including the kidneys! Answer the following questions to find out if you understand the buffering process.

16. Draw a diagram of the process called isohydric buffering.

17. Explain how the lungs can compensate for increased production of fixed acids.

18. Buffers are composed of what two components? _____

_____

19. What happens when you add the acid hydrogen chloride to the base sodium bicarbonate?

20. Describe the two general types of buffering systems in the body, and give examples of each system and what general type of acid (fixed or volatile) they buffer in the body (check out Table 13-2 in *Egan's* for an example).

	Blood Buffers	Acid Buffered
A.		
B.		

21. What does ventilation remove from the body to help eliminate acid? Support your answer with information from the text.

22. Why are buffers in the kidney essential for the secretion of excess hydrogen ions (why can't the lung do it alone)?

When you're healthy, the lungs, kidneys, and buffers work together to keep your pH normal so that enzyme systems can function and homeostasis is maintained. The system responds pretty rapidly to local or systemic changes. As long as the ratio of HCO_3^- buffer to dissolved CO_2 is 20:1, your pH will be about 7.40. A variety of conditions can cause the balance to shift. Increases in ventilation will result in respiratory alkalosis. Increases in HCO_3^- (or other base buffers) will result in metabolic alkalosis. These changes are referred to as acute if they take place over a short period of time. If they become chronic, the body will try to compensate to bring the pH back to normal. Of course, the respiratory system responds rapidly to metabolic disturbances, but the kidney takes time to adjust the HCO_3^-. Answer these questions to test your understanding of simple acid-base disturbances.

23. List the normal range of values for pH, $PaCO_2$, and HCO_3^-. (You MUST memorize these values!)

	Low Normal	**High Normal**
A. pH		
B. $PaCO_2$		
C. HCO_3^-		

24. Write out the Henderson-Hasselbalch equation.

25. Complete the primary acid-base and compensation chart below. Try Table 13-3 if you get stuck.

	Disorder	**Primary Defect**	**Compensation**
A.	Respiratory acidosis		
B.	Respiratory alkalosis		
C.	Metabolic acidosis		
D.	Metabolic alkalosis		

26. What is the *Rule of Thumb* for determining the expected increase in HCO_3^- for any acute increase in CO_2?

27. How much will HCO_3^- increase with a chronic increase in CO_2?

There is a simple four-step method for interpreting blood gas values.

Step 1: Determine the pH first.
1. >7.45 = alkalosis
2. <7.35 = acidosis
3. 7.35 to 7.45 = normal (or fully compensated)

Step 2: Evaluate respiratory status ($PaCO_2$) to see if it agrees with the pH.
1. <35 = alkalosis
2. >45 = acidosis

Step 3: Evaluate metabolic status (HCO_3^-) to see if it agrees.
1. >26 = alkalosis
2. <22 = acidosis

Step 4: Evaluate compensation.
1. Complete: pH is normal with abnormal levels of CO_2 and HCO_3^-. (Even with complete compensation, the pH will tend to be on the primary disorder's side of 7.40.)
2. Partial: pH is abnormal, but not as much as expected.

TRY IT, YOU'LL LIKE IT!

Interpret the following blood gas results. See the example done for you.

pH	7.30
$PaCO_2$	60 mm Hg
HCO_3^-	26 mEq/L

The pH is below 7.35, so the overall state is acidosis. The $PaCO_2$ is above 45 mm Hg, which represents *acidosis*. The pH and the $PaCO_2$ agree! We have *respiratory acidosis*. The HCO_3^- has risen 2 mEq/L above normal. This elevation is most likely due to the increased CO_2 (remember, bicarbonate level goes up 1 mEq/L for each 10–mm Hg acute increase in CO_2). So, we have **acute (uncompensated) respiratory acidosis.**

28. pH   7.34

    $PaCO_2$ 60 mm Hg

    HCO_3^- 31 mEq/L

29. pH   7.36

    $PaCO_2$ 60 mm Hg

    HCO_3^- 33 mEq/L

Stop right there! We're going to continue interpreting blood gas results in the case studies and board exam review questions, but hopefully you can see how the HCO_3^- will be creeping up as the CO_2 rises and the pH returns to low normal to achieve compensation.

WELCOME TO THE GAP!

When a patient has a metabolic acidosis, it can be life-threatening, so we need to try to establish the cause. One way to do this is through history. For example, we know the patient took an aspirin overdose. Another method for determining the type of metabolic acidosis is by looking at the difference between our positive and negative ions. Of course, you need the electrolyte values to do this calculation. Here's how you do it:

$$\text{Sodium (Na}^+) - \text{chloride (Cl}^-) + \text{bicarbonate (HCO}_3^-) \text{ or } 140 - (105 + 24) = 11$$

A normal range for the gap is 9 to 14 mEq/L. Usually, potassium is ignored. When the body loses HCO_3^- through diarrhea, chloride increases and the gap remains normal. When HCO_3^- is used to buffer excess fixed acids, the gap will increase.

30. Name the three common causes of anion gap metabolic acidosis.

    A. _____

    B. _____

    C. _____

31. What are the signs of respiratory compensation for metabolic acidosis?

    _____

32. What are the neurologic symptoms of severe acidosis?

    _____

MATHEMATICS

There have been several math calculations in this chapter. You will have to use a calculator to solve some of them—probably a scientific one. The steps of the H-H equation can be tricky, so pay close attention and DO THE STEPS EXACTLY IN ORDER.

Bicarbonate Blues

Calculate the new HCO_3^- (assume 24 mEq/L as the starting point) level for an acutely elevated $PaCO_2$ of 50 mm Hg (assume it started at 40 mm Hg). You could use the *Rule of Thumb* like this:

$$\text{Formula predicted } HCO_3^- = 24 + (\text{measured } PaCO_2 - \text{normal } CO_2)/10$$

$$\text{Solution predicted } HCO_3^- = 24 + (50 - 40)/10$$

$$\text{Answer predicted } HCO_3^- = 24 + 1$$

You try.

33. Calculate the new HCO_3^- (assume 24 mEq/L as the starting point) level for an acutely elevated $PaCO_2$ of 70 mm Hg (assume it started at 40 mm Hg).

    Formula _____

    Solution _____

    Answer _____

34. Calculate the new HCO_3^- (assume 24 mEq/L as the starting point) level for a *chronically* elevated $PaCO_2$ of 70 mm Hg (assume it started at 40 mm Hg; use the other *Rule of Thumb* to make the new formula).

Formula _____

Solution _____

Answer _____

Hassle? Use the H-H Equation for This

35. Calculate pH if HCO_3^- is 30 mEq/L and $PaCO_2$ is 40 mm Hg.

Formula _____

Solution _____

Answer _____

36. Calculate pH if HCO_3^- is 24 mEq/L and $PaCO_2$ is 40 mm Hg.

Formula _____

Solution _____

Answer _____

37. Calculate pH if HCO_3^- is 24 mEq/L and $PaCO_2$ is 60 mm Hg.

Formula _____

Solution _____

Answer _____

Gap?

38. Calculate anion gap if Na^+ is 144 mEQ/ml, Cl^- is 100 mEQ/ml, and HCO_3^- is 22 mEQ/ml.

Formula _____

Solution _____

Answer _____

39. Calculate anion gap if Na^+ is 135 mEQ/ml, Cl^- is 105 mEQ/ml, and HCO_3^- is 26 mEQ/ml.

Formula _____

Solution _____

Answer _____

The following case studies will systematically take you through the major acid-base disorders. Let's start with some simple, acute states and move into the compensated ones. Remember to evaluate using the four-step process.

Case 1

Mrs. Betty Maladie was depressed and took too much diazepam (Valium). She is found *shortly* thereafter in a coma breathing slowly and shallowly. ABG results reveal pH of 7.28, $PaCO_2$ of 60 mm Hg, and HCO_3^- of 26 mEq/L.

40. How would you interpret this ABG? _____

_____

41. What is the primary cause of the disorder? _____

Case 2

Mrs. M's husband, Bob, is very worried about her condition. He complains of dizziness and tingling in his hands. ABG results reveal pH of 7.58, $PaCO_2$ of 25 mm Hg, and HCO_3^- of 23 mEq/L.

42. How would you interpret this ABG? _____

43. What is the primary cause of the disorder? _____

Case 3

The couple's young son, Billy, has been sick with the stomach flu. ABG results reveal pH of 7.60, $PaCO_2$ of 40 mm Hg, and HCO_3^- of 38 mEq/L.

44. How would you interpret this ABG? _____

45. What is the primary cause of the disorder? _____

Case 4

The couple's diabetic teenage daughter, Lizzy, has not been taking her insulin. ABG results reveal pH of 7.25, $PaCO_2$ of 40 mm Hg, and HCO_3^- of 17 mEq/L.

46. How would you interpret this ABG? _____

47. What is the primary cause of the disorder? _____

Of course, blood gases, like children, don't stay simple for long. Partial or complete compensation may occur.

Case 5

Grandpa Maladie has smoked for years, and now he has COPD. ABG results reveal pH of 7.37, $PaCO_2$ of 50 mm Hg, and HCO_3^- of 28 mEq/L.

48. How would you interpret this ABG? _____

49. What is the source of compensation? _____

As soon as Lizzy Maladie's brain realizes the acute nature of her illness (case 4), compensation begins. ABG results now reveal pH of 7.35, $PaCO_2$ of 25 mm Hg, and HCO_3^- of 13 mEq/L.

50. How would you interpret this ABG? _____

51. What is the source of compensation? _____

Grandma Maladie has congestive heart failure. She takes furosemide (Lasix) to reduce extra water in her body. ABG results now reveal pH of 7.46, $PaCO_2$ of 45 mm Hg, and HCO_3^- of 31 mEq/L.

52. How would you interpret this ABG? _____

53. What is a possible cause of the primary disorder? _____

WHAT DOES THE NBRC SAY?

Blood gas (acid-base) analysis is one of the largest areas in all of the exams. The Entry-Level examination will focus on simple interpretations, whereas the Registry Examinations will ask you for higher order thinking. Here are some examples.

Circle the best answer to the following multiple-choice questions.

54. A 17-year-old girl is brought to the emergency department by paramedics. Her mother states she is a diabetic. Room air ABGs reveal the following:

pH   7.26
$PaCO_2$ 16 mm Hg
HCO_3^- 8 mEq/L
PaO_2 110 mm Hg

This information indicates which of the following?
1. Partly compensated metabolic acidosis is present.
2. This PaO_2 is not possible on room air.
3. Respiratory alkalosis is present.
  A. 1 only
  B. 3 only
  C. 1 and 2 only
  D. 1 and 3 only

55. Interpret the following ABG results:

F_iO_2 0.21
pH   7.36
$PaCO_2$ 37 mm Hg
HCO_3^- 22 mEq/L
PaO_2 95 mm Hg

  A. acute respiratory alkalosis
  B. acute metabolic alkalosis
  C. compensated respiratory alkalosis
  D. normal ABG

56. During CPR, blood gases are drawn. The results are as follows:

F_iO_2 1.0
pH   7.15
$PaCO_2$ 55 mm Hg
HCO_3^- 12 mEq/L
PaO_2 210 mm Hg

What action should be taken to correct the acid-base abnormality shown here?
A. Increase the rate of ventilation.
B. Decrease the F_iO_2.
C. Administer sodium bicarbonate intravenously.
D. Add positive end-expiratory pressure (PEEP) to the ventilation system.

57. The results of an arterial blood gas are shown.

F_iO_2 0.21
pH   7.55
$PaCO_2$ 25 mm Hg
HCO_3^- 24 mEq/L
PaO_2 105 mm Hg

These data indicate which of the following?
A. metabolic acidosis
B. metabolic alkalosis
C. uncompensated hyperventilation
D. uncompensated hypoventilation

58. A 72-year-old man with a history of renal failure is seen in the emergency department. The respiratory therapist notes that the patient is taking 28 very deep breaths per minute. Which of the following accurately describes this breathing pattern?
A. Cheyne-Stokes breathing
B. ataxic breathing
C. Kussmaul breathing
D. eupneic breathing

EXERCISE YOUR MENTAL MUSCLES

In later chapters, you will be called on to use your newfound blood gas interpretation skills to make many clinical decisions about patient care. *If you are having difficulty interpreting the acid-base status, you should take time to solidify these skills now!*

Here are some suggestions.

- **Get access to blood gas interpretation software.** Your instructors probably have a program that will give you sample after sample to interpret. (Or use the Web, see later.)
- **Make flash cards.** Take some 3 × 5 inch cards. Write high, normal, and low values for pH, $PaCO_2$, and HCO_3^-. Make two extra cards for pH that will represent compensation. Use 7.36 for compensated acidotic states and 7.44 for alkalotic states. On the back of each card write out the name of the state. For example, on the $PaCO_2$ 50 mm Hg card, write "respiratory acidosis." You get the idea? Now proceed through the combinations using the four-step method of interpretation. Pretty soon you will be an ace!
- **Drill, drill, drill until you have mastered basic blood gas interpretation!**

Blood gas disorders can get really complicated at times. Just like life. In some cases, a patient will have one disorder superimposed on another. Take the continuing saga of the following older patient...

Grandpa Maladie, discussed in Case 5, acquired a lung infection after visiting his daughter in the hospital. ABG results now reveal pH of 7.46 (pH previously 7.37), $PaCO_2$ of 55 mm Hg (previously 50 mm Hg), PaO_2 of 57 mm Hg, and HCO_3^- of 38 mEq/L (previously 28 mEq/L).

59. How would you interpret this ABG?

_____

60. Why did the blood gas values change from those in the case?

61. State how Stewart's strong ion difference approach to acid-base differs from the Henderson-Hasselbalch approach.

_____

Chapter **13** **Acid-Base Balance**

14 Regulation of Breathing

The brain is a wonderful organ. It starts working the moment you get up in the morning and doesn't stop until you get to the office.

Robert Frost

You are getting sleepy, very sleepy… You didn't stop breathing did you? In just one year as an adult, you will breathe more than *7 million times!* Most of those breaths will be automatically initiated by your brainstem. Just like clockwork. Good thing, eh? It makes sense that respiratory care practitioners would need to know how this system works and what happens when it doesn't. Chapter 14 is a fitting end to the section on anatomy and physiology, because it summarizes the control mechanisms that regulate the respiratory system.

WORD WIZARD

The brain and nervous system have a language all their own. Learning these terms will make it easier to understand concepts in this chapter. (And you can impress your friends with your linguistic abilities!)
Finish the following sentences by filling in the correct term(s).

1. _____ occurs when there is no breathing at all.

2. Many important responses involve the vagus nerve and are called _____ reflexes.

3. The _____ center in the pons is ill-defined, but gasping inhalations take place when it is out of control.

4. The _____ barrier prevents many substances from entering the cerebrospinal fluid.

5. The _____ center in the pons helps increase rate and control depth of ventilation and inspiratory time.

6. _____ respond to changes in O_2 and pH to signal the need to breathe.

WHERE'S THE ACTION?

Input into how we breathe comes from many areas. Conscious thought, receptors throughout the body, and reflexes all play important roles. The medulla's job is to organize the information and send messages to the motor fibers that innervate the muscles of the airway and chest (sort of a mental air-traffic controller). The medulla is located in your brainstem just above your spinal cord. If you cut the brainstem (don't try this at home) below the medulla, all ventilatory effort ceases. Another structure, the pons, sits on top of the medulla.

7. Label the parts of these central controlling bodies.

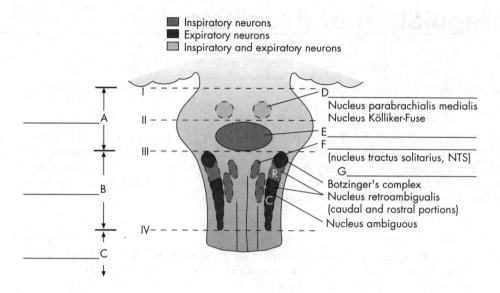

8. Briefly explain the role of the two primary respiratory groups in the medulla.

9. Compare and contrast the two primary centers in the pons.

10. What diseases or conditions might affect the performance of the brainstem's respiratory controllers?

AUTOMATIC PILOT

Respiratory reflexes are involuntary nervous responses located in airways, muscles, and tissues that influence breathing by sending information directly to the medulla (mostly via the vagus nerve). You'll need to be able to identify the most important reflexes, so here goes. Each reflex goes with a particular stimulus and has a response from receptors in a specific location.

Later on, let's apply some of these reflexes to the clinical setting and bring them to life.

	REFLEX	STIMULUS	RESPONSE	LOCATION
11.	Hering-Breuer			
12.	Deflation			
13.	Head			
14.	Vagovagal			
15.	C fiber			
16.	Proprioceptors			

BETTER LIVING THROUGH CHEMISTRY

Regulating ventilation ensures that tissues are exposed to just the right amount of oxygen (O_2), carbon dioxide (CO_2), and hydrogen ions. Blood carries these substances to specialized nerve structures called chemoreceptors that are strategically placed in the brainstem, carotid bodies, and arch of the aorta. All these chemoreceptors will respond in some way to decreased levels of O_2 and pH or increased CO_2 in the blood (or vice versa).

Central Chemoreceptors

Central chemoreceptors sit in the medulla, taking a bath in the cerebrospinal fluid (CSF). They are not in direct contact with the blood because of the blood-brain barrier, a semipermeable membrane that surrounds the brain.

17. Explain the process that allows CO_2 to stimulate the central receptors.

18. Describe the stimulating effects of CO_2 on the receptors in terms of the immediate response to increased CO_2 in the blood. What happens when this goes on for 1 or 2 days?

Peripheral Chemoreceptors

Someone thought it would be a good idea to monitor the chemical composition of blood leaving the heart and heading toward the brain. Pretty smart!

19. Describe the peripheral receptor response to decreased arterial O_2 levels. What do the receptors actually respond to when O_2 levels drop?

20. What specific range of PaO_2 values causes the greatest response when CO_2 and pH are normal?

21. How does altitude modify the receptor's response to hypoxemia?

22. Describe the peripheral receptor response to increased arterial CO_2 and H^+ ions. How is it different than the central chemoreceptor response?

NO ONE UNDERSTANDS ME!

Here goes something… Some patients, especially those with chronic obstructive pulmonary disease (COPD), become chronically hypoxic and hypercapnic. This happens when a high arterial CO_2 level persists over time. The kidneys compensate, which restores pH. Some of the bicarbonate diffuses into your head and corrects the pH in the CSF. The central receptors are fooled into thinking everything is fine. Because they are low on O_2, the hypoxic stimulus drives their ventilation.

So far, so bad. When someone intervenes and administers O_2 to this special type of patient, the patient may experience an *acute rise in arterial CO_2*. The simple explanation is that the patient is no longer driven by the peripheral receptors to breathe because of low O_2 levels. Though true, this explanation is too simple. We're not sure exactly what happens, but I follow the theory that increased O_2 also worsens the ventilation/perfusion ($\dot{V}/\dot{Q}$) relationship in the lung by increasing blood flow to poorly ventilated areas and through absorption atelectasis. Ventilation is decreased in the low–$\dot{V}/\dot{Q}$ areas and increased in the high–$\dot{V}/\dot{Q}$ regions. The drive to breathe is probably also blunted. It helps if the patient is exhausted or had medications that further depress the central nervous system (CNS). The result is an increased arterial P_{CO_2} in any case.

The point is that CO_2 in high concentrations in the blood is bad for you. It further decreases drive to breathe by depressing the CNS. So don't give the patient too much O_2, but **never withhold O_2 from a hypoxic patient!**

23. What concentration of O_2 is usually given to chronically hypercapnic patients? _____

_____

24. What is the best way to monitor oxygenation in these patients?

25. Why do low concentrations of O_2 usually result in adequate improvement?

OUCH!

Obviously if the brain is physically or physiologically injured, abnormal breathing patterns will occur. When you observe these patterns, you know something is wrong with the controller.

100

26. Describe Cheyne-Stokes breathing (use words or draw a picture). State two important causes of this distinctive pattern.

27. How does Biot breathing differ from Cheyne-Stokes in terms of pattern and origin?

28. Describe apneustic breathing. What does this pattern indicate?

29. What are the two central neurogenic breathing patterns. State three events that could cause these patterns.

CASE STUDIES

Case 1

Your patient rode his motorcycle without a helmet. He sustained a closed head injury during an accident that results in a subdural hematoma. He is intubated by the paramedics with an endotracheal tube.

30. Hyperventilation may lower the intracranial pressure of a patient with traumatic brain injury. What rules should you follow if you decide to do this procedure?

A. When:

_____

B. Lowest safe CO_2 value:

_____

C. Length of time you can safely hyperventilate:

_____

31. Why is lowering the CO_2 level controversial in traumatic brain injury?

Grandpa Maladie, COPD patient from Chapter 13, is back in the hospital. He became short of breath at home, and his family increased his O_2 from 2 to 6 L/min. When he arrives at the hospital, he is somnolent (sleepy) and difficult to arouse. ABG results reveal that pH is 7.25, $PaCO_2$ is 75 mm Hg, PaO_2 is 90 mm Hg, and HCO_3^- level is 37 mEq/L on 6 L/min by nasal cannula.

32. What changes should you make in the patient's therapy? Why?

33. What target PaO_2 would be more appropriate for this patient? (Consider the PO_2 where the receptors kick in...)

WHAT DOES THE NBRC SAY?

The NBRC won't exactly ask you direct questions about the information in this chapter, but they do love COPD patients with CO_2 retention and problems with hypoxic drive. See below for example variations on this theme.

Circle the best answer for each of the following multiple-choice questions.

34. A patient who has had COPD for many years is admitted for an acute episode of dyspnea. An arterial blood gas is drawn on room air with these results:

pH	7.50
$PaCO_2$	48 mm Hg
PaO_2	44 mm Hg
HCO_3^-	36 mEq/L
SaO_2	84%

What therapy do you recommend at this time?
A. 28% Venturi mask
B. 35% Venturi mask
C. nasal cannula delivering O_2 at 5 L/min
D. simple mask delivering O_2 at 10 L/min

35. A cooperative elderly patient with chronic asthma presents at her pulmonologist's office. You observe the following findings:

Pulse	94
RR	28
Temperature	36.5° C
BP	135/90
F_iO_2	0.21
pH	7.33
$PaCO_2$	70
PaO_2	35
HCO_3^-	34 mEq/L

What action would you take at this time?
- A. Administer bronchodilator therapy via MDI.
- B. Administer O_2 via cannula at 2 L/min.
- C. Administer O_2 via cannula at 6 L/min.
- D. Administer O_2 via non-rebreathing mask.

36. A patient with COPD and a history of hypercapnia is receiving O_2 via simple mask at 10 L/min in the recovery room following admission for pneumonia. Upon transfer to the medical floor, he is noted to be increasingly drowsy and difficult to arouse. The nurse requests that you give him a breathing treatment with a bronchodilator. The most appropriate action would be to
- A. Administer the breathing treatment as requested.
- B. Obtain an arterial blood gas sample.
- C. Change the O_2 to 2 L/min via nasal cannula.
- D. Change the O_2 to 40% via Venturi mask.

There are many variations of this type of question regarding chronic hypercapnia and O_2 administration on both the Entry Level and Registry examinations
You may also expect:

37. A patient is being mechanically ventilated following craniotomy. During a suctioning procedure, the intracranial pressure monitor shows a sudden increase in intracranial therapist. The patient becomes restless and agitated. What is the most appropriate immediate action for the respiratory therapist in this situation?
- A. Increase the F_iO_2 on the ventilator to deliver 100% O_2.
- B. Recommend administration of a sedative.
- C. Increase rate and volume of ventilation with a resuscitation bag.
- D. Ask the registered nurse to page the physician "STAT."

This type of question about head injuries is a hot topic right now clinically. We'll have to keep a close watch on the NBRC to see what they say on the subject in the next revision of the tests. Currently, the boards still favor reducing the CO_2 to lower intracranial pressure.

EXPERIMENT

This exercise will seem simple, but it will help you understand control of breathing. It's even better if you have a pulse oximeter.
- Put the oximeter probe on your finger.
- Breathe normally.
- Now inhale deeply and hold your breath.
- Time how long you can hold your breath.
- Next, inhale and exhale deeply several times. Fill your lungs and time how long you can hold your breath. (Remember to be seated and have a partner...)
- Answer the following questions.

38. How long could you hold your breath the first time? _____ What about the second try?

_____

39. What were the pulse oximetry readings before _____, during _____,

and at the end of breath holding? _____

40. Compare the results and explain the differences in the breath holding time and why you had to breathe. What is the meaning of the pulse oximetry readings?

41. Central chemoreceptors stimulate ventilation in response to the formation of _____ by CO_2 and water.

42. _____ increases the peripheral receptor response to arterial pH.

43. The primary stimulus for breathing in healthy individuals is arterial _____.

44. The secondary stimulus for breathing is arterial _____.

45. The breathing of patients with chronic hypercapnia is driven more by _____ stimulus than in patients with normal acid-base status.

46. _____ therapy is associated with acute arterial CO_2 retention in patients with chronic

_____.

FOOD FOR THOUGHT

The reflexes and receptors that control breathing are important. So is the input of conscious thought. The higher brain centers have a definite impact on how we breathe.

47. Why do we take the patient's respiratory rate without telling them we are doing it?

48. Name as many factors as you can that involve the higher brain centers increasing the rate of ventilation. (Hint: How do you breathe when a police car pulls up behind you and turns on the flashing lights?)

A Little More Food for Thought
Ascending to altitude can have profound consequences on ventilation.

49. An astronomy student goes to the volcano observatory (elevation, 11,000 feet) for his first clinical assignment. What is likely to happen to his breathing pattern as he goes higher up the mountain? What causes this to happen?

50. What would happen over the next 24 hours and why?

15 Bedside Assessment of the Patient

As I grow older, I pay less attention to what men say. I just watch what they do.
Andrew Carnegie

Patient assessment is the compass we steer by in the clinical setting. Chapter 15 helps you learn the fundamentals and help you identify the basics of the boards. Only bedside practice will give you mastery, and I think you'll have a lot of fun learning assessment. Your ability to evaluate using your senses will make all the difference in your career. The role of the respiratory therapist (RT) is evolving as we play an increasingly important part in in-house medical emergency response teams. Assessment skills are the KEY to everything from passing your boards to making lifesaving interventions at the bedside. Before you can go out and do that, you need to learn the material in this chapter.

WORD WIZARD

Chapter 15 starts off with an impressive list of more than 40 new words for you to learn. Power up your medical terminology by reading the chapter and making a match with this top 20 list.

Definitions	Terms
1. _____ musical expiratory sound associated with asthma	A. angina
2. _____ difficulty breathing when lying supine	B. barrel chest
3. _____ shape of thorax associated with emphysema	C. bradycardia
4. _____ chest pain typical of acute coronary syndromes	D. breathlessness
5. _____ physical wasting associated with chronic lung disease	E. cachexia
6. _____ blood pressure that is too low	F. crackles
7. _____ the sitting position that emphysema patients use when they are in trouble	G. cyanosis
8. _____ drop in blood pressure on inhalation associated with asthma and hyperinflation	H. dyspnea
9. _____ inspiratory sound associated with atelectasis, pneumonia, and fibrosis	I. febrile
10. _____ upper airway sound that may indicate life-threatening obstruction	J. orthopnea
11. _____ soft tissue sucking in around ribs and neck when a patient has severe distress	K. pulse deficit
12. _____ dizziness associated with drop in blood pressure	L. pulse pressure
13. _____ a rapid heart rate that may indicate a low blood oxygen level	M. pulsus paradoxus
14. _____ presence of a fever	N. retractions
15. _____ difference between systolic and diastolic blood pressure	O. shock
16. _____ a slow heart rate that may result in poor perfusion of tissues	P. stridor
17. _____ bluish discoloration of skin that could mean hypoxemia	Q. syncope
18. _____ heart rate auscultated in chest is different than pulse rate felt in arm	R. tachycardia
19. _____ difficulty breathing	S. tripodding
20. _____ sensation of suffocation	T. wheezes

105

Successful assessors develop a systematic way of evaluating patients. Except in life-threatening emergencies, most practitioners begin by interviewing the patient. The interview may be short or long depending on the situation. The increasing use of protocols requires respiratory therapists to conduct more in-depth interviews. There is some evidence that clinicians who are trained in interpersonal communication are better able to gain valuable information from patients. Let's review the essentials of interviewing and history-taking.

21. What information would you gather before entering the patient's room? Hint: *Egan's* doesn't get to this for several pages, so use your common sense to come up with an answer, then check Boxes 15-3 and 15-4 in "Format for the Medical History."

22. Describe how to *start* the ideal interview. Be sure to discuss space, privacy, and introductions. Now you can go back to "Structure and Technique for Interviewing" at the beginning of the chapter.

    A. Space: _____

    B. Privacy: _____

    C. Introductions: _____

23. Circle the *best approach* from each set of choices in the following list:
    A1. "Hi, Bob, good morning."
    A2. "Good morning Mr. Johnson."

    B1. Stand at the foot of the bed.
    B2. Sit in a chair at the bedside.

    C1. Make room for your notes on the bedside table.
    C2. Keep your clipboard on your lap.

    D1. "Do you need anything right now?"
    D2. "I'll tell your nurse to check on you."

    E1. "I'll be back to see you in one hour."
    E2. "I'll return in a while to check on you."

ARE YOU ASKING THE QUESTIONS CORRECTLY?

The way you ask questions will determine your relationship with the patient and the amount and quality of the information you gather.

24. Circle the best approach from each set of choices in following list:
    A1. "What are you coughing up?"
    A2. "You didn't cough up blood, did you?"

    B1. "I understand you don't like your breathing treatments."
    B2. "Why don't you like these treatments?"

    C1. "How is your breathing today?"
    C2. "Is your breathing better today?"

25. When are "closed" questions most useful? Give an example.

SIGNS AND SYMPTOMS OF CARDIOPULMONARY DISEASE

"I Feel Short of Breath..."

26. Describe the dyspnea (Borg) scale. Try to think of several reasons why this would be useful.

27. How else can you identify the degree of dyspnea a patient feels? Explain the difference between dyspnea and breathlessness.

"Cough It Up!"

28. What are the possible causes of these common types of cough?

	Cough	Cause(s)
A.	Dry	
B.	Loose, productive	
C.	Acute, self-limiting	
D.	Chronic	

29. What is the difference between mucus and sputum?

30. What are the three characteristics of sputum that should be documented and reported to the physician and other members of the health care team?

_____

_____

_____

31. Define *nonmassive* hemoptysis and give three common causes.

32. Define *massive* hemoptysis and give three possible causes.

"It Hurts When I Take a Deep Breath!"

33. What is the most serious (and famous) kind of nonpleuritic chest pain?

_____

_____

34. How does pleuritic chest pain differ from nonpleuritic pain?

"Hot Stuff!"

35. Significant elevation of temperature will have what result on metabolic rate, oxygen consumption, carbon dioxide production, and breathing pattern?

_____

_____

36. Along with fever, what are two signs that are highly suggestive of respiratory infection?

A. _____

B. _____

Whether you personally take medical histories or not, you will need to be familiar with the standard format used in this process that is *always* conducted at some point (usually early on) during a patient's admission to the formal health care setting.

37. What do the initials "CC" and "HPI" stand for? List at least five important areas described in the HPI.

   A. CC = _____

   B. HPI = _____

      1. _____

      2. _____

      3. _____

      4. _____

      5. _____

38. What do the initials "PMH" stand for? List at least five important areas described in the PMH.

   A. PMH = _____

      1. _____

      2. _____

      3. _____

      4. _____

      5. _____

General appearance is assessed during the first few seconds of *every* encounter with a patient. During the first encounter, always look at their body as a whole, facial expression, anxiety level, positioning, and personal hygiene. (You may smell and hear information, too!)

39. Describe the significance of the findings for each of the areas of general appearance listed below.

	FINDING	SIGNIFICANCE
1.	Weak, emaciated, and diaphoretic	
2.	Appears anxious	
3.	Sitting up, leaning with arms on table	

LEVEL OF CONSCIOUSNESS

What's the difference between stuporous and lethargic? Obtunded and comatose? Alert and confused? These are not completely subjective terms, and you will see them used frequently in the medical record. After taking a look at the overall appearance, you need to determine the level of consciousness. For starters, the patient is either obviously conscious or not. If he or she is conscious, you have to find out the level of alertness. If the patient does not seem to be obviously conscious, you need to find out how depressed the sensorium is and describe this with commonly accepted terms.

40. What does the phrase "oriented × 3" mean?

_____

41. Compare and contrast the terms "lethargic" and "obtunded."

42. What is the difference between a "stuporous" patient and a "comatose" patient?

43. What is the first thing a respiratory therapist should evaluate in cases of a depressed level of consciousness?

_____

There are special rating systems like the Glasgow Coma Scale (Chapter 46) to help further identify the degree of coma. You also need to keep in mind that there are special circumstances that may make assessment more difficult, such as a hearing-impaired patient.

VITAL INFORMATION

Temperature, pulse, respiratory rate, and blood pressure are the traditional vital signs. These are useful, and easy to obtain. (People call pulse oximetry the "fifth vital sign" because it is taken so often.) Vital signs offer great clues about response to therapeutic interventions, but they're not as simple as you might think considering how often they are measured. Let's start with the basics.

44. Fill in the correct normal values (or terms) for an adult in the chart below.

	SIGN	AVERAGE NORMAL	LOWEST NORMAL	HIGHEST NORMAL
A.	Temperature			
B.	Heart rate			
C.	Respiratory rate			
D.	Systolic blood pressure			
E.	Diastolic blood pressure			

45. Name the four common sites for temperature measurement. Give a disadvantage of each site. Which site most accurately reflects core temperature?

A. _____ _____

B. _____ _____

C. _____ _____

D. _____ _____

46. Match these pulsating terms to their throbbing definitions.

Terms	Definitions
A. _____ tachycardia	1. palpable vibrations in pulse
B. _____ bruits	2. strength of pulse
C. _____ amplitude	3. pulse rate below 60 beats/min
D. _____ paradoxical pulse	4. drop in amplitude with inspiration
E. _____ pulsus alternans	5. pulse rate greater than 100 beats/min
F. _____ bradycardia	6. alternating strong and weak pulses

47. Match these flowing respiratory patterns to their whooshing definitions. Hint: When in doubt, try the glossary in the back of the book!

Terms	Definitions
A. _____ tachypnea	1. difficulty breathing in a supine position
B. _____ eupnea	2. abnormally low respiratory rate
C. _____ orthopnea	3. deep breathing
D. _____ platypnea	4. normal breathing pattern
E. _____ hyperpnea	5. abnormally high respiratory rate
F. _____ bradypnea	6. labored breathing in an upright position

48. How can you prevent the patient from becoming aware (and consciously altering) that you are taking their respiratory rate?

49. What condition may result in syncope in the hypovolemic patient? How can you prevent this from happening? How is it treated medically?

A. Condition: _____

B. Prevention: _____

C. Treatment: _____

Chapter **15** **Bedside Assessment of the Patient**

50. What does it mean when patients show larger (>6 to 8 mm Hg) than normal drop in systolic pressure during inspiration?

EXAMINING THE CHEST AND LUNGS

The Big Four
- Inspect the chest!
- Palpate the chest!
- Percuss the chest!
- Auscultate the chest!

Sounds so easy when you put it that way, doesn't it? Before you start to assess, make sure you have enough **light,** enough **privacy,** enough **time,** and enough **quiet.** Chapter 15 describes the *ideal* evaluation of a patient. You will have to modify to meet the circumstances every time!

Inspection

There's a lot you can see when you take a quick look at the patient. Practice looking. Let's find out if you know what to look for in a patient with respiratory problems.

51. Write a description for the following 6 abnormal chest shapes.

Bad Chests	Description
A. Barrel	_____
B. Kyphosis	_____
C. Kyphoscoliosis	_____
D. Pectus carinatum	_____
E. Pectus excavatum	_____
F. Scoliosis	_____

52. Breathing patterns are important too. Describe the pattern that goes with these six conditions.

Condition	Pattern of Breathing
A. Asthma	_____
B. Atelectasis	_____
C. Chest trauma	_____
D. Epiglottitis	_____
E. Increased ICP	_____
F. Metabolic acidosis	_____

Experiment

To get good at this, you might try the mall. Yes, the mall. Or a coffee shop or market with Wi-Fi! If you sit with a nice cup of espresso, you can see chest shape, breathing pattern, and all the rest. Compare adult patterns with those of children. Compare the chest shape of an elderly person to that of a young adult. If you can't go to the mall, search the Internet; but there is no substitute for really looking. After you try this exercise, answer the following questions.

53. Did you observe anyone breathing with their diaphragm? How could you tell? _____

_____

54. Did you observe the use of accessory muscles? How could you tell? _____

_____

55. How does the chest shape of a young adult differ from that of a senior? _____

_____

56. What unusual chest shapes did you observe? Anyone on portable oxygen? _____

_____

Palpation

Palpation is the art of touching the chest wall. Palpation is an art (and a useful one) because it's so subjective. You have to get a feel for it.

57. Explain the difference between vocal, tactile, and bronchial fremitus.

58. Describe the difference in fremitus between emphysema and pneumonia.

59. How does subcutaneous emphysema form? What is the feeling of air under the skin called?

Experiment

You should learn palpation in the laboratory setting of your program. Because disrobing may be necessary, gowns, privacy, and professionalism are needed.

- Assess tactile fremitus by asking your classmate to repeat the word "ninety-nine" while you palpate under the clavicles, between the shoulder blades, along the sides, and over the lower lobes.
- Measure chest expansion as demonstrated in Figure 15-4, "Estimation of thoracic expansion," in your text. Now answer these questions:

113

60. Describe the temperature of your partner's skin. _____

_____

61. Were there any areas of abnormal fremitus? Why (why not)?

62. Estimate the amount of chest expansion in centimeters. What is normal adult expansion? Was the expansion equal on both sides?

Percussion

Diagnostic percussion of the chest is another art form that is rarely practiced these days. Still, it can be useful in detecting some important abnormalities, and the NBRC expects you to be able to interpret the results of percussion findings!

63. Complete the following chart by identifying the percussion notes for these conditions.

Condition	Percussion Note
A. Emphysema	_____
B. Atelectasis	_____
C. Pleural effusion	_____
D. Pneumothorax	_____
E. Pneumonia	_____

64. What are the limitations of percussion? What can't you feel? _____

_____

Experiment

You should do this in the lab while you are performing the palpation and auscultation (see following section) exercises.
- Place your left middle finger on the intercostal space on the side of the chest.
- Rapidly strike it with your index finger or middle finger of your right hand. Do this on both sides of the chest.
- Repeat over the lower lobes in the back.
- Have your partner take a really deep breath and hold it while you tap.
- Have them exhale fully, then tap.
- Try tapping over something solid like the scapula.
- Try tapping over the abdomen.
- Tap on your own head.
- It takes practice to get good at percussion.

Don't include this procedure in a routine examination of a patient unless other observations suggest an appropriate problem. Have an expert present when you try this in the clinical setting!

65. What happened to the resonance when your partner inhaled deeply? On exhalation?

By the way, percussion is the method many people use to assess the ripeness of a watermelon! You can, in fact, practice on watermelon quite nicely.

Auscultation

This is it. This is the big one. Auscultation seems so easy, and identifying breath sounds so difficult. Follow these 10 steps to improve your technique.

1. Sit the patient up whenever you can.
2. Turn off the TV, radio, or other external sources of noise.
3. Ask the patient to breathe slowly and deeply through his or her mouth.
4. Listen to skin whenever you can.
5. Listen to the lower lobes first.
6. Listen to one full inspiration and exhalation in each spot.
7. Listen to both sides in each spot.
8. Auscultate lower, middle, and upper portions of the lung.
9. Listen to front and back of the chest.
10. Compare right and left lungs and compare upper and lower lobes.

Experiment

You should try this in the laboratory before going to the bedside. You can listen at home, too. The more normal sounds you auscultate, the better you will be at recognizing abnormal sounds. All you need is your stethoscope, a partner (you can even start on yourself), and a quiet place to listen. Adjust the earpieces on your stethoscope so they are pointing slightly forward, not straight into your ears. (If your scope is adjustable, check to make sure the diaphragm is "on," not the bell.) Now, listen.

- Place your partner in a sitting position (or high Fowler).
- Ask your partner to breathe in and out slowly through the mouth.
- Listen on skin over the posterior lower lobes (below the shoulder blade).
- In and out, right side and left side!
- Listen on the side of the chest (still lower lobes).
- Listen between the shoulder blades (not over the spine!).
- Listen on the front to the middle lobe and lingula (anterior, below nipple).
- Listen on the front below the collar bone (above nipples).
- Listen over the trachea.

Look in your text at Figure 15-6. You can auscultate 20 or more places on the chest, but we don't usually do this much auscultation in the clinical setting. It takes too long for a routine evaluation. Always listen to upper, middle, lower, front, and back. Count 10 spots that MUST be listened to in the routine screening of breath sounds. When you hear abnormal sounds or have a critically ill patient, you should expand your assessment.

Now that you've read the chapter and practiced, try answering these questions:

66. Fill in the chart below with descriptions of your favorite breath sounds.

	BREATH SOUND	PITCH	INTENSITY	LOCATION
A.	Vesicular			
B.	Bronchial			
C.	Bronchovesicular			

67. Compare the mechanisms and causes of coarse, low-pitched crackles and fine end-inspiratory crackles.

68. Contrast monophonic and polyphonic wheezes in terms of mechanisms, phase of ventilation, and conditions that produce these different musical sounds.

69. What's up with that rhonchi thing?

EXTREMITY EXAM

You will almost always want to take a look at a patient's fingers. For one thing, it goes hand in hand with pulse oximetry. Cardiopulmonary disease may alter the fingers and other extremities.

70. How do you test for capillary refill? (Test your own while you're at it.) What is a normal capillary refill time?

71. Where should you check for edema caused by heart failure? Why? _____

_____

72. Cyanosis is a bluish discoloration of the skin. Answer the following questions about cyanosis.

    A. What is the specific cause of cyanosis? _____

_____

    B. What is peripheral cyanosis? _____

_____

    C. What is the main cause of peripheral cyanosis? _____

_____

Case 1

An alert 67-year-old politician is admitted for dyspnea and hemoptysis. While interviewing the patient you discover that he has been coughing up small amounts of thick, blood-streaked mucus several times per day for the last few days. He has a history of 100 pack-years of cigarette smoking. Physical examination reveals a barrel chest, use of accessory muscles, and digital clubbing.

73. The patient's history and chest configuration suggest what primary pulmonary disorder?

_____

_____

74. Along with enlargement of the ends of the fingers, what sign helps you recognize clubbing?

_____

_____

75. What does the presence of clubbing suggest in this case?

_____

_____

Case 2

A 47-year-old homemaker is admitted for a systemic infection 3 days after cutting herself in the kitchen while preparing some chicken. She complains of dyspnea and has a fever. Her vital signs are pulse 110 beats/min, respiratory rate 28 breaths/min, and blood pressure 76/58 mm Hg. The nurse's notes reveal that the patient was alert on admission, but she is now confused and anxious. Her extremities are warm and capillary refill is normal.

76. Why do you think the patient's mental status has deteriorated?

77. What other "vital sign" should be evaluated? _____

_____

78. Which abnormal vital sign has the most clinical significance in this case?

_____

_____

You are called to the ward to evaluate a 29-year-old medical student who was admitted for shortness of breath and is now complaining of chest pain. The patient tells you that the pain came on suddenly and is worse when he inhales. Your interview reveals that this pain is on the right side and feels like a sharp, stabbing sensation. His temperature is normal, but blood pressure, heart rate, and respiratory rate are elevated. Palpation reveals crepitus over the right lateral chest wall.

79. What other physical assessments would be useful in determining the nature of the problem?

_____

_____

80. What immediate treatment should you initiate in this situation?

_____

_____

_____

81. What diagnostic test would be helpful in determining the cause of the pain?

_____

_____

82. What does the finding of crepitus on palpation indicate?

_____

_____

_____

A 59-year-old rock star, is recovering from open heart surgery performed 2 days earlier. He is alert and oriented × 3. He complains of dyspnea (a lot of people seem to complain about that) and a dry cough. Vital signs reveal a pulse of 104 beats/min and a respiratory rate of 32 breaths/min with a shallow pattern. The patient tells you that his difficulty breathing started yesterday and has been gradually getting worse. Auscultation reveals decreased breath sounds in both bases with end-inspiratory crackles.

83. What is the most likely cause of the dyspnea?

_____

_____

118

84. What diagnostic test is indicated to confirm the diagnosis?

_____

_____

85. What respiratory care intervention(s) is indicated?

WHAT DOES THE NBRC SAY?

Killer. Whole sections of each test are devoted to this subject.

The NBRC exam matrix is filled with "assess by inspection," "assess by palpation," "assess by auscultation," and "interview the patient." There are additional questions in the therapy section of the test where you need the results of percussion or auscultation to come up with the right procedure. The effort you put into this one chapter will pay off more than any other. You will need to look at this subject more closely later on as you prepare for your boards. For now, here are some sample questions.

86. During a chest examination of an intubated patient, the RT palpates vibrations on exhalation over the upper chest. What action should be taken at this time?
   A. The patient should be given a bronchodilator.
   B. The patient should be suctioned.
   C. The patient should be given supplemental oxygen.
   D. The patient should be placed on mechanical ventilation.

87. A patient's medical record indicates that he has orthopnea. Which of the following best describes this condition?
   A. difficulty breathing at night
   B. difficulty breathing when upright
   C. difficulty breathing on exertion
   D. difficulty breathing when lying down

88. A child is brought to the emergency department for severe respiratory distress. Upon entering the room, the RT hears a high-pitched sound when the child inhales. This is most likely
   A. wheezing
   B. stridor
   C. rhonchi
   D. crackles

89. An RT is asked to evaluate a patient for oxygen therapy. She notices that the patient is sleepy but arouses when questioned. This level of consciousness is best described as
   A. confused
   B. obtunded
   C. stuporous
   D. lethargic

Chapter **15** **Bedside Assessment of the Patient**

90. Which of the following breath sounds is most likely to be heard during acute exacerbation of asthma?
    A. wheezes
    B. crackles
    C. stridor
    D. rhonchi

91. All of the following physical findings are consistent with pneumonia *except*
    A. dull percussion note
    B. presence of inspiratory crackles
    C. bronchial breath sounds over the affected area
    D. bradypnea

92. Which of the following findings suggest that a patient is oriented?
    1. awareness of the correct date
    2. ability to correctly state his own name
    3. awake when you enter the room
    4. cooperation with the treatment
        A. 1 and 2
        B. 2 and 3
        C. 1 and 4
        D. 3 and 4

93. During an interview, the patient states he has been coughing up thick, foul-smelling sputum. This finding is most consistent with
    A. a bacterial infection of the lung
    B. a diagnosis of lung cancer
    C. obstructive lung disease
    D. pulmonary tuberculosis

94. An RT is inspecting the chest of a child with respiratory distress. The practitioner notes that the child has a large concave depression of the sternum. This finding should be documented as
    A. barrel chest
    B. pectus carinatum
    C. pectus excavatum
    D. kyphoscoliosis

95. All of the following physical findings are consistent with complete upper airway obstruction *except*
    A. inability to speak
    B. stridor
    C. supraclavicular retractions
    D. flaring of the nostrils

96. While assessing a patient who is dyspneic and tachypneic, an RT notices a bluish discoloration of the lips and oral mucosa. The practitioner should document which of the following in the medical record?
    A. cyanosis
    B. hypoxemia
    C. increased work of breathing
    D. orthopnea

16 Interpreting Clinical Laboratory Data

A little learning is a dangerous thing, but a lot of ignorance is just as bad.

Bob Edwards

In the clinical setting, laboratory assessment directly follows the interview and physical assessment. The NBRC's Clinical Simulation Examinations often follow a similar format. So it seems natural for Chapter 16 to follow Chapter 15! A lot of students struggle with this topic because it is outside our usual realm, but you'll be on it when you finish these exercises. Remember, these tests are a lot harder on the patient than on you!

WORD WIZARD

The words sound so similar, it's easy to get confused. *Leuko* means "white," *erythro* means "red," and *thrombo* means "blood clot"—at least they do in Latin. Now finish these words.

_____ ology is the study of blood. The CBC, or complete _____

_____, is a test used to establish the overall picture of the blood. A _____ test value is significantly outside the normal range and may be life-threatening to the patient. White blood

cells are called _____ cytes. When the white blood count goes up in infection, we call it

_____ cytosis. If the white count goes down, the new name is _____

penia. Hemoglobin is found in the _____ cyte and can carry oxygen. Your blood won't clot without

the smallest formed element, the _____ cytes. A condition of _____ penia may result in bleeding if you suction or draw a blood gas!

LAB TESTS

Certain laboratory test results are very useful to the respiratory therapist (RT). You will need to learn the normal values and what abnormal results mean if you want to pass your boards or get the big picture in the hospital. Let's start with complete blood counts.

White

1. What does a large elevation in white blood cell (WBC) count suggest?

   A. _____

   B. _____

   C. _____

2. Name three common causes of low WBC count.

   A. _____

   B. _____

   C. _____

3. What specific type of WBC is elevated in bacterial pneumonia? Viral?

   A. Bacterial: _____

   B. Viral: _____

   Remember this one. We want to know if we need to give antibiotics. Also watch for bands and segs.

4. Which WBCs are involved in problems like allergic asthma?

Red

5. What term describes a low red blood cell (RBC) count? What is the treatment for this disorder?

   A. Term: _____

   B. Treatment: _____

   _____

6. What is a normal hemoglobin level, and why are RTs especially interested in hemoglobin levels?

   A. Normal: _____

   B. Respiratory role: _____

   _____

7. What blood abnormality is caused by chronic hypoxemia? _____

   _____

   Anyone with this RBC count either has a lung problem or lives at altitude. Pumping this thick blood through the lung contributes to right-sided heart failure.

8. Before performing an arterial blood gas (ABG), you would be wise to check what two *specific* laboratory values?

   A. Blood count _____

   B. Blood chemistry test _____

ELECTROLYTES

RTs are interested in electrolyte values because they affect acid-base balance and muscle function. A "chemistry panel" is the name of the test ordered by the physician to determine the values. Electrolytes were covered in Chapter 12. See how much you remember.

9. What is the normal range for serum potassium?

   _____

122

10. Why is potassium of particular interest in patients being weaned from mechanical ventilation?

11. Give at least one clinical example of how a patient develops a very high or very low potassium level.

   A. Hyperkalemia _____

   B. Hypokalemia _____

12. What value on the venous chemistry panel represents bicarbonate?

   _____

13. Low chloride levels occur for what two primary reasons?

   A. _____

   B. _____

14. Why is the chloride level in sweat so important? What is the critical value?

   A. Importance: _____

   B. Value: _____

   Sweat-chloride, an older test, is still useful, but genetic testing is able to give a better picture of the disease.

15. What other test is indicated when a chemistry panel shows abnormal anion gap? *This is an important idea on your board exams. If the electrolytes are off, the RT should recommend...*

   _____

16. What are the two tests that together indicate renal function?

   _____

ENZYMES

Enzymes are present everywhere in the body. They make reactions happen. (Remember carbonic anhydrase?) Specific enzymes are released when tissues are damaged, so you can track down the origin of the problem. The liver and the heart are good examples of organs that release enzymes when injured.

17. Name the two common liver enzymes that might be elevated in patients with hepatitis. Give the old names and the new names.

	OLD	NEW
A.		
B.		

Chapter **16** **Interpreting Clinical Laboratory Data**

18. CPK is an example of an enzyme that can show you specific injury to brain, lungs, heart, or muscles. Describe the three types of CPK and what they mean.

A. CPK-BB _____

B. CPK-MM _____

C. CPK-MB _____

19. Discuss troponin I and explain why it would be important in emergency medicine.

20. Another interesting chemical can tell you if the patient has heart failure, rather than a heart attack. What does BNP stand for and how do we use this test?

A. BNP = _____

B. What does it show us? _____

C. Name another condition that can elevate BNP. _____

CLOTTING IS COOL

Most of the time, the respiratory therapist is happier if the blood clots than if it does not! Arterial blood gases, suctioning, and other procedures may result in bleeding, and a little pressure will usually stop the bleeding after 3 to 5 minutes. Patients with clotting disorders and certain medications may not stop bleeding as expected! Other patients are likely to get clots in blood and the brain, so RTs medicate them to "thin" the blood or lengthen clotting times. A pulmonary embolus, or clot in the lung, is a common cause of death. You need to know the drugs and the tests so you will recognize which patients are at risk.

Coagulation studies are done to check clotting. Explain PT and PTT so we know you've got it.

21. PT

A. Full name _____

B. When is it used? _____

22. PTT

A. Full name _____

B. When is it used? _____

C. Explain the difference in the two tests.

D. Name medications associated with PTT.

23. Explain the D-dimer test and how it is useful to respiratory therapists.

24. What blood cell is vital to clotting, and what are the normal values?

SPUTUM IS OUR BREAD AND BUTTER

You will probably be asked to obtain many sputum specimens during your career. Sputum samples are needed when lung infections are suspected. Gram stain, culture, and sensitivity are almost always performed, but only if you get the right stuff!

25. Why would the laboratory reject your beautiful sputum specimen? Give me specific reasons and include numerical values.

   A. Pus _____

   B. Epithelials _____

   How can you improve the quality? Have patients rinse out their mouth and pharynx before you have them cough.

26. What is the purpose of growing the bacteria on a culture plate?

   _____

   _____

CASE STUDIES

Case 1

A patient presents in the emergency department complaining of shortness of breath, fever, and productive cough. A chest radiograph reveals pneumonia in the right lower lobe.

27. What blood test is indicated?

   _____

28. What specific finding would suggest bacterial pneumonia?

   _____

29. What would you like to do about the sputum?

A 60-year-old, two-pack-per-day smoker has a complete blood count ordered, and his WBC count is 9000. His hematocrit is 60%, and his hemoglobin is 20 g/dL.

30. What is the name for this elevation of red blood cells?

_____

31. What respiratory problem is indicated by the high hematocrit and hemoglobin?

_____

WHAT DOES THE NBRC SAY?

There aren't too many lab questions on the CRT or Written Registry Examinations. But the NBRC makes it clear you need to know every scrap of information in this chapter! Sounds confusing, but the lab values and tests will be inside the questions and especially the cases in the Clinical Simulation Examination. You may get to "order" a CBC on the exam. You'll need to be able to interpret the results. You will see some multiple-choice questions like these. Circle the best answer.

32. Sputum culture and sensitivity would be indicated for which of the following conditions?
    A. ST segment elevation
    B. pleural effusion
    C. pneumothorax
    D. bronchitis

33. A patient presents in the emergency department with vomiting. Blood gas results reveal a metabolic alkalosis. Based on this information, you would also suggest
    A. a STAT chest radiograph
    B. an electrolyte analysis
    C. a complete blood count
    D. clotting time

34. A Chem 7 panel was ordered for a patient in the emergency department and hypokalemia is present. What test should the RT recommend?
    A. STAT chest radiograph
    B. arterial blood gas
    C. sputum culture
    D. complete blood count

35. A sputum culture that is sent to the lab is likely to be rejected as saliva if
    A. less than 25 epithelial cells are present
    B. less than 25 pus cells are present
    C. more than 25 epithelial cells are present
    D. more than 25 pus cells are present

FOOD FOR THOUGHT

36. A young adult male patient presents with symptoms of hypoxemia and signs of pneumonia. What are several possible reasons the WBC count is severely depressed?

> *There is only one thing worse than hardness of heart and that is softness of head.*
>
> Theodore Roosevelt

In the clinical setting, a lot of respiratory therapists (RTs) perform electrocardiography procedures as part of their jobs. Advanced life support certification requires knowledge of heart rhythms, and so do your board examinations. We discuss cardiac care in respiratory care because of the close relationship between the heart and the lungs. A lot of students struggle to learn arrhythmias, so I've tried to help you figure out what to emphasize and what the classic patterns look like on tests. The "real world" of electrocardiography is wonderfully complex and specialized, so you can spend many years learning the finer points after you graduate.

A PICTURE IS WORTH...

There are no new words that we haven't already covered, so why not go right to the picture? Label all these heart parts and conduction clues.

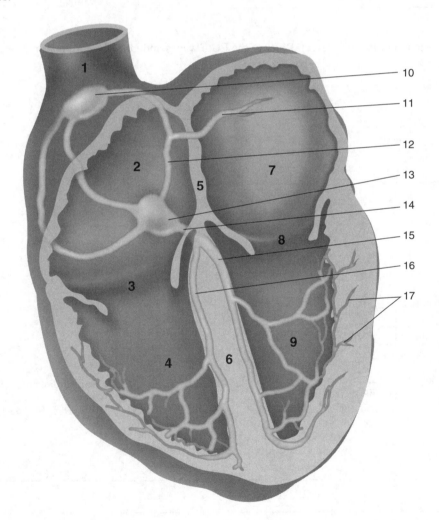

Anatomy of the impulse-conducting system of the human heart.

Heart Parts	Conduction Clues

1. _____

2. _____

3. _____

4. _____

5. _____

6. _____

7. _____

8. _____

9. _____

10. _____ natural "pacemaker" of the heart

11. _____ conducts impulses through the atria

12. _____ carries impulses across the right atrium

13. _____ "backup pacemaker"

14. _____ why not "hers"?

15. _____ carries impulse to the left ventricle

16. _____ carries impulse to the right ventricle

17. _____ fingerlike projections penetrate the ventricles

18. Let's get the basic identification perfect. Refer to the ECG waves and label the four common waves and indicate the event they represent.

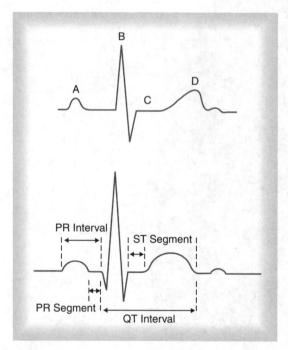

Normal configuration of electrocardiographic waves, segments, and intervals. (Modified from Wilkins RL, Krider SI, Sheldon RL: *Clinical Assessment in Respiratory Care,* ed 5, St. Louis, 2005, Mosby.)

Wave

A. _____

B. _____

C. _____

D. _____

Represents

_____

_____

_____

_____

Now answer the following questions about ECG waves.

19. Where is atrial repolarization?

_____

20. What is the maximum duration of the P–R interval?

_____

21. What pathologic abnormality results in a depressed or elevated ST segment?

_____

MAKING MEASUREMENTS

The ECG paper is made up of tiny boxes or grids that allow you to measure time on the horizontal axis and millimeters of deflection on the vertical axis. A darker line occurs every five boxes.

22. What is the normal paper speed for an ECG?

_____

23. The time (horizontal) represented by one small box is _____ seconds and by one

    large box is _____ seconds.

24. One millivolt of electrical energy will produce a deflection of _____ small boxes

    or _____ large boxes.

START AT THE BEGINNING

Because many RTs perform ECGs on patients or take care of monitored patients, you will need to be able to evaluate the rhythms you see to maintain safe patient care. Successful assessors have developed a systematic way of evaluating the ECG.

Step 1: Evaluate the Rate

You can do this manually, or rely on the electronic data. There are time marks every 3 seconds. So, the number of QRS complexes in 6 seconds can be multiplied by 10. When the rate is regular, you can divide 300 by the number of large boxes between two QRS complexes.

Try It, You'll Like It!

Count the rate in pattern 1 by both manual methods.

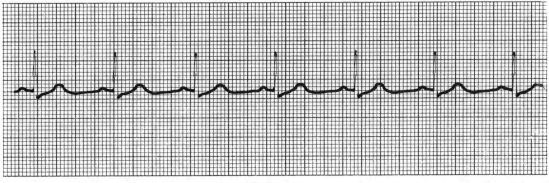

Pattern 1

Chapter **17** **Interpreting the Electrocardiogram**

25. The number of QRS complexes in this 6-second strip is _____. Multiply by 10

    to get a rate of _____.

26. There are _____ heavy lines between complex A and complex B; 300 divided

    by this number is _____. That's the average rate!

    Is every P wave followed by a QRS complex? That indicates a sinus rhythm!

27. If the rate is below 60 beats/min, it is called sinus _____.

28. If the rate is above 100 beats/min, it is called sinus _____.

Step 2: Measure the P–R Interval

Count the number of small boxes between the start of the P wave and the start of the QRS complex. Remember the normal value of less than 0.20 second (five small boxes). AP wave, followed by a QRS, but separated by a prolonged P–R interval, represents a delay at the AV node. This is called a first-degree heart block. No treatment is usually needed. We just monitor for a worsening block.

Try It, You'll Like It!

Measure the P–R interval in pattern 2.

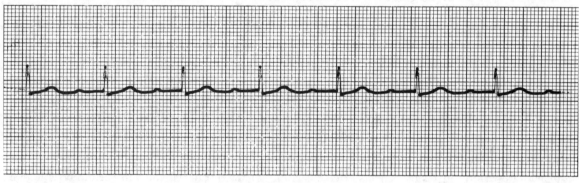

Pattern 2

29. The time from the P wave to the QRS complex is _____ second(s).

30. What arrhythmia does this represent?

    _____

Step 3: Evaluate the QRS Complex

The normal QRS complex is no more than 0.12 second (three small boxes) in width. Wide QRS complexes are abnormal and do not result in good ventricular contractions.

Try It, You'll Like It!

Measure the QRS complex in pattern 3.

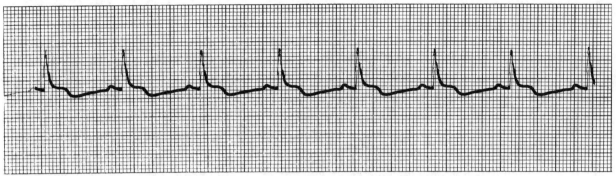

Pattern 3

31. The duration of the QRS complex is _____ second(s).

Step 4: Evaluate the T Wave

Normal T waves are upright and rounded. Inverted T waves represent poor blood flow to the heart muscle. Strangely shaped T waves may be caused by hyperkalemia.

32. The T wave in pattern 1 is (circle one)
    upright
    inverted

Step 5: Evaluate the ST Segment

A normal ST segment is basically flat-isoelectric. Elevated or depressed ST segments are bad. They represent oxygenation problems and are seen in conditions like myocardial infarction (MI).

Try It, You'll Like It!

Evaluate the ST segment seen in pattern 4.

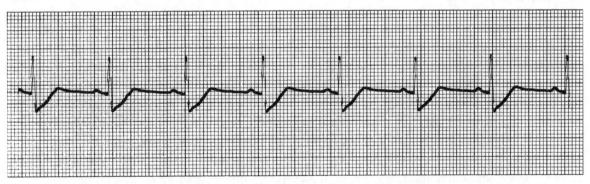

Pattern 4

33. The ST segment in pattern 4 is (circle one)
    elevated
    flat
    depressed

Step 6: Identify the RR Interval

You are looking for a regular relationship. If the Rs are not the same distance apart, you have an irregular rhythm.

Try It, You'll Like It!

Evaluate the RR interval seen in pattern 5.

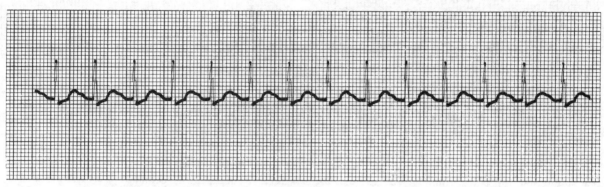

Pattern 5

34. The RR interval in this pattern is (circle one)
    regular
    irregular

RECOGNIZING ARRHYTHMIAS

Now that you have the basic idea, let's take a look at the major dysrhythmias that you will encounter. This is pattern recognition, so look for the "picture" each rhythm shows.

Normal Sinus Rhythm

Pattern 6

- The P wave is upright.
- The P–R interval is normal.
- Each P wave is followed by a normal QRS complex.
- RR intervals are regular, and the rate is between 60 and 100 per minute.
  No treatment is needed for this rhythm!

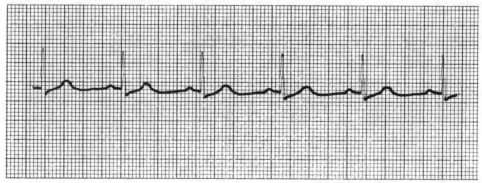

Pattern 6

Sinus Bradycardia

Pattern 7

- Upright P wave.
- Normal P–R interval.
- Each P wave is followed by a normal QRS complex.
- RR intervals are regular, *but the rate is less than 60 per minute.*

This is **absolute bradycardia.** It is only a problem if the blood pressure drops. You might see this rhythm during suctioning as a result of vagal stimulation. Stop suctioning! Intravenous atropine is a treatment for this arrhythmia.

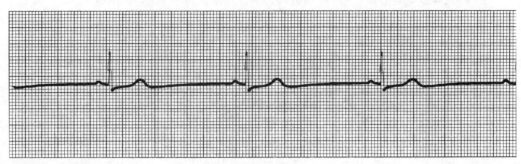

Pattern 7

Sinus Tachycardia

- The P wave is upright.
- The P–R interval is short.
- Each P wave is followed by a normal QRS complex.
- RR intervals are regular, *but the rate is over 100 per minute!*

This is sinus tachycardia. Tachycardia is the first sign of hypoxemia in most patients. Consider whether you are doing something to cause it, like suctioning. Look back at pattern 5 to see an example of sinus tachycardia.

First-Degree Heart Block

- The P wave is upright.
- The P–R interval is *prolonged.*
- Each P wave is followed by a normal QRS complex.
- RR intervals are regular.

This is only a problem if signs and symptoms, such as low blood pressure, chest pain, and so on, come with it. It may be caused by drugs or a myocardial infarction. Look back at pattern 2 to see an example of a first-degree block.

Second-Degree Heart Block

Our block is moving lower down the conduction pathway. Not good! There are two types.

Second-Degree Type I

This one is called Wenckebach or Mobitz type I. The P waves have a progressively prolonged transmission (prolonged P–R interval) followed by a P wave with no QRS complex. There is usually a repeated pattern, like three P waves and one lost QRS complex (pattern 8).

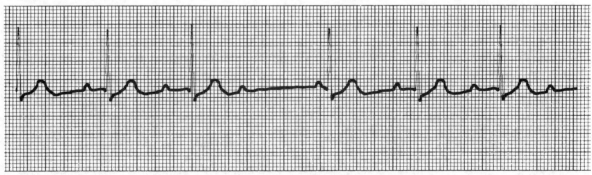

Pattern 8

Second-Degree Type II

This is Mobitz type II. It is definitely not a good sign. This block is worse. You will see some P waves conducted (followed by a QRS complex) and some P waves with no QRS complex following (pattern 9).

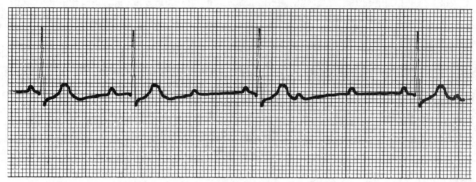

Pattern 9

Third-Degree Block

Also called complete heart block, this rhythm is definitely life-threatening. No impulses from the SA node are conducted. Because the ventricles have their own intrinsic rate, you will see the atria paced by the SA node (P waves) and the ventricles (QRS complex) pacing themselves (pattern 10). These QRS complexes are often wide. Blood pressure is poor, and an artificial pacemaker is needed.

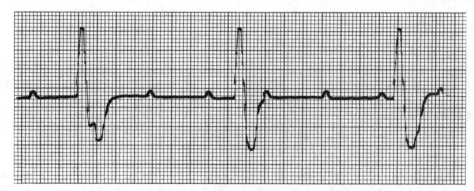

Pattern 10

Atrial Dysrhythmias

Atrial fibrillation is an erratic quivering of the atria that does not deliver a good preload to the ventricles (pattern 11). Also, clots may form in the atria. Sometimes the ventricle responds to fibrillation with a rapid rate as well. No P wave is seen, but the QRS complexes probably look OK. Drugs (like digitalis) or cardioversion are possible treatments. (Notice the RR intervals.)

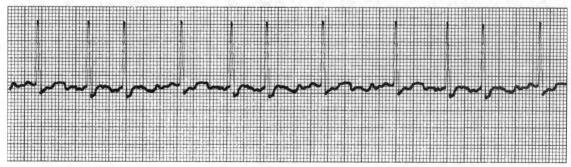

Pattern 11

Atrial flutter is a very rapid (250 per minute) atrial rate. You can spot it every time by noting the "sawtooth" or "picket fence" pattern of the atrial discharge (pattern 12). Drug or electrical treatments can help.

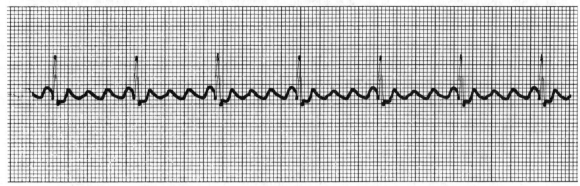

Pattern 12

Premature Ventricular Contractions

You will want to notice these abnormal QRS complexes (pattern 13) because they are often caused by hypoxemia. In other words, if you are suctioning and the patient gets premature ventricular contractions (PVCs), STOP! Oxygenate the patient. There are other causes, like stress, caffeine, and nicotine. No big deal. Intravenous lidocaine is one therapy for too many PVCs (usually more than 6 per minute).

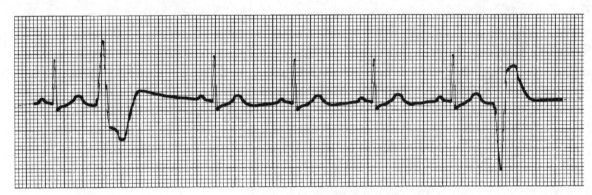

Pattern 13

Ventricular Tachycardia

Tachycardia, of course, is a rate above 100 beats/min. But this rhythm shows no P waves and shows wide QRS complexes and does not usually have a pulse (pattern 14). **This condition is life threatening!** Stop, call for help, check for a pulse, and act appropriately. Drugs or defibrillation are needed.

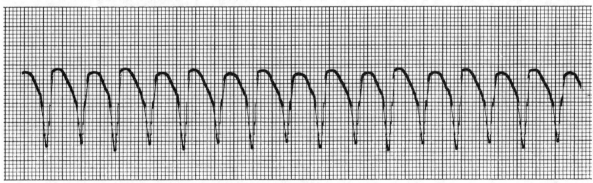

Pattern 14

135

Ventricular Fibrillation

The only rhythm worse than this is a flatline (asystole) (pattern 15). There is no pulse, cardiac output, or blood pressure. Only defibrillation will really help, but you can do CPR and give oxygen and drugs as well (pattern 16).

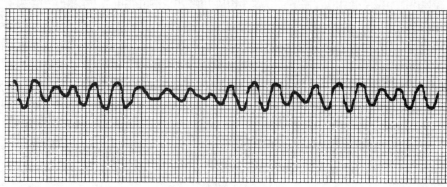

Pattern 15

Practice recognizing the important arrhythmias. After a while, these basic patterns will be easy to spot, just like a van Gogh painting, and you won't have to think too hard!

CASE STUDIES

Case 1

A student is suctioning a patient orally with a tonsil suction. The monitor shows sinus bradycardia. Blood pressure is falling. Alarms are sounding.

35. What should the student do?

36. What physiologic mechanism was responsible for the drop in rate?

_____

Case 2

A student is suctioning a patient via the endotracheal tube. The monitor shows sinus tachycardia with frequent premature ventricular contractions. Alarms are sounding. The patient is agitated.

37. What should this student do about the arrhythmias? _____

38. What physiologic mechanism was responsible for the increased rate and arrhythmias?

_____

Case 3

While performing a ventilator check on a patient in the coronary care unit, a student observes the rhythm on the monitor has changed from atrial fibrillation to ventricular fibrillation.

39. What should the student do first?

40. Name at least three responses indicated to treat this rhythm.

WHAT DOES THE NBRC SAY?

Actual pictures of ECG rhythms usually appear in the Clinical Simulation Exam and occasionally on the other written exams. Cardioversion and defibrillation are on the Written Registry as well. You will need to supplement the text with more information to understand these subjects. The Advanced Cardiac Life Support material from the American Heart Association is a good resource. The Entry-Level Exam doesn't have too much on the heart ECG interpretation, but they do like to ask about performing ECGs. That isn't covered in this chapter, but you need to know about the specific lead placements for the diagnostic 12-lead ECG you see in Figure 17-3. Here are some sample questions from Chapter 17 that you might run into on the subject of ECG interpretation. Circle the best answer.

41. An RT is suctioning a patient on a ventilator and observes the following rhythm on the monitor:

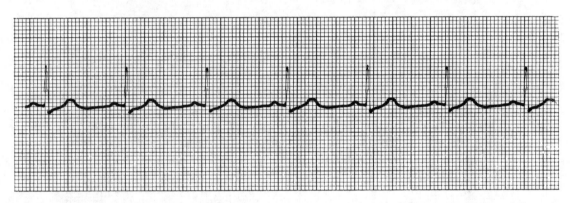

In regard to this pattern, the RT should
A. continue to suction the patient
B. stop and administer 100% oxygen
C. recommend atropine administration
D. defibrillate the patient

42. An RT is preparing to perform an arterial puncture when the following rhythm is observed on the monitor:

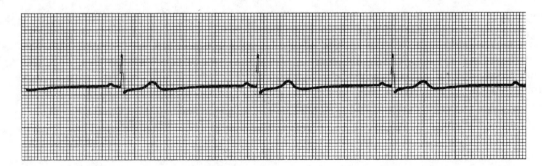

In regard to this pattern, the RT should
A. continue to suction the patient
B. stop and administer 100% oxygen
C. recommend atropine administration
D. defibrillate the patient

137

43. During a routine suctioning procedure, an RT notes the following rhythm on the cardiac monitor:

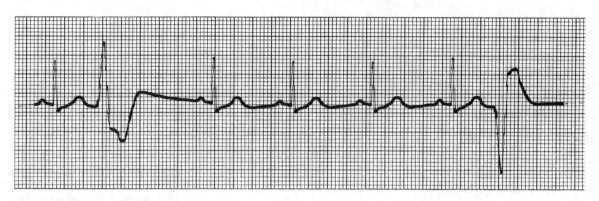

In regard to this pattern, the RT should
A. continue to suction the patient.
B. stop and administer 100% oxygen.
C. recommend atropine administration.
D. defibrillate the patient.

44. During a routine suctioning procedure, an RT notes the following rhythm on the cardiac monitor:

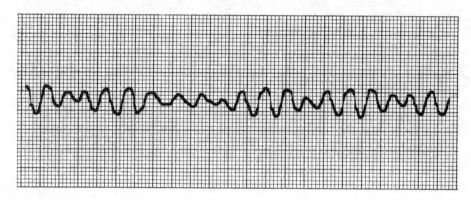

In regard to this pattern, the RT should
A. continue to suction the patient
B. stop and administer 100% oxygen
C. recommend atropine administration
D. defibrillate the patient

45. A respiratory therapist is called to perform a STAT ECG on a patient with chest pain in the emergency department. Proper placement of chest lead V6 is the
A. fourth intercostal space, left sternal margin
B. fourth intercostal space, right sternal margin
C. fifth intercostal space, left midaxillary line
D. fifth intercostal space, left midclavicular line

Performing ECGs can be embarrassing and awkward. You'll get over it. Is this a good time to ask you a few personal questions?

46. Have you ever had to disrobe at the physician's office or clinic? How did you feel? How do you think patients feel when you ask them to disrobe?

47. How will you ensure that your patients don't feel awkward or embarrassed when you do ECGs or chest exams?

Analysis and Monitoring of Gas Exchange

Vision is the art of seeing the invisible.
Jonathon Swift

Analyzing and monitoring gas exchange is one of the most important areas of the respiratory care profession. After all, gas exchange is the number one function of the lungs. Chapter 18 begins to put together concepts you've learned in other parts of *Egan's,* like gas exchange and perfusion. In Chapter 13 we talked about interpreting the acid-base balance of arterial blood gases. Naturally, there's more to it than that. Chapter 18 covers the equipment used to analyze blood and much more. For example, there are noninvasive methods to monitor gas exchange like capnometry and pulse oximetry. So whether you're talking about clinical practice or thinking about credentialing examinations, you're going to need a clear view of these methods of detection.

WORD WIZARD

Learning the specialized terminology of invasive and noninvasive monitoring will help you get a better picture of this topic. Quality is the name of the game. You would not want to give the physician bad data about gas exchange when you're trying to save a critically ill patient.

1. Match these eight quality terms to their definitions:

Definitions	Terms
1. _____ examining the repeatability of results	A. Quality control
2. _____ comparing the values with a known value	B. Bias
3. _____ errors of precision	C. Imprecision
4. _____ another term associated with errors of precision	D. Random error
5. _____ a trend or abrupt shift in data outside the limits	E. Systematic error
6. _____ an abrupt shift in data outside the limits	F. Preanalytical error
7. _____ problems that occur prior to testing a sample	G. Precision
8. _____ CLIA standards are an important example	H. Accuracy

FIRST THINGS FIRST

First, you have to make a choice between analysis and monitoring. Analysis usually means obtaining a sample of body fluid and putting it in some type of lab analyzer to get results. Properly done, these measurements have a high degree of accuracy. Unfortunately, they are like a snapshot of a single event. Monitoring is usually done at the bedside and is a continuous process—more like watching a video. Next, you have a choice of invasive or noninvasive techniques. Invasive techniques are probably more accurate, but they also have a greater risk of harm to the patient. Good way to establish a baseline. Noninvasive methods are often used for monitoring and are especially useful when used together with invasive techniques. What is the conclusion? No one method is best. Your role as a clinician is to get the right balance.

Answer the following questions and you will get a grip on the good stuff. Relax, get some coffee or soda; this is going to take a little time.

2. In your own words, explain how an electrochemical analyzer converts the number of O_2 molecules (PO_2) into a measurable reading.

3. There are two common types of electrochemical analyzers. Name them.

   A. _____

   B. _____

4. Explain the differences between the two types of analyzers in terms of principle of operation and response time.

5. Describe the two-step process for calibrating an O_2 analyzer.

6. What is the gold standard of gas exchange analysis? What does this mean?

7. List four reasons why the radial artery is the preferred site for ABG sampling?

   A. _____

   B. _____

   C. _____

   D. _____

8. Describe the modified Allen test, and give the definition of a positive result.

   A. _____

   B. _____

9. Name four other sites you can use if the radial artery is unavailable or has a poor pulse.

A. _____

B. _____

C. _____

D. _____

10. How long should you wait after changing the F_IO_2 before performing an ABG on a patient with healthy lungs? A patient with COPD?

A. _____

B. _____

11. What technique can help prevent hyperventilation from pain or anxiety from altering the sample results?

12. AARC's ABG sampling guidelines describe several medications that may result in prolonged bleeding. These are anticoagulants (clot preventers) and thrombolytics (clot busters). Give two examples of each of these classes of drugs.

A. Anticoagulants

1. _____

2. _____

B. Thrombolytics

1. _____

2. _____

13. Name the four things you can do to avoid most preanalytical sampling errors. Hint: Check Table 18-1 in your text.

A. _____

B. _____

C. _____

D. _____

14. What precaution should you take when handling any laboratory specimen?

15. What are the three primary parameters measured by a blood gas analyzer?

A. _____

B. _____

C. _____

16. If you wanted to measure actual hemoglobin saturation, what type of analyzer would be needed?

_____

17. What is the range of accuracy for most commercially available pulse oximeters?

_____

18. Describe three noninvasive ways you can determine the reliability of a pulse oximeter at the bedside.

A. _____

B. _____

C. _____

19. According to the AARC guidelines, what action should you take to verify the results when pulse oximetry is unreliable or does not confirm suspicions about the patient's clinical state?

20. Describe the three main quality assurance procedures used to maintain consistently accurate blood gas results.
A. Automated calibration

B. Control media

C. Proficiency testing

21. For which patients is capillary sampling appropriate? _____

_____

22. What are the two most common errors committed during capillary sampling?

    A. _____

    B. _____

23. Explain what variables are reliable and unreliable in capillary sampling compared to arterial sampling.

24. What are the primary advantages and disadvantages of transcutaneous gas monitoring over arterial sampling?
    A. Advantages

        1. _____

        2. _____

    B. Disadvantages

        1. _____

        2. _____

25. When would you choose a pulse oximeter for monitoring an infant's oxygenation status over a transcutaneous monitor?

26. When would the transcutaneous monitor be preferred over the pulse oximeter?

27. Describe proper placement of a capnometer sampling chamber or adaptor for a patient who is being mechanically ventilated.

145

28. What are the normal values for end-tidal CO_2 for health individuals and how do they compare with values for arterial CO_2?

29. An end-tidal CO_2 of "0" may indicate a serious problem. Name two life-threatening causes of a "0" value for end-tidal CO_2.

    A. _____

    B. _____

30. While performing end-tidal CO_2 measurements, you notice that the baseline does not return to "0" on inspiration. Interpret this result.

31. While performing end-tidal CO_2 measurements, you notice that no real plateau is reached. Give two possible interpretations of this result.

    A. _____

    B. _____

SUMMARY CHECKLIST

The questions you just answered covered just the objectives; however, this chapter was really crammed with details. Here are a few more questions that highlight some of the main points we haven't already covered.

32. What are the three most common causes of O_2 analyzer malfunctions?

    A. _____

    B. _____

    C. _____

33. Blood gases provide more information than other methods of gas exchange analysis. What are the three general areas that a blood gas helps to assess?

    A. _____

    B. _____

    C. _____

146

34. What is the maximum ideal time between ABG sampling and analysis?

_____

35. What are the two primary benefits and hazards of indwelling peripheral arterial lines?
   A. Benefits

   1. _____

   2. _____

   B. Hazards

   1. _____

   2. _____

36. What is point-of-care testing, and what are the potential benefits of this method of testing blood samples? Name a potential problem or drawback.

37. What is the difference between capnography and capnometry?

38. Indwelling arterial, central venous, or pulmonary artery catheters are widely used in the ICU. Please list the two main benefits and two main drawbacks of these invasive lines.
   A. Benefits

   B. Drawbacks

CASE STUDIES

Now that you have the information, let's see if you can apply it to the following scenarios.

Case 1

A 34-year-old firefighter is brought to the emergency department for treatment of smoke inhalation while fighting a house fire. His heart rate is 126 beats/min, and respirations are 28 breaths/min and labored. SpO_2 is 100% on 6 L/min via nasal cannula. Blood pressure is 145/90 mm Hg. Breath sounds are coarse with inspiratory crackles in both bases. The patient's face is smudged with soot, and he is coughing up sputum with black specks in it.

39. What clinical signs of hypoxemia does the patient display?

40. Explain why the pulse oximeter is reading 100% despite these signs?

41. What is the most probable cause of the hypoxemia?

42. What blood test would you recommend to confirm your suspicions?

Case 2

A premature infant is receiving supplemental O_2. Her physician is concerned about the effects of hyperoxia on her lungs and eyes. The infant is being monitored by a pulse oximeter, which shows a saturation of 100%.

43. What range of PO_2 is possible with an SpO_2 of 100%?

44. What type of noninvasive monitoring would you recommend in this situation?

Case 3

An elderly patient is admitted for acute exacerbation of his long-standing COPD. He is wearing a nasal cannula at 2 L/min.

45. What is the simplest way to quickly assess his oxygenation status?

46. Why would you recommend arterial blood gas sampling for this patient?

A patient was riding his motorcycle without a helmet when he crashed. Now he has a head injury and is being mechanically ventilated. His physician asks you to make recommendations regarding monitoring his gas exchange.

47. What are the advantages of using capnometry to monitor carbon dioxide in this situation?

48. Where would you place the capnometer probe in the ventilator circuit?

49. During monitoring, you notice that the capnograph does not return to "0" when the patient inhales. What does this indicate?

50. A few minutes later, the patient's exhaled CO_2 levels begin to rise. So does his blood pressure. The patient becomes agitated. What action would you take?

51. Why do rising CO_2 levels cause increases in intracranial pressure?

WHAT DOES THE NBRC SAY?

The NBRC has a strong affinity for monitoring gas exchange. So should you! You will find pulse oximeters and O_2 analyzers on the Entry-Level Exam. Capnography and transcutaneous monitoring go into the Registry Exams, as does mixed venous sampling, co-oximetry, blood gas analyzers, and quality control. Here's a baker's dozen of what you can expect. Circle the best answer.

52. A respiratory therapist is preparing to perform pulse oximetry. Which of the following would be *least* beneficial for assessing accuracy of the device?
    A. checking the capillary refill time
    B. assessing skin color and temperature
    C. performing an Allen test on the patient
    D. assessing pulse rate

53. Which of the following would you perform after obtaining an arterial blood gas sample?
    1. Remove air bubbles from the sample.
    2. Mix the sample by rotating the syringe.
    3. Maintain site pressure for at least 1 minute.
    4. Add heparin to the sample.
       A. 1 only
       B. 1 and 2 only
       C. 1, 2, and 3 only
       D. 1, 2, 3, and 4 only

54. A pulse oximeter is being used to monitor a patient who was rescued from a fire. The SpO_2 is 90%; however, the patient is unconscious and shows signs of respiratory distress. What additional test should the RT recommend?
    A. CT scan
    B. electrolyte measurement
    C. co-oximetry
    D. hemoglobin and hematocrit levels

55. A polarographic O_2 analzyer fails to calibrate when exposed to 100% O_2. The first action the respiratory therapist should take would be to
    A. replace the battery
    B. replace the membrane
    C. replace the fuel cell
    D. try another O_2 source

150

56. An infant is placed on a transcutaneous O_2 monitor. The TcPO$_2$ is reading 40 mm Hg less than the PaO$_2$ obtained from an arterial sample. All of the following could cause this problem *except*
    A. improper calibration of the transcutaneous electrode
    B. room air contamination of the transcutaneous electrode
    C. inadequate heating of the skin at the electrode site
    D. inadequate perfusion of the skin at the electrode site

57. Which of the following analyzers is calibrated to a value of zero when exposed to room air?
    A. Clark electrode
    B. galvanic O_2 analyzer
    C. capnometer
    D. Geisler type of nitrogen analyzer

58. Which of the following would be most useful in assessing proper tube placement following endotracheal intubation?
    A. transcutaneous monitoring
    B. arterial blood gas analysis
    C. pulse oximetry
    D. end-tidal CO_2 monitoring

59. Complications of arterial puncture include all of the following *except*
    A. pulmonary embolus
    B. hematoma
    C. infection
    D. nerve damage

60. A galvanic O_2 analyzer is being used as a check of the ventilator system to measure the delivered F_IO_2. The set F_IO_2 is 40%; however, the analyzer is reading 32%. Which of the following is the most likely cause of this discrepancy?
    A. The batteries in the analyzer need to be changed.
    B. The electrode membrane has water condensation on its surface.
    C. The analyzer needs to be calibrated.
    D. The ventilator requires servicing.

61. Which of the following will affect the accuracy of pulse oximeter measurements?
    1. increased bilirubin levels
    2. decreased hematocrit levels
    3. dark skin pigmentation
    4. exposure to sunlight
       A. 1 and 2 only
       B. 2 and 3 only
       C. 3 and 4 only
       D. 2, 3, and 4 only

62. An arterial blood gas sample is drawn from a patient who is breathing room air. Analysis reveals the following results:

pH	7.45
PaCO$_2$	35 mm Hg
PaO$_2$	155 mm Hg

    Which of the following best explains these results?
    A. Too much heparin was added to the sample.
    B. An air bubble has contaminated the sample.
    C. Analysis of the sample was delayed for more than 60 minutes.
    D. The patient was hyperventilating during the puncture.

63. Which of the following sites would be the best for continuous monitoring of exhaled carbon dioxide during mechanical ventilation?
   A. exhalation valve
   B. inspiratory side of the ventilator circuit
   C. expiratory side of the ventilator circuit
   D. endotracheal tube connector

64. Which of the following is true concerning the use of a transcutaneous PO_2 monitor?
   A. $TcPO_2$ should be checked with arterial blood samples.
   B. The skin temperature control should be maintained at 37° C.
   C. The site should be changed every 24 hours.
   D. The low calibration point is determined using room air.

FOOD FOR THOUGHT

65. How would you modify your technique if you had to perform ABGs on a patient receiving anticoagulants?

66. Discuss the problems you might encounter with MRI or electrocautery.

67. Why can you use a capnometer during CPR but not a pulse oximeter?

19 Pulmonary Function Testing

Most teachers would continue to lecture on navigation while the ship is going down.

James Boren

Remember when you were little, and blowing out those candles on your birthday cake was an exciting but difficult task? That was your first pulmonary function test (PFT). If you could blow out the candles, you passed and got your wish. Pulmonary function testing has always been important in the diagnosis, assessment, and treatment of lung disease. PFTs come in three flavors: assessment of flow rates, volumes (and capacities of course), and diffusion of gases in and out of the lung. In the last few years, lung testing has taken on even greater importance. Multiskilling, assessment-based protocols, increased interest in asthma, disability and legal issues, and a strong focus on the credentialing examinations are just a few reasons for the resurgence of interest in the science of diagnosing and quantifying pulmonary disorders.

WORD WIZARD

A quick glance at the key terms in Chapter 19 should leave you breathless with desire (or despair) to know what all those abbreviations mean. In fact, it would be pretty difficult to have a conversation with a pulmonary function technologist without speaking in acronyms. Match the right terms or abbreviations with the correct definition.

Terms/Abbreviations	Definitions
1. _____ DL	A. volume inspired with a normal breath
2. _____ ERV	B. greatest amount of air you can breathe in 12 to 15 seconds
3. _____ VT	C. largest amount of air the lungs can hold
4. _____ IRV	D. fastest flow rate generated at the very beginning of forced exhalation
5. _____ RV	E. milliliters of gas the lung can transfer to the blood
6. _____ TLC	F. amount of air you can exhale after a maximum inspiration
7. _____ VC	G. ratio of volume exhaled in 1 second to total volume exhaled
8. _____ IC	H. average expiratory flow during the early part of forced exhalation
9. _____ FRC	I. amount of air you can inhale after a normal exhalation
10. _____ MVV	J. amount of air you can inhale after a normal inspiration
11. _____ FVC	K. air left in the lungs after a maximum exhalation
12. _____ PEF	L. air left in the lungs after a normal exhalation
13. _____ $FEF_{200-1200}$	M. amount of air you can forcefully exhale after a maximum inspiration
14. _____ FEV1	N. average expiratory flow during the middle part of forced exhalation
15. _____ $FEF_{25\%-75\%}$	O. volume of air you can forcefully exhale in 1 second
16. _____ FEV_1/FVC	P. amount of air you can exhale after a normal exhalation

As if learning all those acronyms wasn't enough, we can't really go on until you put the four lung volumes and four lung capacities into perspective with their normal values in a healthy adult. Use the box provided. MEMORIZE this information! It will serve you well on your board exams!

A	E	C	B
	F		
	G	D	
	H		H

17. Fill in the names and normal values that go with each letter in the box. See Figure 19-10 in your text if you need help.

	VOLUME/CAPACITY	**VALUE**
A.		
B.		
C.		
D.		
E.		
F.		
G.		
H.		

Now see if you can draw the box and fill in the values on a separate sheet of paper without looking. Check your answers. Do this until you have it down! These are the same values the NBRC uses for normal subjects. Note the way it progresses from 1.2 to 2.4, etc., to make your memorizing easier.

MEET THE OBJECTIVES

Answer these questions to find out if you have grasped the important points for each area of lung testing.

Lung Volumes

Lung volume measurement is an important adjunct to spirometry and helps quantify and determine a diagnosis of restriction or obstruction. Specialized equipment is needed to perform these tests.

18. Which volumes *cannot* be measured with a spirometer?

_____

19. Which capacities *cannot* be measured with a spirometer?

_____

20. Name the three tests used to determine the volumes and capacities that cannot be measured.

    A. _____

    B. _____

    C. _____

21. What is thoracic gas volume?

22. How will volumes or capacities for a patient with air trapping obtained by helium dilution or nitrogen washout differ from those obtained with a body plethysmograph?

23. What effect will an air leak have on the values obtained by helium dilution or nitrogen washout?

Spirometry

Spirometry is the most commonly performed pulmonary function test, and vital capacity (also known as forced vital capacity) is the most commonly obtained value. Many types of spirometers exist, but any one that meets the standards and is working properly can be used.

24. What four variables are used to calculate normal values for spirometry?

    A. _____

    B. _____

    C. _____

    D. _____

25. You must produce acceptable results that provide valid, reliable information based on how long the patient exhales, how closely multiple tests correlate, and how fast the patient starts the maneuver. Fill in the details for each of the criteria below:

    A. duration: _____

    B. variance of two best FVCs: _____

    C. satisfactory start: _____

    D. minimum number: _____

26. Which FVC should you report? Which FEV_1?

    A. FVC: _____

    B. FEV_1: _____

27. Which flow rate is the greatest? _____

28. Which flow rate represents large airways? _____

29. Which flow rate represents the middle range? _____

30. A spirometer is considered accurate if the volume is verified to be within what percentage of a known value? Hint: Check out "Quality Control" in the AARC CPG on Spirometry, or look at Table 19-3 in *Egan's*.

31. What device is used to verify the volume of a spirometer? _____

32. What is the normal value for MVV? How is this test performed? _____

Diffusion

Diffusing capacity represents the ability of the lung to transfer gas into the blood. This test requires breathing a special gas mixture.

33. What gas is usually used to measure the lung's ability to transfer gas to the blood?

    _____

34. What other special gas is used in this test? Why?

    _____

    _____

35. What blood test results are needed to ensure accuracy of diffusion studies?

_____

_____

INTERPRETATION FUNDAMENTALS

In a minute, we'll go to our case studies and board exam questions to test your ability to put all the information together. First, see if you have the basic ideas straight.

36. What are the two major categories of pulmonary disease classification? Fill in the chart below to compare the effects of each category. Hint: See Table 19-1!

	CATEGORY	ANATOMY	PHASE	PATHOLOGIC CONDITION	MEASURE
A.					
B.					

37. Fill in the corresponding percent of predicted for the degrees of impairment.

Degree of Impairment   **% Predicted Value**

A. Normal   _____

B. Mild   _____

C. Moderate   _____

D. Severe   _____

38. The original normal values for pulmonary functions were probably based on a 6-foot-tall, 20-year-old white male. How are normal values corrected for nonwhites?

_____

39. Compare the FEV_1/FVC ratios you would see in normal, obstructed, and restricted patients. Hint: Take a look at Table 19-2 in your text.

A. Normal: _____

B. Obstructed: _____

C. Restricted: _____

CASE STUDIES

Now that you have the information, let's see if you can apply it to the following scenarios. Use the algorithm in Figure 19-16 until you have the basics down pat. Remember, the LLN, or lower limit of normal, is 80% for the vital capacity, and the lower limit of normal for FEV_1/FVC is 70% for case purposes.

Chapter **19** **Pulmonary Function Testing**

Spirometry is performed on a 24-year-old woman who complains of a "tight chest" and cough. Simple spirometry shows the following:

Test	Actual	Predicted	% Predicted
FVC	3.2 L	4 L	80%
FEV_1	1.6 L	3.2 L	50%
FEV_1/FVC	50%	70%	

40. Interpretation? _____

41. What test should be performed in light of the results and the clinical information? (If you're not sure, check out PFT Report No. 2 in the Mini-Clini that starts on page 447.)

_____

A 34-year-old respiratory care student is required by his instructor to undergo pulmonary function testing as part of a course. Here are the results:

Test	Actual	Predicted	% Predicted
FVC	3.9 L	4.8 L	81%
FEV_1	3.1 L	4.1 L	76%
FEV_1/FVC	79%	70%	

42. Interpretation? _____

43. What pulmonary function test does the algorithm suggest using now?

A 60-year-old shipyard worker complains of dyspnea on exertion and dry cough. Here are his spirometry results.

Test	Actual	Predicted	% Predicted
FVC	2 L	4 L	50%
FEV_1	1.5 L	3.4 L	44%
FEV_1/FVC	75%	70%	
TLC	2.4	4.8	50%

44. Interpretation? _____

Chapter **19** **Pulmonary Function Testing**

45. What additional test would be helpful?

46. What additional history would be helpful?

Case 4

Case 4

A woman presents in her physician's office complaining of dyspnea on exertion. Spirometry and lung volume results show the following.

Test	Actual	Predicted	% Predicted
FVC	1.5 L	3 L	50%
FEV$_1$	0.75 L	2.5 L	30%
FEV$_1$/FVC	50%	70%	
TLC	2.6 L	3.8 L	68%

47. Interpretation? _____

48. What additional history would be helpful?

Case 5

A 70-year-old man with a 100-pack-year smoking history complains of a dry cough and dyspnea on exertion. Results of lung tests show the following.

Test	Actual	Predicted	% Predicted
FVC	2.9 L	4.4 L	65%
FEV$_1$	1.3 L	3.7 L	35%
FEV$_1$/FVC	59%	70%	
TLC	6.6 L	5.5	120%
FRC	4.5 L	2.2	
RV	3.7 L	1.1 L	
DLCO	16	25	64%

49. Interpretation? Be complete; what specific type of disease is suggested?

50. What disease state do the lung volumes and history suggest?

_____

51. Why is the vital capacity lower than predicted?

_____

For additional practice, be sure to check out the case studies in Chapter 19 of your textbook!

WHAT DOES THE NBRC SAY?

If you look at the board exam matrix, you'll see things like "PFT studies (e.g., flows, volumes, diffusion, prebronchodilator and postbronchodilator)" and "perform FVC and FEV_1," and, of course, the equipment, such as body boxes, spirometers, and pneumotachometers. Try your hand at some questions in the good old NBRC style. Circle the best answer.

52. Which of the following tests would be helpful in assessing the effects of cigarette smoking on the smaller airways?
   A. FVC
   B. $FEF_{25\%-75\%}$
   C. FEV_1
   D. $FEF_{200-1200}$

53. A patient's physician asks you to recommend a pulmonary function test to help assess the effects of a possible tumor in the trachea. Which of the following would you recommend?
   A. spirometry with volume-time curves
   B. spirometry before and after bronchodilator
   C. lung volume studies via nitrogen washout
   D. spirometry with flow-volume loops

54. A pulmonary function technologist tests a spirometer by injecting 3.0 L of air from a large-volume syringe. The spirometer measures a result of 2.90 L. Which of the following is true regarding this situation?
   A. The results are within normal limits.
   B. The spirometer is not ready to use.
   C. The air was injected too slowly.
   D. The BTPS corrections were not made properly.

55. Which of the following values could be incorrectly calculated?

Test	Actual	Predicted	% Predicted
FVC	4.4 L	4.8 L	92%
FEV_1	3.5 L	4.1 L	80%
FEV_1/FVC	80%	70%	
TLC	5.2 L	5.5	
FRC	2 L	2.4	
ERV	1.2 L	1.2 L	
RV	1 L	1.2 L	

   A. TLC
   B. FVC
   C. FRC
   D. RV

56. Which of the following pulmonary measurements is usually the smallest?
    A. inspiratory capacity
    B. vital capacity
    C. functional residual capacity
    D. total lung capacity

57. The following results were obtained from spirometry of an adult female smoker with chronic bronchitis. What is the correct interpretation?

Test	Actual	Predicted	% Predicted
FVC	3.9 L	4.8 L	81%
FEV$_1$	3.1 L	4.1 L	76%
FEV$_1$/FVC	79%	70%	

    A. Results indicate a mild diffusion defect.
    B. Results are within the normal range.
    C. A mixed obstructive/restrictive defect is present.
    D. Results show obstructive lung disease.

58. What percent increase in forced spirometric volumes or flow rates after a bronchodilator is administered is the *minimum* indication that reversible airway obstruction is present?*
    A. 5%
    B. 10%
    C. 15%
    D. 20%

59. Which of the following can be measured during spirometric testing?
    A. residual volume
    B. tidal volume
    C. total lung capacity
    D. functional residual capacity

60. An increased total lung capacity combined with a decreased diffusing capacity is strongly indicative of which of the following conditions?
    A. emphysema
    B. pneumonia
    C. pulmonary fibrosis
    D. pleural effusion

61. A patient reports tightness in his chest and wheezing at different times throughout the day. The wheezing is not associated with exercise. His primary provider sends him to your laboratory for evaluation. The initial spirometry is normal. What test might help determine the cause of the pulmonary symptoms?
    A. body plethysmography
    B. pre- and post-bronchodilator studies
    C. bronchial challenge studies
    D. diffusion capacity

62. What drug is used in the test in question 61?
    A. carbon monoxide
    B. oxygen
    C. albuterol
    D. methacholine

---

*In *Egan's* you will find the answer under the topic of reversibility. Unfortunately, the new ATS standard is 12% and at least 200 ml. The boards will give a hearty increase in reversible cases so you don't get confused.

We have just scratched the surface of a complex area of testing. Entire textbooks are devoted to pulmonary function testing! Here are a few more questions to fill up the corners of your brain.

63. What effect does smoking have on the results of a diffusion test? Why?

64. What lung volume or capacity is useful in predicting normal values for incentive spirometry?

_____

65. Calculate your normal values for FVC, FEV_1, and $FEF_{25\%-75\%}$ using Table 19-4 in your text. Do it using the regression equation.

A. FVC _____

B. FEV_1 _____

C. $FEF_{25\%-75\%}$ _____

Show your work for the regression equation (be sure to use a calculator!).

Formula: _____

Calculation: _____

66. You should look at Table 19-2 in *Egan's*. This is a severity rating scale based on percent predicted. You will want to know this for your boards, but it also helps when you take care of patients. Moderately severe and severe COPD might be treated with different medications than mild COPD, for example. So what would a patient have if his FEV_1 was 55% of the predicted value?

20 Review of Thoracic Imaging

In the field of observation, chance favors the prepared mind.

L. Pasteur

Thoracic imaging provides a window for the practitioner to view structures and events inside the chest that they normally cannot see. The chest radiograph is especially important to the respiratory therapist for the purpose of confirming placement of tubes or for diagnosis of certain conditions like pneumothorax. Neck films might help diagnose croup or epiglottitis. You should also understand the usefulness of other common imaging techniques you will encounter in clinical practice such as computed tomography and magnetic resonance imaging. Perhaps you will even unlock the mysteries of the infamous Kerley B lines!

WORD WIZARD

Complete the following paragraph by writing the correct term(s) in the blank(s) provided. You have been provided with part of the word to help you on your way.

The chest _____ ogram _____ is more commonly called a chest film, or x-ray. It is one of the most common methods for evaluating the lungs and other structures in the thorax. Air-filled lung tissue appears mostly dark on the film because it is easily penetrated by x-rays. We describe this effect by saying the tissue is

_____ radio _____. The dense bone tissue of ribs appears white. Dense matter that

is not easily penetrated is referred to as _____ opaque _____. Fat is pretty dense so it appears whiter than air or tissues. A female patient's breast tissue will alter the appearance of film. Obesity has the same effect. Soft tissues like blood vessels appear more grayish because they have an intermediate density.

Abnormal conditions may be spotted through observation of certain densities in the wrong location. Accumulation

of fluid in the pleural space, or _____ thorax _____, appears white and may

obscure the angle where the ribs meet the diaphragm. If pus collects in the pleura, we call it _____

em _____. Alveoli appear white when filled with pus or blood. On the chest film these white areas

are called pulmonary _____ in _____. If alveoli are filled with fluid but the airways

around them are open, you will see _____ air _____ that may indicate pneumonia.

Air in the pleural space, or _____ thorax _____, is another example of an abnormal density. This condition appears as a black area with none of the usual grayish markings of blood vessels in the lung tissue.

OVERVIEW

1. Describe the four tissue densities you can see on a chest radiograph.

   A. Air: _____

   _____

   B. Fat: _____

   _____

C. Tissue: _____

_____

D. Bone: _____

_____

2. Physicians may order, but RTs recommend; we all work toward good care of the patient. The National Board for Respiratory Care (NBRC) thinks you should know when to suggest a chest film in a variety of settings. Let's call them inpatient and outpatient but you could use these criteria in any setting. Name three indications for a chest radiograph.

Outpatient (clinic or office setting)

A. _____

B. _____

C. _____

Inpatient (ED, ICU, or medical/surgical patient)

A. _____

B. _____

C. _____

3. Explain lag time in reference to the chest x-ray.

STEP-BY-STEP

Every primer on chest radiograph interpretation recommends you develop a systematic method for approaching interpretation. If you are handling an actual film as opposed to a digitized one, make sure it is placed on the viewer correctly. The "left" side of the film (usually where the heart is) should be facing your right-hand side—as if the patient was standing facing you. A marker is normally placed on the film to indicate the left side.

4. The two basic ways to shoot a plain chest film are anterior to posterior (AP) and posterior to anterior (PA). You'll want to know which method was used before you continue. Explain the differences between AP and PA.

A. Where does the film go in relationship to the chest, and where is the energy beam (x-ray machine)?

1. PA

2. AP

B. What might happen to the heart in an AP film?

C. If PA films are so much better in quality, why do most of our patients have AP chest x-rays?

5. What structures offer clues to help identify whether the patient is straight or rotated?

6. What appearance of the vertebral bodies suggests underexposure?

7. What effect does underexposure have on the appearance of lung tissue?

8. The pleura appear at the edge of the chest wall (although the pleura themselves are usually difficult to see). What are the two major pleural abnormalities detected on the chest film?

A. _____

B. _____

ADVANCED CHEST IMAGING

Regular old radiographs are great for initial evaluation or in the ICU when you can't move the person easily, but more advanced techniques can provide vital information. RTs are often involved in the transport and management of patients to and from specialized imaging procedures like computed tomography (CT) and magnetic resonance imaging (MRI).

9. CT = _____

What's the advantage over regular radiographs?

What is CT angiography used for?

Chapter **20** **Review of Thoracic Imaging**

10. HRCT = _____

Explain the thing about slices, and what is this thing good for anyway?

11. MRI = _____

What type of tissue in the chest is imaged with this technique?

IDENTIFYING ABNORMALITIES

The second part of Chapter 20 covers evaluation of abnormalities seen in the three major anatomic portions seen in chest imaging. After you read the material, answer the following questions that highlight the important points.

Evaluation of the Pleura

12. What is the costophrenic angle? _____

13. Describe how you recognize the presence of fluid in the pleural space; what does that angle look like?

14. What view is most sensitive for detecting pleural fluid? How is the patient positioned to obtain this view?

15. When is sonography (ultrasound) indicated in the evaluation of pleural abnormalities?

16. What other imaging procedure may be helpful? _____

_____

17. Air in the pleural space is always abnormal. Name three common causes of this condition.

    A. _____

    B. _____

    C. _____

18. What breathing maneuver will help identify a small pneumothorax on a chest film? _____

    _____

19. Tension pneumothorax is immediately life threatening. Name at least two radiographic signs of tension pneumothorax.

    A. _____

    B. _____

20. What is the treatment for tension pneumothorax? _____

    _____

Evaluation of Lung Parenchyma

21. What are the two components of the lung parenchyma?

    A. _____

    B. _____

22. How will alveolar infiltrates appear on the chest film?

    _____

23. What is the difference between the radiographic appearance of pneumonia and pulmonary hemorrhage?

    _____

24. What causes airways to become visible, and what is this sign called?

    _____

25. Honeycombing, nodules, and volume loss are all radiographic hallmarks of what type of lung disorder?

    _____

26. Describe the silhouette sign. Discuss the difference between a right lower and right middle lobe infiltrate as seen on a chest film.

Let's Get Wet!

27. List some of the causes of pulmonary edema.

    Vascular

    A. _____

    B. _____

    C. _____

28. Describe Kerley B lines. When do you see them?

29. What are "bat's wings"? _____

Lost Volume

30. List five important indirect signs of volume loss, or atelectasis, seen on the chest radiograph. Check the Rule of Thumb on page 466 if you get lost.

    A. _____

    B. _____

    C. _____

    D. _____

    E. _____

31. You can count on your ribs to tell you about lung volumes. Fill in the chart below based on what anterior ribs you would see above the diaphragm depending on the degree of lung inflation.

	LUNG VOLUME	ANTERIOR RIBS
A.	Poor inspiration	
B.	Good effort	
C.	Hyperinflation	

32. Ribs aren't the only way to assess COPD with hyperinflation. List the two primary and three secondary radiographic signs seen with emphysema.

    A. Primary

    1. _____

    2. _____

B. Secondary

   1. _____

   2. _____

   3. _____

33. Compare the sensitivity of the chest radiograph and computed tomography for detection of obstructive airway disease.

Catheters, Lines, and Tubes

Checking placement of tubes and lines is key for RTs.

34. The endotracheal tube is made of soft plastic. How can the chest film be useful in deciding correct tube position after intubation?

35. Where is the distal tip of an ideally placed endotracheal tube in relation to the carina?

_____

36. Where will the endotracheal tube usually end up if it is placed too far into the trachea?

_____

37. What pulmonary complication may be identified on a chest film when a CVP catheter is placed via the subclavian vein?

_____

38. A pulmonary artery catheter (Swan-Ganz) that is seen to extend too far into the lung fields of a chest radiograph may have what unwanted results?

_____

The Mediastinum

39. Where does the mediastinum lie within the chest?

_____

40. What imaging technique is most favored for assessing mediastinal masses?

_____

Case 1

You are asked to perform postural drainage and clapping on a patient with a large right-sided pulmonary infiltrate. Evaluation of the chest radiograph shows a patchy white density with air bronchograms in the right lung. The right border of the heart is visible in the film.

41. Based on your knowledge of the silhouette sign, in what lobe is the infiltrate located?

_____

42. What diagnosis does the presence of air bronchograms suggest?

_____

43. What physical assessments could confirm the information in the chest film?

_____

Case 2

An elderly man presents in the emergency department with acute exacerbation of his long-standing COPD. A decision is made to intubate him. It is difficult to auscultate breath sounds, and chest movement is minimal; however, your impression is that breath sounds are more diminished on the left. A chest radiograph is obtained, which shows the tip of the endotracheal tube 1 cm above the carina. The left lung field is slightly smaller than the right. Both diaphragms appear flat, and you are able to count eight anterior ribs above the diaphragms.

44. Where should the tip of the tube be in relation to the carina?

_____

45. With regard to the endotracheal tube, what action should you take?

_____

46. What is the significance of the flattened diaphragms and number of ribs seen above the diaphragm?

_____

WHAT DOES THE NBRC SAY?

No one textbook contains all of the radiograph information indicated to be part of the examinations! Chapter 20 covers some of this material, and you will find much of the rest in later chapters on lung diseases and pediatric/neonatal respiratory care.

Below are some sample questions based on the material covered in this chapter, but you will need to carefully review each examination matrix to identify all the areas you need to know. Both the Certification and the Written Registry Examinations require you to "Review the chest radiograph to determine the position of endotracheal or tracheostomy tube." You must also know when to "recommend a chest radiograph" and when to "review existing data in the patient

170

record" such as the "results of chest radiographs." The examinations agree on content, including asking you to "review the chest radiograph to determine":
1. pneumothorax or subcutaneous air
2. consolidation or atelectasis
3. diaphragm position
4. hyperinflation
5. pleural fluid
6. pulmonary infiltrates
7. position of chest tubes and pulmonary artery catheters are items on the Written Registry

You will also be asked to "review the lateral neck radiograph to determine":
1. presence of epiglottitis and subglottic edema
2. presence of foreign bodies
3. airway narrowing

The main difference between the two tests is the difficulty level and depth of the questions. There's more! How many questions will you see on this topic? The matrix doesn't really say, but review of available practice exams suggests one to three on the Certification Exam and up to five on the Registry. Each examination can vary considerably, but you are guaranteed to be tested on this material in some fashion! Try these on for size. Circle the best answer.

47. A patient has dyspnea and tachycardia following thoracentesis to treat a pleural effusion. Evaluation of this patient should include a(n) _____.
    A. CT scan.
    B. MRI.
    C. chest radiograph.
    D. bronchoscopy.

48. A pneumothorax would appear on a chest radiograph as a _____.
    A. white area near the lung base
    B. white area that obscures the costophrenic angle
    C. dark area without lung marking
    D. dark area with honeycomb markings

49. The medical record of an intubated patient indicates that the morning chest film shows opacification of the lower right lung field with elevated right diaphragm and a shift of the trachea to the right. These findings suggest _____.
    A. left-sided pneumothorax
    B. right-sided pleural effusion
    C. right mainstem intubation
    D. right-sided atelectasis

50. On a chest radiograph, the tip of the endotracheal tube for an adult patient should be _____.
    A. 2 cm above the vocal cords
    B. 2 cm above the carina
    C. at the carina
    D. 2 cm below the carina

51. A patient is believed to have a pleural effusion. Which of the following radiographic techniques would be most useful in making a confirmation?
    A. CT
    B. decubitus radiograph projection
    C. MRI
    D. AP radiograph projection

52. What specific technique may be useful in evaluating pleural effusion?
    A. lateral decubitus position
    B. apical lordotic position
    C. lateral upright
    D. PA expiratory film

171

53. A patient with a history of hypertension presents in the ED with headache, slurred speech, and left-sided weakness. What diagnostic imaging procedure would the respiratory therapist recommend to further evaluate this patient according to the ACLS guidelines?
   A. computed tomography (CT)
   B. ultrasound
   C. angiography with contrast
   D. magnetic resonance imaging (MRI)

54. A patient with a history of pulmonary pathology and cancer presents with a suspicious mediastinal mass on the chest x-ray. What diagnostic imaging procedure would be useful in gathering further information about the mass?
   A. computed tomography (CT)
   B. ultrasound
   C. angiography with contrast
   D. magnetic resonance imaging (MRI)

55. Ultrasound is useful in the cardiopulmonary setting for
   1. guiding catheter placement
   2. evaluation of pleural effusion
   3. evaluation of pneumonia
   4. diagnosis of myocardial infarction
      A. 1 and 2
      B. 1 and 3
      C. 2 and 4
      D. 3 and 4

56. A respiratory care practitioner is treating a child with respiratory distress in the emergency department. Which type of diagnostic imaging procedure may be useful for differentiating between epiglottitis and croup in children?
   A. AP chest x-ray
   B. lateral neck x-ray
   C. MRI
   D. ultrasound

57. The respiratory therapist is making a patient-ventilator system check in the medical intensive care unit when the high pressure alarm begins to sound. Breath sounds are absent on the left with good tube placement. Blood pressure is 80/50 mm Hg. SpO$_2$ is 86% and falling. The heart rate is 160 beats/min. There is a hyperresonant percussion note on the left upper chest. The patient has lost consciousness. What action should the respiratory therapist take at this time?
   A. Call for a STAT portable chest x-ray.
   B. Remove the patient from the ventilator and begin manual ventilation.
   C. Remove the endotracheal tube and begin manual ventilation.
   D. Recommend immediate needle decompression of the chest.

Naturally, chest film interpretation will appear as part of the information in questions that are not specifically about radiographs (same as blood gases). Remember: Chest radiographs are diagnostic, not therapeutic! If a patient is circling the drain from a tension pneumothorax, the radiograph will not be lifesaving—a chest tube will!

FOOD FOR THOUGHT

58. The author states that head position is important in assessing the tip of an endotracheal tube on a radiograph. What happens to the tube if the head moves up (extension) or the chin goes down (flexion)? How far can the tube move?

21 Nutrition Assessment

To eat is human. To digest divine.
Mark Twain

Hospitals put a tremendous effort into providing nourishing, specialized diets, with about as much public relations success as the airlines. When was the last time you heard anyone raving about the three-star meal they had after surgery? Dietary habits have far-reaching consequences in terms of overall health, so it should come as no surprise that nutrition plays a role in cardiopulmonary function (or that respiratory therapists would get involved).

WORD WIZARD

The language in Chapter 21 reads like a French menu—incomprehensibly. You may need to look up some of these terms before you can match them up with their definitions.

Terms	Definitions
_____ 1. anergy	A. excess nitrogenous waste in the blood
_____ 2. anthropometry	B. relationship of weight to height
_____ 3. azotemia	C. so thin that ribs stick out in persistent malnutrition
_____ 4. basal metabolic rate	D. daily resting energy consumption
_____ 5. body mass index	E. impaired immune response
_____ 6. indirect calorimetry	F. science of measuring the human body
_____ 7. cachexic	G. hypercatabolic form of malnutrition
_____ 8. kwashiorkor	H. hourly resting energy consumption after fasting
_____ 9. marasmus	I. energy measurement based on O_2 consumption and CO_2 production
_____ 10. normometabolic	J. malnutrition associated with starvation
_____ 11. protein-energy malnutrition	K. calorimetry REE within 10% of predicted
_____ 12. resting energy expenditure	L. wasting condition resulting from a deficient diet

MEET THE OBJECTIVES

13. Describe the "most helpful" technique for nutrition assessment performed by dietitians in the acute care setting.

14. What does BMI stand for, and what two variables are measured?

   A. BMI = _____

   B. Variable 1: _____

   C. Variable 2: _____

15. State the range of normal for BMI. (How is *your* BMI? What about your loved ones?)

   _____

16. State the formula for calculating ideal body weight.

   A. Males: _____

   B. Females: _____

   C. Calculate your own ideal body weight:

17. Compare starvation and hypercatabolism malnutrition. Be sure to give at least two clinical examples of each that a respiratory therapist might encounter. Check out Table 21-3 on page 481 of your text if you get lost.

   A. Kwashiorkor (starvation) _____

   B. Marasmus (malnutrition) _____

18. Lab studies could help restore nutrients to achieve respiratory muscle function and homeostasis. Test yourself on these meanings!

	MEANING	TEST
A.	Cheap, effective method for long-term assessment	
B.	Might help predict a compromised immune system	
C.	An acute phase protein monitored in trauma and illness	
D.	Indicator of catabolism	

19. How do patients with persistent malnutrition look? What is the funny sounding name for this appearance?

   A. How do they look? _____

   _____

   B. What is it called? _____

174

20. Good nourishment begins inside the womb, but that's a huge public health issue in the United States, so let's move on to children. What are the key influences that determine a child's lifetime eating habits?

21. What are some of the hallmark changes in eating patterns seen in the teen years?

22. Name the four diseases that now plague U.S. adults who eat too much fat and sugar.

    A. _____

    B. _____

    C. _____

    D. _____

23. Elderly patients might not eat well because of a variety of reasons. List some examples under each topic.

    A. Age-related change in senses

    B. Socioeconomic issues

C. Health

MACRONUTRIENTS

24. Name the three macronutrients that supply your body's energy requirements. State the kilocalories per gram for each.

	MACRONUTRIENT	KILOCALORIES PER GRAM
A.		
B.		
C.		

25. Write the Harris-Benedict prediction equation for estimating REE. Calculate yours (be sure to use the right one for your gender!).

A. Formula: _____

B. Calculation:

26. How many calories will an average man who weighs 80 kg need per day to maintain his body weight? Hint: Use

the Rule of Thumb on page 487. _____

27. State the effect of decreases in the following micronutrients through disease or malnutrition. (Just a few examples; this is a really huge subject!)

A. Zinc _____

_____

B. Magnesium _____

_____

C. Hypophosphatemia _____

_____

28. What percentage of patients with acute respiratory failure suffer from malnutrition?

_____

29. Give two reasons why malnourished patients are difficult to wean from the ventilator.

   A. _____

   B. _____

30. Why are COPD patients often malnourished?

31. What are the consequences of malnutrition on respiratory muscles and response to hypoxia and hypercapnia?

INDIRECT CALORIMETRY

32. List three conditions where indirect calorimetry may be indicated. (See Box 21-3.)

   A. _____

   B. _____

   C. _____

33. What are the contraindications to indirect calorimetry in mechanically ventilated patients? (See the Clinical Practice Guideline.)

34. According to the AARC Clinical Practice Guidelines, closed-circuit calorimeters may reduce alveolar volume or increase work of breathing. Explain how these two hazards occur.

35. What actions should be taken to prepare a patient for indirect calorimetry? (See Box 21-4.)

A. 4 hours before the test: _____

B. 2 hours before the test: _____

C. 1 hour before the test: _____

36. Describe the most significant problem in performing indirect calorimetry on mechanically ventilated patients.

37. Interpret the following RQs and identify the general nutritional strategy. (See Table 21-6.)

	VALUE	INTERPRETATION	STRATEGY
A.	>1		
B.	0.9 to 1		
C.	0.7 to 0.8		

38. State the formula for calculating REE using a pulmonary artery catheter. _____

_____

39. What factors are used to adjust predicted REEs in patients? Give one example. (Go to Table 21-5.)

RESPIRATORY CONSEQUENCES

40. How many patients in respiratory failure have malnutrition?

_____

41. COPD patients have special dietary problems. Identify four factors that lead to poor intake in these patients.

A. _____

B. _____

C. _____

D. _____

42. What is the effect of high-carbohydrate loads on COPD patients?

_____

ENTERAL, PARENTERAL

43. What do the terms "enteral" and "parenteral" mean?

A. Enteral: _____

B. Parenteral: _____

44. Explain what is meant by the following tube feeding regimens:

A. Bolus: _____

B. Intermittent: _____

C. Drip: _____

45. How would the respiratory therapist confirm suspected aspiration of tube feedings? How is this complication avoided?

A. Confirmation: _____

B. Prevention: _____

_____

_____

46. Explain what happens when patients receive too much of the following substrates. Give a pulmonary example, please.

A. Protein: _____

B. Carbohydrates: _____

C. Fat: _____

179

47. Approximately how many people with COPD have poor nutrition? _____

48. Which disease often shows progressive severe weight loss? _____

49. In general, COPD patients eat to optimize nutrition.

    A. How often? _____

    B. Calories? _____

50. Asthmatics may greatly benefit from what specific type of fatty acids? _____

51. In addition to a lot of calories, what supplements do CF patients need? _____

SUMMARY CHECKLIST

Complete the following sentences by writing in the correct term(s) in the blank(s) provided.

52. The _____-_____ equations estimate daily resting energy expenditure.

53. _____ is a state of impaired metabolism in which the intake of nutrients falls short of the body's needs.

54. For the patient with pulmonary disease, high _____ loads can increase carbon dioxide production.

55. Whenever possible, the _____ route should be used for supplying nutrients.

56. The likelihood of _____ during tube feedings can be minimized by _____ the head of the bed by _____.

CASE STUDY

A thin, undernourished COPD patient tells you that he has difficulty eating because he gets tired and short of breath during meals. Besides, food just doesn't taste as good now.

57. What eating pattern should be emphasized to this patient?

_____

_____

58. Make some suggestions that would increase his nutrient intake.

_____

_____

59. What other big problem might interfere with the patient's appetite?

_____

_____

WHAT DOES THE NBRC SAY?

Though muscle wasting and general appearance do show up in the matrix, and RTs are very involved in indirect calorimetry in many institutions, this information has not made it to the boards yet. However, it is known that nutrition can affect weaning, and the CRT and both Registry Examinations are specific about the RT participating in patient education and disease management. COPD and cystic fibrosis are conditions where nutrition is an issue. So you may see a few questions like these:

60. A respiratory therapist is caring for a 66-year-old male patient with acute exacerbation of COPD. The therapist notes the patient is extremely thin, with ribs obviously showing on his chest. What term should the therapist use to document the patient's appearance?

    A. malnourished

    B. cyanotic

    C. cachexic

    D. wasted

61. Cystic fibrosis patients may need what dietary supplement to be able to absorb nutrients?

    A. calcium

    B. amino acids

    C. enzymes

    D. vitamin C

62. A patient with COPD is being counseled in a pulmonary rehabilitation program. What general nutrition recommendation would you recommend for this individual?

    A. eat frequent small meals

    B. restrict sodium intake

    C. restrict carbohydrate intake

    D. increase whole grain and fiber intake

FOOD FOR THOUGHT

63. What type of nutritional strategy may help in the weaning of COPD patients from the ventilator?

22 Pulmonary Infections

Captain of the men of death . . .
Sir William Osler

More than one hundred years after these words were said, pneumonia is still a leading cause of death. In fact, it is the eighth leading cause of death in the United States and the single most common cause of infection-related death in the United States. It is interesting to note that author John Bunyon (1680) had said tuberculosis (TB) was the Captain of the Men of Death. Osler (1901) was saying that pneumonia was taking over. Tuberculosis is still a big problem in developing countries. In those countries, pneumonia is the number one killer and TB is number seven! There is a tremendous clinical interest in ventilator-associated pneumonia right now. Respiratory therapists (RTs) play a key role in the research and prevention of this serious complication of life in the intensive care unit. Pneumonia is simple to understand, right? There are only two types: community and nosocomial. Or is it viral and bacterial? Acute and chronic? Typical and atypical? Ventilator associated . . . or perhaps aspiration pneumonia . . . Read on, and you will meet "the old man's friend" in its many forms.

WORD WIZARD

Ok, we're on an acronym hunt. You need to know your VAPS from your CAPS! Write out the definition for each acronym.

CAP _____

HCAP _____

HAP _____

VAP _____

Ok, now put the right acronym next to these statements:

This patient got sick in their home. _____

This patient got sick on life support. _____

This patient got sick in the hospital. _____

This patient got sick in a nursing home. _____

1. What does the term "empirical therapy" mean?

2. The textbook definition of nosocomial pneumonia is now subdivided into HAP and VAP. Please describe these new terms *in depth* using the textbook criteria, because they are critical to your understanding of this life-threatening illness.

   A. HAP

   B. VAP

3. How common is hospital-acquired pneumonia, and what are the costs and mortality?

   A. Prevalence: _____

   _____

   B. Cost: _____

   _____

   C. Mortality: _____

   _____

4. List two patient populations that are at special risk for fatal forms of nosocomial pneumonia.

   A. _____

   B. _____

5. Name four diseases acquired via inhalation of infectious particles.

A. _____

B. _____

C. _____

D. _____

6. List four of the patient populations at risk for aspiration of large volumes of gastric fluids.

A. _____

B. _____

C. _____

D. _____

7. State the two novel strategies mentioned in the book to reduce HAP or VAP in ventilated patients.

A. _____

B. _____

8. Describe the role of suctioning as a cause of lower respiratory tract inoculation.

9. Give the prime example of reactivation of a latent infection. _____

_____

MICROBIOLOGY

10. Why is it so important to know what organisms are commonly associated with pneumonia?

11. What organism is most commonly identified as the cause of community-acquired pneumonia? _____

_____

12. Name the two most common atypical pathogens.

    A. _____

    B. _____

13. Why is no microbiologic identification made in so many cases of pneumonia?

14. Name two viruses associated with pneumonia. What time of year are they encountered?

    A. Viruses:

        1. _____

        2. _____

    B. Time of year: _____

CLINICAL MANIFESTATIONS

15. Patients with community-acquired pneumonia typically have fever and what three respiratory symptoms?

    A. _____

    B. _____

    C. _____

16. What two other common respiratory problems show the same symptoms?

    A. _____

    B. _____

17. What is the classic, typical presentation of community-acquired pneumonia? _____

_____

_____

18. In intubated patients, VAP usually shows up as what three changes in the patient's condition?

    A. _____

    B. _____

    C. _____

19. Describe the common radiograph abnormalities associated with pneumonia.

20. Why is the chest film of limited use in diagnosing pneumonia in critically ill patients?

RISK FACTORS

21. Fill in the data for each of the following risk factors for mortality associated with community-acquired pneumonia (see Box 22-1).

	FACTOR	DESCRIPTION
A.	Age	
B.	Gender	
C.	Vital signs	
D.	Arterial pH	
E.	High-risk causes	
F.	Comorbid illness	

22. A number of factors predispose the hospital patient to pneumonia, such as poor host defenses from underlying illness. Name five such "comorbidities." Hint: Table 22-5!

    A. _____

    B. _____

    C. _____

    D. _____

    E. _____

23. List four factors that expose the lungs to large numbers of microorganisms.

A. _____

B. _____

C. _____

D. _____

DIAGNOSTIC STUDIES

24. Why is determining the predominant causative organism via sputum Gram stain, culture, and sensitivity so useful in pneumonia patients?

25. Describe the process for collecting a good specimen by expectoration.

26. Describe the satisfactory specimen. (This is board exam material!)

27. Name the organism identified by each of the following specialized tests.

	TEST	ORGANISM
A.	Acid-fast stain	
B.	Direct fluorescent stain	
C.	Toluidine blue	
D.	Potassium hydroxide	

28. When should HIV testing be recommended in cases of community-acquired pneumonia?

29. When should fiber-optic bronchoscopy be recommended in cases of community-acquired pneumonia?

30. Name four techniques useful in confirming the diagnosis of nosocomial pneumonia.

A. _____

B. _____

C. _____

D. _____

Diagnosing VAP is a big challenge for everyone in the ICU. Regular sputum specimens just don't seem to get us the right antibiotics for those bugs. New techniques have had some success.

31. Direct visualization of the lower airway is helpful in diagnosing VAP. What are the three criteria?

A. _____

B. _____

C. _____

32. What do the initials BAL stand for? Describe BAL.

A. BAL = _____

B. Description: _____

_____

_____

189

33. What is mini-BAL, and what health care professional performs the procedure?

THERAPY

34. What is the primary medical treatment for pneumonia? _____

_____

35. What is the agent of choice for treating the following organisms? Hint: See Table 22-8 in your text.

	ORGANISM	AGENT OF CHOICE
A.	Pneumococcus	
B.	*Mycoplasma*	
C.	*Pneumocystis carinii*	
D.	*Legionella*	

36. How long is a typical course of treatment for pneumonia? _____

37. How long does it take for the radiograph to show resolution of pneumonia in young individuals? What about older patients?

   A. Young patients: _____

   B. Older patients: _____

PREVENTION

38. Immunization is one of the primary strategies for preventing community-acquired pneumonia. Individuals are immunized against what two organisms?

   A. _____

   B. _____

39. Identify three groups that should be immunized.

   A. _____

   B. _____

   C. _____

40. Identify the three "probably effective" strategies for the prevention of nosocomial pneumonia.

A. _____

B. _____

C. _____

41. What positioning technique is useful in preventing pneumonia in patients? _____

_____

42. What is the current medication for gastrointestinal bleeding prophylaxis that may be effective in preventing

pneumonia? _____

CASE STUDIES

Case 1

A 55-year-old man arrives at the clinic complaining of chills, fever, and chest pain on inspiration. He is coughing up rusty-colored sputum. He admits to a history of heavy smoking and regular use of alcoholic beverages. Physical examination reveals a heart rate of 125 beats/min, respiratory rate of 30 breaths/min, and temperature of 104° F. He has inspiratory crackles in the right lower lobe. Blood gases reveal a pH of 7.34, $PaCO_2$ of 50 mm Hg, and PaO_2 of 58 mm Hg.

43. What is the most likely diagnosis? Support your answer based on the clinical signs and symptoms.

44. What immediate treatment should you initiate? _____

_____

45. Give at least five reasons why the patient is at risk of dying from his condition.

A. _____

B. _____

C. _____

D. _____

E. _____

191

A patient is intubated and on the ventilator following a head injury. On the third day following his craniotomy, he develops a fever. During routine suctioning, you notice his secretions are thick and yellow. Breath sounds are decreased in the left lower lobe.

46. What is the role of the artificial airway in development of pneumonia?

47. What test would you recommend at this time to help confirm a diagnosis?

WHAT DOES THE NBRC SAY?

Interestingly enough, they don't say much about pneumonia! Certain lung infections may appear on the boards in the context of their *treatment and recognition,* such as the use of ribavirin to treat respiratory syncytial virus (RSV). Or, inhaled pentamidine in HIV patients with pneumonia. Isolation procedures for tuberculosis patients is a possible area of testing as well as general methods to prevent the spread of infection. You should certainly recognize when a patient has a lung infection, and *pay attention to basic microbiology.* The new matrix states that a respiratory therapist should be able to implement a VAP protocol. In summary, you will need to know the diagnostic tests and therapies that go with all lower respiratory tract infections regardless of whether pneumonia is present or not.

48. A patient is seen in the ED with fever, chills, and tachypnea. He states he feels weak and short of breath. The vitals are T 101.4 ° F, f 28, HR 121, BP 140/96, and SpO_2 88% on room air. What should the respiratory therapist do first?

    A. Obtain a sputum specimen.

    B. Request a chest x-ray.

    C. Place the patient on antibiotics.

    D. Place the patient on oxygen.

49. A 14-year-old is admitted to the medical floor with "acute exacerbation of asthma secondary to lung infection." While administering bronchodilator therapy, the respiratory therapist observes the patient producing moderate amounts of thick yellow phlegm. What should the therapist recommend at this point?

    A. Obtain a sputum specimen.

    B. Request a chest x-ray.

    C. Place the patient on antibiotics.

    D. Place the patient on oxygen.

50. The gold standard for confirming diagnosis of pneumonia in an acutely ill patient is
    A. sputum culture
    B. chest x-ray
    C. blood cultures
    D. CT scan

51. A person with AIDS presents in the ED with profound hypoxemia, shortness of breath, and nonproductive cough. Physical exam findings suggest bilateral lower lobe pneumonia. Which of the following organisms is most likely to be seen in this particular individual?
    1. *Pneumocystis jiroveci*
    2. *Streptococcus pneumoniae*
    3. *Mycobacterium tuberculosis*
        A. 1
        B. 2 and 3
        C. 1 and 3
        D. 1, 2, and 3

52. New onset of fever accompanied by purulent secretions and a new infiltrate on the chest film in an intubated patient are strongly suggestive of
    A. VAP
    B. HAP
    C. CAP
    D. HCAP

53. The respiratory therapist suspects that one of her ventilator patients is at high risk for developing pneumonia. What general action should the therapist take?
    A. Request a chest x-ray
    B. Elevate the head of the bed
    C. Implement the VAP protocol
    D. Implement an in-line suction catheter

FOOD FOR THOUGHT

54. What is the role of the RT in educating at-risk populations about methods to prevent pneumonia?

55. Have you had your flu shot? What about your updated whooping cough (pertussis) vaccine?

Chapter **22** **Pulmonary Infections**

Obstructive Lung Disease: Chronic Obstructive Pulmonary Disease (COPD), Asthma, and Related Diseases

Human action can be modified to some extent, but human nature cannot be changed.

Abraham Lincoln

The conditions discussed in Chapter 23 are so common that you probably know someone who has them too. (Famous people get chronic obstructive pulmonary disease [COPD] as well. If "honest Abe" had Marfan syndrome, he might have developed emphysema!) Respiratory therapists spend a lot of their time working with COPD patients. Pay special attention to the information in this chapter, as you get to know the "pink puffers" and "blue bloaters."

WORD WIZARD

Before we start on the long dark journey into the lungs, take a shot at the COPD crossword puzzle on the following page.

CHRONIC OBSTRUCTIVE PULMONARY DISEASE

If you talk about each type of COPD as if it was "pure emphysema," you would be oversimplifying in many cases. The Venn diagram shown in Figure 23-1 in *Egan's* demonstrates this nicely. Many patients show signs of having mixed disease states. Asthma is classified as separate from COPD, but those with long-standing, poorly controlled asthma often present with signs of COPD later in life. So though it is convenient to talk about (or test about) emphysema, chronic bronchitis, or asthma as if they were pure and separate entities, in the clinical setting you will see patients who have varying degrees of pathology that represent each of these important components of the spectrum of COPD. Remember that most COPD patients have a smoking history, so you will want to explore this issue. (You can calculate pack-years by multiplying packs-per-day by the number of years the patient smoked.)

Overview

COPD is so pervasive in the United States and worldwide that we need to start off with some definitions and demographics so you can get a clear picture of the conditions that RTs treat almost constantly.

1. *Chronic obstructive pulmonary disease* is defined by the American Thoracic Society in four key concepts. Please elaborate on the following.

   A. Limitation: _____

   B. Progressive: _____

   C. Inflammatory: _____

   D. Systemic: _____

2. According to the NHANES data, what percentage of the U.S. population has mild *or* moderate COPD (add the two populations)?

   _____

3. How does COPD rank as a leading cause of death, and why is this condition strikingly different from heart disease or stroke?

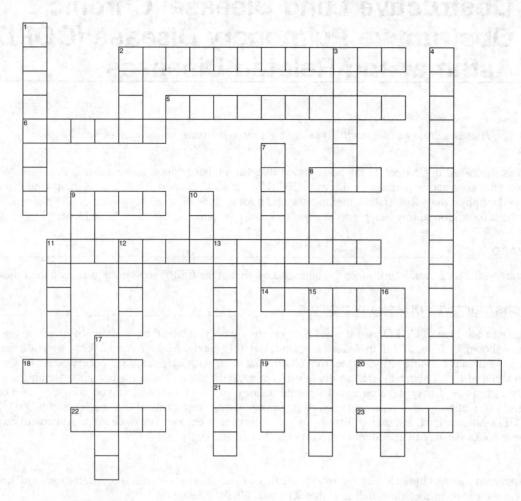

ACROSS

2. Smooth muscle contraction in the airways
5. Chronic form shows productive cough for 3 months in 2 consecutive years
6. The only thing that increases survival of end-stage COPD patients
8. Late asthma response
9. Another four letter word for COPD
11. Results in permanent dilation of the airways
14. This fibrosis is the most frequently lethal genetic disease of white children
18. _____ one antitrypsin deficiency, a genetic form of emphysema
20. Where COPD stands as a killer
21. Asthma you get when you exercise
22. Common bedside test used to manage asthma
23. These puffers really have emphysema

DOWN

1. Cystic _____, known in Europe as mucoviscidosis
2. Bloater, or patient with chronic bronchitis
3. Complex lung disease associated with wheezing and airway inflammation
4. Drug that opens the airways
7. Passed on from parents to children via DNA
8. Abbreviation for surgery that removes part of the emphysematous lung
9. _____ pulmonale, the heart failure associated with hypoxemia
10. Most common way to deliver drugs to the airway
11. COPD chest shape
12. Famous oxygen therapy study that proved increased survival with oxygen
13. Enlargement and destruction of the distal airways and alveoli
15. Stop it
16. The "C" in COPD
17. Lung butter
19. Early asthma response

4. What is the approximate cost of health care associated with COPD in the 2000s?

    A. Hospitalizations (1993 = $500,000): _____

    B. Office visits: _____

    C. Emergency department visits: _____

    D. Total health dollars (1993 = $24 billion): _____

Risk Factors and Pathophysiology

5. OK, so cigarette smokers get COPD. What is the other major cause of emphysema? _____

_____

6. Describe the "susceptible smoker."

7. Briefly explain the protease-antiprotease hypothesis of emphysema.

8. Describe the three mechanisms of airflow obstruction in COPD.

    A. _____

    B. _____

    C. _____

Clinical Signs

9. Name four common symptoms of COPD.

    A. _____

    B. _____

    C. _____

    D. _____

10. Compare the onset of dyspnea in typical cases of COPD with that of α_1-antitrypsin deficiency.

Chapter **23** **Obstructive Lung Disease**

11. What physical change in the chest wall occurs as a result of prolonged hyperinflation? _____

_____

12. Name three other late signs of COPD.

A. _____

B. _____

C. _____

13. Compare chronic bronchitis, emphysema, and α_1-antitrypsin deficiency in terms of the following features.

	FEATURES	CHRONIC BRONCHITIS	EMPHYSEMA	α_1-ANTITRYPSIN DEFICIENCY
A.	Age of onset			
B.	Family history			
C.	Smoker			
D.	Lung volume			
E.	DLCO			
F.	FEV$_1$/FVC			
G.	Radiograph			

Management

Your text lists five general goals of management for COPD. In addition, we need to think about how to avoid complications when the patient has an acute exacerbation of their condition.

14. Why would it be important to differentiate asthma from other forms of COPD? List some features that favor each.

A. Why differentiate?

B. Features that favor COPD

C. Features that favor asthma

15. Reversible airflow obstruction is defined as an increase of what amount?

A. Percentage: _____

B. Milliliters: _____

16. Why is bronchodilator therapy recommended for COPD? What types of drugs are used? What is the effect on decline of lung function and survival?

A. Why? _____

B. Types of drugs? _____

C. Lung decline and survival? _____

17. Discuss the role of inhaled steroids in COPD. Which group should receive glucocorticosteroids according to the GOLD guidelines/ATS guidelines?

18. What is the primary effect of theophylline (methylxanthines) on patients with COPD? What serum blood levels are currently recommended to avoid side effects?

19. Name the four important elements of managing an acute exacerbation of COPD due to purulent bronchitis.

A. _____

B. _____

C. _____

D. _____

20. When hypercapnia and respiratory failure are present (and pH is <7.3) you might want to avoid intubation with noninvasive ventilation. What are some of the criteria of a good candidate for this lifesaving therapy?

21. What is the primary goal of pulmonary rehabilitation? _____

_____

22. What is the effect of pulmonary rehabilitation programs on survival and pulmonary function?

23. A comprehensive smoking cessation program usually includes what three elements?

A. _____

B. _____

C. _____

24. Only three treatments for COPD have been shown to prolong survival. Please elaborate.
A. Oxygen:

B. Quitting smoking:

C. LVRS

25. What is the relationship between bronchodilator therapy and home oxygen therapy?

26. You need to know the indication for continuous oxygen. Please give the correct values for

A. Resting PaO_2: _____

B. Hematocrit: _____

C. ECG: _____

27. What two vaccines are recommended for patients with COPD? Which one is given annually?

A. _____

B. _____

28. Describe the two surgical options for end-stage COPD. Discuss the outcomes of each of these options.

A.

B.

ASTHMA

All that wheezes is not asthma.
Anonymous RTs

Asthma is on the rise, and all of our drugs and technology have not been able to solve the problem. A number of interesting theories exist to explain why industrialized countries are experiencing worse problems than underdeveloped nations. For RTs, many of whom are certified by the National Asthma Educator Certification Board (NAECB), the situation is a wonderful opportunity to apply our special expertise to help educate the public and our clients regarding prevention, treatment, and control.

Overview

29. What is the difference between older definitions and the more current view of asthma?

30. What percentage of people in the United States is believed to have asthma? (In 2002, it was estimated to be 5%!)

_____

Etiology and Pathogenesis

31. Airway inflammation and bronchial hyperreactivity result in airflow obstruction. Name four triggers:

A. _____

B. _____

C. _____

D. _____

32. What happens when a patient with asthma inhales an allergen to which he or she is sensitized?

33. Describe the early and late asthmatic reactions (EAR and LAR, respectively).

   A. EAR

   B. LAR

Clinical Signs

34. What factor plays a key role in suggesting and establishing a diagnosis of asthma? _____

   _____

35. What are the four classic symptoms of asthma?

   A. _____

   B. _____

   C. _____

   D. _____

36. List five conditions that can mimic the wheezing of asthma.

   A. _____

   B. _____

   C. _____

   D. _____

   E. _____

37. What change in values determines reversibility of airflow obstruction?

202

38. Bronchial provocation is the specialized test regimen used to demonstrate obstruction in suspected asthmatics who are symptom-free at the time of testing. Name the drug used for this test and what response indicates hyperresponsiveness.

A. Drug: _____

B. Response: _____

39. Describe the role of arterial blood gases in the diagnosis *and* assessment of asthma.
A. Diagnosis

B. Assessment

Management

The goal of asthma management is to maintain a high quality of life without symptoms or limitations. The goal is to reduce death (mortality) and lost time from work and school, pneumonia, and other consequences of asthma (morbidity). The patient should be relatively free of side effects from treatment. To achieve this, a four-step approach has been recommended by the National Institutes of Health National Expert Panel.

40. Complete the chart below to show your understanding of the stepwise approach. Table 23-2 in your text will help.

	SEVERITY	SYMPTOMS	LONG-TERM MEDICATIONS
A.	1: Intermittent		
B.	2: Mild persistent		
C.	3: Moderate persistent		
D.	4: Severe persistent		

41. Explain control of asthma in terms of the following criteria:

A. Symptoms: _____

_____

B. β_2-Agonists: _____

_____

_____

C. Exercise: _____

_____

D. PEFR/FEV$_1$: _____

_____

_____

E. Exacerbations: _____

_____

42. Give the criteria and actions for green, yellow, and red peak flow zones.

	ZONE	PEFR % PREDICTED	TREATMENT/ACTION
A.	Green		
B.	Yellow		
C.	Red		

43. Compare the use of inhaled corticosteroids and bronchodilators in treating asthma.

44. Name the two common side effects of inhaled steroids and two ways to control them.

    A. _____

    B. _____

    C. Control/reduce side effects:

        1. _____

        2. _____

45. Discuss the use of cromolyn/nedocromil sodium in asthma treatment.
    A. Indications

        1. Adults: _____

        2. Children: _____

    B. Acute attacks: _____

    C. What three problems could cromolyn protect against?

        1. _____

        2. _____

        3. _____

46. Leukotriene modifiers like montelukast sodium (Singulair) are popular and useful for what specific type of asthmatic? Do these drugs replace steroids?

    _____

47. What type of drug is the first-line treatment for all types of acute bronchospasm? _____

    _____

48. Name the two long-acting β-agonists, and explain the new FDA warnings.

49. Describe the use of methylxanthines such as theophylline in the treatment of asthma. What's a good dose, and how do you check?

50. What is the benefit of using anticholinergics like ipratropium in the day-to-day management of asthma?

For a Good Time, Meet Me in the Emergency Department

The goal is to reduce death (mortality), time lost from work and school, pneumonia, and other consequences of asthma (morbidity).

51. Name three factors you should monitor in a patient hospitalized with acute asthma.

A. _____

B. _____

C. _____

52. Give the criteria for hospital discharge for each of the following:

A. PaO$_2$: _____

B. PEFR: _____

C. Symptoms: _____

_____

D. Discharge medications: _____

_____

Chapter **23** **Obstructive Lung Disease**

53. Management of asthma should be aggressive, including two specific types of medications along with oxygen. Discuss the use of β-agonists and steroids in this specific situation.

A. β-Agonists: _____

_____

B. Steroids: _____

_____

54. How can you prevent allergic reactions in asthmatic patients through immunotherapy?

55. Name some common outdoor and indoor allergens. Then give suggestions for control.

		ALLERGEN	CONTROL
A.	Outdoor		
B.	Indoor		

56. What is EIA? List three prophylactic drug treatments.

A. EIA = _____

B. Prophylaxis:

1. _____

2. _____

3. _____

57. Define occupational asthma. What is the most common cause?

58. What is the only way to eliminate occupational asthma once an individual is sensitized?_____

_____

59. What drug is particularly helpful in the treatment of cough-variant asthma?

_____

60. List three medications that may be helpful in treating nocturnal asthma.

   A. _____

   B. _____

   C. _____

61. What recommendations would you make to a patient who has aspirin sensitivity?

62. What is the effect of pregnancy on asthmatics?

63. Discuss the use of asthma medications during pregnancy.

64. GER (most of us call it GERD) can also play a role in asthma. Any ideas on how to help?

65. A surprising number of asthmatics have trouble with the nose and sinuses. No surprise really, the nose and sinuses are part of the respiratory system! What types of inhalers are needed here?

BRONCHIECTASIS

Bronchiectasis is a condition where airways are deformed and destroyed by chronic inflammation.

66. What is the clinical hallmark of bronchiectasis?

   _____

67. What test is now considered definitive for diagnosing bronchiectasis?

   _____

68. List the causes of local and diffuse bronchiectasis.
   A. Local

   1. _____

   2. _____

   B. Diffuse

   1. _____

   2. _____

   3. _____

69. Name the two primary treatments for bronchiectasis.

   A. _____

   B. _____

And if these don't work, the patient needs to have _____.

CASE STUDIES

Case 1

A 70-year-old man's chief complaint is dyspnea on exertion. He has a smoking history of two packs per day for the past 50 years. He has a barrel-shaped chest and much decreased breath sounds. His chest radiograph shows hyperinflation, especially in the apices; flattened diaphragms; and a small heart. He admits to a morning cough but denies significant sputum production.

70. What is the most likely diagnosis?

   _____

71. Calculate the patient's pack-years. _____.

72. What factor should you focus on to help the patient control his condition? _____

   _____

Case 2

A 60-year-old man has smoked a pack of cigarettes per day since he was a teenager. He complains of a chronic productive cough that is producing thick, yellow sputum. He is admitted to the medical floor with a fever and shortness of breath. Blood gases reveal pH of 7.35, $PaCO_2$ of 50 mm Hg, and PaO_2 of 57 mm Hg. Physical exam shows pedal edema, distended neck veins, and use of accessory muscles of ventilation. He has scattered wheezing and rhonchi on auscultation.

73. What type of COPD is most likely in this case?

   _____

74. What should you do with his sputum the next time he coughs productively?

75. What is the immediate respiratory treatment in this case?

76. What respiratory medications would you recommend?

Case 3

A 44-year-old man complains of dyspnea on exertion. He is a nonsmoker but drinks wine with his meals. He has a barrel-shaped chest and very decreased breath sounds. His chest radiograph shows hyperinflation, especially in the bases. History reveals that his father and uncle both died of "lung problems."

77. What is the most likely cause of the patient's COPD symptoms? Justify your answer based on the information presented.

78. What treatments are available for this condition?

Case 4

A 15-year-old boy complains that he cannot catch his breath when he exercises. He states that he coughs a lot, especially in the winter. His breath sounds are clear, and his physical examination is unremarkable.

79. What do you suspect is the problem? _____

_____

80. How could a definitive diagnosis be made?

WHAT DOES THE NBRC SAY?

It will come as no surprise that the board exams place a special emphasis on COPD and asthma. The Clinical Simulation Examination Matrix states that you will see at least "two problems involving adult patients with COPD." You may also see a pediatric patient with asthma. *All* aspects of managing these patients may be included, from pulmonary function testing to rehabilitation. Multiple choice exams, like the Written Registry and Entry-Level Examinations, do not specifically mention COPD or asthma in the matrices; however, diagnosis and management of these patients are heavily tested. Here are some sample questions. Circle the best answer.

Use the following data to answer questions 81 through 86.

A 20-year-old woman who has a history of asthma is brought to the emergency department in respiratory distress. Your assessment of the patient reveals the following:

pH	7.47
$PaCO_2$	33 mm Hg
PaO_2	72 mm Hg
HCO_3^-	23 mEq/L
RR	28
HR	115
PEFR	200 L/min

81. Which of the following breath sounds would you expect to hear in this patient?
    A. inspiratory crackles
    B. expiratory wheezing
    C. inspiratory stridor
    D. expiratory rhonchi

82. The arterial blood gas results indicate the presence of
    A. acute respiratory alkalosis
    B. acute metabolic alkalosis
    C. chronic respiratory acidosis
    D. acute respiratory acidosis

83. You are asked to initiate oxygen therapy. What would you recommend?
    A. simple mask at 10 L/min
    B. non-rebreathing mask at 15 L/min
    C. nasal cannula at 2 L/min
    D. air-entrainment mask at 50% F_IO_2

84. What therapy would you recommend after the oxygen is in place?
    A. 2 puffs ipratropium (Atrovent) via MDI
    B. 0.5 ml albuterol (Proventil) via SVN
    C. intravenous aminophylline (theophylline) administration
    D. intravenous antibiotics

85. Blood gases are repeated 30 minutes after the oxygen therapy is initiated.

pH	7.42
$PaCO_2$	38 mm Hg
PaO_2	86 mm Hg
HCO_3^-	23 mEq/L
RR	24
HR	88
PEFR	210 L/min

Which of the following has shown significant improvement based on this information?
A. compliance
B. resistance
C. oxygenation
D. ventilation

86. Intravenous steroids and repeated bronchodilators have been given. The patient is now receiving 40% oxygen.

pH	7.34
$PaCO_2$	53 mm Hg
PaO_2	74 mm Hg
HCO_3^-	26 mEq/L
RR	18
HR	125
PEFR	110 L/min

What would you suggest at this point?
A. increase of F_1O_2 to 50%
B. continuous nebulization of bronchodilators
C. administration of intravenous bicarbonate
D. intubation and mechanical ventilation

87. A patient with COPD and CO_2 retention is admitted for an acute exacerbation of her disease. The physician requests your suggestion for initiating oxygen therapy. Which of the following would you recommend?
A. nasal cannula at 6 L/min
B. air-entrainment mask at 28%
C. simple mask at 2 L/min
D. partial rebreathing mask at 8 L/min

88. A PFT on a 65-year-old woman indicates airflow obstruction with mild air-trapping. The patient is coughing up thick sputum. Which of the following diagnoses is most likely?
A. cystic fibrosis
B. pneumonia
C. pulmonary fibrosis
D. bronchiectasis

89. A PFT on a 56-year-old man with a history of smoking shows increased TLC and RV. The DLCO is reduced. What diagnosis is suggested by these findings?
A. emphysema
B. pneumonia
C. sarcoidosis
D. pneumoconiosis

90. Spirometry is performed before and after bronchodilator administration. Which of the following indicates a therapeutic response?
1. FEV_1 increased by 10%
2. FVC increased by 300 ml
3. PEFR increased by 5%
    A. 1 only
    B. 2 only
    C. 1 and 2 only
    D. 1 and 3 only

211

91. Because only 15% of smokers actually show big declines in airflow, why should we encourage all patients to quit smoking?

92. Patients with α_1-antitrypsin deficiency can now benefit from therapy. What is needed?

93. What is omalizumab (Xolair), and how does it work for asthma?

24 Interstitial Lung Disease

There is a remedy for everything; it is called death.
Portuguese Proverb

There are an unbelievable number of interstitial lung diseases (ILDs). Individually, they are not common, but as a group, they represent a significant set of lung disorders. Sooner or later, you will encounter some of the members of this broad category of restrictive conditions. Fortunately there are many common elements in the clinical signs, pulmonary function test (PFT) abnormalities, and treatment of most forms of ILD.

WORD WIZARD

Because there are so many new terms related to ILD in Chapter 24, a quick review will probably help you keep them straight. Match the correct definition with the correct term.

Terms	Definitions
_____ 1. asbestosis	A. formation of scar tissue in the lung without known cause
_____ 2. corticosteroids	B. respiratory disorder characterized by fibrotic infiltrates in the lower lobes
_____ 3. drug-related lung disease	C. inflammatory reaction provoked by inhalation of organic dusts
_____ 4. lymphangioleiomyomatosis	D. lung disease caused by chemotherapy agents, for example
_____ 5. hypersensitivity pneumonitis	E. interstitial lung disease associated with tobacco smoke
_____ 6. idiopathic pulmonary fibrosis	F. restrictive disorder associated with pleural abnormalities and lung tumors
_____ 7. interstitial lung disease	G. disorder of unknown origin that results in formation of epithelioid tubercles
_____ 8. connective tissue disease	H. hormones associated with control of body processes
_____ 9. occupational ILD	I. bone growth associated with numerous histiocytes and specific white blood cells (WBCs)
_____ 10. organizing pneumonitis	J. abnormal airway smooth muscle growth
_____ 11. pulmonary Langerhans histiocytosis	K. lupus is a good example of this type of ILD
_____ 12. sarcoidosis	L. disorder caused by long-term exposure to sand and stone dust
_____ 13. silicosis	M. star-shaped areas of disease associated with smoking

CLINICAL SIGNS AND SYMPTOMS OF ILD

14. Patients with ILD of many different etiologies will usually present with which two common complaints?

    A. _____

    B. _____

15. Describe the breath sounds usually heard in ILD. _____

    _____

16. What two explanations does *Egan's* give for wheezing heard in patients with ILD?

    A. _____

    B. _____

213

17. Name at least two of the late signs of ILD.

A. _____

B. _____

18. Physical signs of underlying connective tissue disease include what three features?

A. _____

B. _____

C. _____

19. Describe the classic and late radiographic findings in idiopathic pulmonary fibrosis; use the colorful descriptive terms from *Egan's*. What are the late-stage findings?

A. Classic: _____

B. Late: _____

20. Discuss the effects of ILD on the following pulmonary function variables.

	VARIABLE	EFFECT OF ILD
A.	FEV_1	
B.	FVC	
C.	FEV_1/FVC	
D.	D_{LCO}	
E.	Lung volumes	
F.	Compliance	

SPECIFIC TYPES OF ILD

Because there are so many causes of ILD, it will help you to look at the primary groupings and some representative examples of each category.

21. What are the three most common types of occupational ILD?

A. _____

B. _____

C. _____

22. What do these examples have in common?

23. Give at least one specific example for each of the following general categories of drugs that are associated with the development of ILD. Hint: Box 24-1 on page 552 of your text is useful.

	CATEGORY	EXAMPLE
A.	Antibiotic	
B.	Antiinflammatory	
C.	Cardiovascular	
D.	Chemotherapeutic	
E.	Illegal drugs	
F.	Miscellaneous agents	

24. Why is pulmonary involvement in connective tissue disorders often undetected until late in the course of the disease?

25. Name three common connective disorders associated with lung disease.

A. _____

B. _____

C. _____

26. What is the name for chronic exposure to inhaled organic material that results in progressive scarring of the

lung? _____

27. What factor is critical to identifying the cause of this condition? _____

_____

Chapter **24** **Interstitial Lung Disease**

28. What is meant by the term "idiopathic"? _____

_____

29. Let's compare the two idiopathic lung diseases discussed in the text.

		Idiopathic Pulmonary Fibrosis (IPF)	Sarcoidosis
A.	Age		
B.	Symptoms		
C.	Treatment		
D.	Prognosis		

30. Discuss the common areas of treatment for hypersensitivity pneumonitis and occupational lung disease.

31. What is the primary drug (traditional) therapy for ILD? _____

_____

32. What is the most common respiratory therapy modality for ILD? _____

_____

33. What two vaccines are recommended to help avoid infections? What about pneumocystosis?

A. Vaccines _____

_____

B. Pneumocystosis: _____

_____

34. What is the only therapy shown to prolong life in end-stage ILD? _____

_____

Case 1

A 48-year-old man is admitted for dyspnea on exertion and a dry cough of unknown origin. The chest radiograph shows bilateral reticulonodular infiltrates. Pulse oximetry indicates mild hypoxemia on room air. History reveals that the patient is a hay farmer.

35. What is the most likely diagnosis?

_____

36. What is the most likely cause of the lung disease? What are some other possible causes?

Case 2

A retired Pearl Harbor shipyard worker states that he has had a cough for some time but recently began expectorating some blood. He has bibasilar inspiratory crackles, with otherwise clear breath sounds. A chest radiograph shows reticulonodular infiltrates in both lower lobes. The radiologist also notes the presence of a small right-sided pleural effusion and the presence of pleural plaques and pleural fibrosis. PFTs reveal a normal FEV_1 %, decreased TLC and RV, and a decreased D_{LCO}.

37. What is the most likely pulmonary diagnosis?

_____

38. What other information would be helpful in making a determination?

39. What type of disorder is suggested by the PFT results?

The NBRC thinks you should know your PFT and physical examination findings pretty well! ILDs don't have a particular category on the boards, but they may be included as side issues to material like interpreting PFT results. Try these on for size.

40. A patient with a history of sarcoidosis presents in the emergency department with shortness of breath. Vital signs are T 99, P 114, f 32, BP 138/88, SpO_2 82%. The respiratory care practitioner would
    A. administer oxygen via nasal cannula at 2 L/min
    B. request a stat portable AP chest x-ray
    C. perform a stat ABG
    D. administer albuterol

FOOD FOR THOUGHT

41. What is the general term for all lung diseases that cause a reduction in lung volumes without a reduction in flow

    rates? _____

25 Pleural Diseases

Some men dream of doing great things. Others stay awake and accomplish them.

Author unknown

Imagine a piece of cake enclosed in Saran Wrap. Or, if you prefer collapsed lungs, a sandwich covered in that thin, tough clear stuff that we use to store food. Pleura can be compared to plastic wrap. Like that clingy food protector, a breach in the pleura has important consequences. You may get a chance to play with some pig lungs while you're in training, but if you don't, you can always head for the kitchen!

WORD WIZARD

Chapter 25 introduces lots of important new terms. Match these pleural puzzlers to their definitions. You're going to need the glossary, but it will be worth it. Many of these words are commonly seen on board exams or in clinical practice.

Terms	Definitions
1. _____ bronchopleural fistula	A. pleural effusion high in protein
2. _____ chylothorax	B. air leak from the lung to the pleural space
3. _____ empyema	C. membrane covering the surface of the chest wall
4. _____ exudative effusion	D. pleural fluid rich with triglycerides from a ruptured thoracic duct
5. _____ hemothorax	E. pleural pain
6. _____ parietal pleura	F. pus-filled pleural effusion
7. _____ pleural effusion	G. blood in the pleural space
8. _____ pleurisy	H. abnormal collection of fluid in the pleural space
9. _____ pleurodesis	I. pneumothorax without underlying lung disease
10. _____ pneumothorax	J. air under pressure in the pleural space
11. _____ primary spontaneous pneumothorax	K. procedure that fuses the pleura to prevent pneumothorax
12. _____ reexpansion pulmonary edema	L. air in the pleural space
13. _____ secondary spontaneous pneumothorax	M. occurs when the lung is rapidly inflated after compression by pleural fluid
14. _____ tension pneumothorax	N. pneumothorax that occurs with underlying lung disease
15. _____ thoracentesis	O. low-protein effusion caused by CHF or cirrhosis
16. _____ transudative pleural effusion	P. chest wall puncture for diagnostic or therapeutic purposes
17. _____ visceral pleura	Q. membrane that lines the lung surface

18. How is the pleura of the American buffalo different from that of humans? What is the clinical significance for the buffalo, and when are humans in the same situation?

19. Describe the so-called pleural space.

20. What is normal intrapleural pressure, and what effect does this have on fluid movement?

21. Explain why pleural pressures are different at the apex and lung bases.

PLEURAL EFFUSIONS

22. Give a brief explanation of how each of the following conditions can cause transudative pleural effusions. If you get lost, refer to Box 25-1 in your text.
    A. CHF:

    B. Hypoalbuminemia:

    C. Liver disease:

D. Lymph obstruction:

E. CVP line:

23. What is the most common cause of clinical pleural effusions?

_____

24. What is the general cause of exudative pleural effusions?

_____

25. Give a brief explanation of the cause of these exudative pleural effusions.
A. Parapneumonic

B. Malignant

C. Chylothorax

D. Hemothorax

26. What change in pulmonary function is associated with pleural effusion?

_____

27. In what specific portion of the upright chest film is pleural effusion visualized?

_____

221

28. Describe the specific type of chest film used to improve visualization of pleural effusions.

29. What type of imaging is the most sensitive test for identification of pleural effusions?

_____

30. What are the three major risks of thoracentesis?

A. _____

B. _____

C. _____

31. Identify the purpose of each of the chambers in the three-bottle chest tube drainage system shown here.

A. _____

B. _____

C. _____

The standard three-bottle system is the basis for all commercial chest tube drainage systems.

PNEUMOTHORAX

32. What two symptoms are common to almost all cases of pneumothorax?

A. _____

B. _____

33. What is the most common type of traumatic pneumothorax, and how is it treated? Give three examples.

34. Compare blunt and penetrating chest trauma as causes of pneumothorax. How does treatment differ in these two situations?

35. What special technique may be helpful to visualize pneumothorax in a newborn?

_____

36. Compare the two major types of spontaneous pneumothorax.

37. Tension pneumothorax can be a life-threatening medical emergency. It is a common board exam item. Please give short clear explanations for items A through D.
   A. Definition

   B. Radiographic finding

   C. Clinical signs

   D. Treatment

223

38. Compare the outcomes of early clinical diagnosis and treatment of tension pneumothorax with delayed diagnosis.

39. How does oxygen administration assist in resolution of a pneumothorax?

40. What is BPF? How does mechanical ventilation perpetuate this problem? What special modes of ventilation may be indicated?

A. BPF = _____

B. Ventilators perpetuate BPF by: _____

C. Adjust ventilator for BPF patient by: _____

CASE STUDIES

Case 1

A mathematics instructor with a history of CHF is admitted with a complaint of pain on inspiration. Her respirations are rapid and shallow, and her heart rate is 104 beats/min. The pulse oximeter shows a saturation of 93% on room air. Breath sounds are very decreased on the right side, with crackles in the left base. Chest wall movement is markedly less on the right. The chest radiograph shows opacification of the right lung, with shift of mediastinal structures to the left. Diagnostic percussion reveals a dull note on the right side.

41. What do you think is wrong with this patient's right lung? Support your conclusion with at least five pieces of information from the case.

A. I think the patient has a _____ because

1. _____

2. _____

3. _____

4. _____

5. _____

42. What would you recommend as the first respiratory intervention?

_____

43. How could this disorder be resolved?

A tall, thin, young male respiratory care instructor is admitted with a complaint of pain on inspiration. His respirations are rapid and shallow, and his heart rate is 104 beats/min. The pulse oximeter shows a saturation of 93% on room air. Breath sounds are very decreased on the right side, and clear in the left base. Chest wall movement is markedly less on the right. The chest radiograph shows a dark area without lung markings on the right side, with a shift of mediastinal structures to the left. Diagnostic percussion reveals increased resonance on the right side.

44. What do you think is wrong with this patient's right lung? Support your conclusion with at least five pieces of information from the case.

  A. I think this patient has a _____ because

    1. _____

    2. _____

    3. _____

    4. _____

    5. _____

45. What would you recommend as the first respiratory intervention?

46. How could this disorder be resolved?

WHAT DOES THE NBRC SAY?

Because pneumothorax can be caused iatrogenically and may be life threatening in mechanically ventilated patients, you will be expected to know how to recognize and treat this problem. Although there is no special category called "pneumothorax," you can expect at least three questions related to this topic. You could almost say the NBRC is obsessed with tension pneumothorax.

In addition, you are expected to understand the causes of pleural effusion and how effusions are diagnosed and treated. Questions on assisting the physician in performing thoracentesis and equipment such as chest tubes and drainage systems are all on the boards because they are all connected to effusions and pneumothorax.

Circle the best answer.

47. Immediately after insertion of a central line via the subclavian vein, an intubated patient becomes dyspneic. The respiratory therapist should recommend which of the following diagnostic tests?
    A. 12-lead ECG
    B. chest radiograph
    C. ABG
    D. bedside spirometry

48. The middle bottle of a three-bottle chest drainage system is used as a _____.
    A. water seal
    B. fluid collection
    C. means of applying vacuum to the chest
    D. measurement of improvement of the pneumothorax

49. A chest tube is placed anteriorly between the second and third ribs. The tube is probably intended to treat a
    A. chylothorax
    B. hemothorax
    C. transudative pleural effusion
    D. pneumothorax

50. A patient is suspected of having a pleural effusion. Which x-ray position is most appropriate to confirm this diagnosis?
    A. AP chest film
    B. lateral decubitus chest film
    C. apical lordotic chest film
    D. PA chest film

51. Thoracentesis is performed and 1500 ml of fluid is removed from the right chest. Which of the following is likely to occur as a result?
    A. pulmonary edema in the right lung
    B. stridor and respiratory distress
    C. pneumothorax in the right lung
    D. atelectasis in the right lung

52. All of the following would be useful in differentiating right mainstem intubation from left-sided pneumothorax *except*
    A. chest radiograph
    B. diagnostic percussion
    C. auscultation
    D. lung compliance measurement

53. Following an IPPB treatment, a COPD patient complains of sudden severe chest pain. What is the respiratory therapist's first priority in this situation?
    A. Notify the physician of the problem.
    B. Initiate oxygen therapy.
    C. Recommend a chest radiograph.
    D. Perform an arterial blood gas.

54. A patient develops subcutaneous emphysema following a motor vehicle accident involving multiple rib fractures. What action should the respiratory therapist take in this situation?
    A. Perform bedside spirometry.
    B. Initiate oxygen therapy.
    C. Recommend a chest radiograph.
    D. Perform an arterial blood gas.

There are *endless* variations on these themes. The subject material in Chapter 25 is limited and probably seems pretty straightforward. Be prepared to encounter this topic many times in both the clinical and board examination settings.

FOOD FOR THOUGHT

55. What is meant by the term "ascites"? Besides causing effusions, how could this affect respiratory function?

56. How is thoracentesis modified to prevent reexpansion pulmonary edema?

57. What is subcutaneous emphysema and what relationship does it have to pneumothorax?

26 Pulmonary Vascular Disease

The person who moves a mountain begins by carrying away small stones.

Chinese Proverb

The invisible miles of delicate vessels in the lung remain hidden and ignored as they play their vital role in gas exchange and pressure regulation. Then a clot breaks loose and lodges in the pulmonary vascular highway, an accident that frequently has fatal consequences. Though rarely recognized, pulmonary embolism results in thousands of deaths each year in the United States. Chapter 26 reviews the incidence, pathophysiology, and treatment of pulmonary embolus and pulmonary hypertension, two conditions the respiratory therapist will encounter many times in the hospital setting.

WORD WIZARD

Complete the following paragraph by writing in the correct term(s) in the blank(s) provided.

When the pressure inside the lung vessels is elevated, a condition called pulmonary _____

exists. Prolonged bed rest could result in formation of a venous _____. Most clots form in the

_____ veins of the lower legs. The blood clot could travel to the lung where it is called a pul-

monary _____, or PE. If this process results in death of the lung tissue, it is called pulmonary

_____. Small particles of fat or air could also form an embolus. Chronic elevation of pulmonary

blood pressure will eventually cause a form of right heart failure known as cor _____.

MEET THE OBJECTIVES

1. How many people develop thromboembolic disease each year in the United States? _____

2. Is a PE likely to be fatal? _____

3. How often is the diagnosis missed? _____

4. How do these clots form? Where are they most likely to form first?

5. What patients or situations have the most risk for this sort of pathology to get started?

6. Explain how pulmonary embolism (PE) affects the heart and lungs as they try to function together. Just give the basic idea.

7. What is the primary hemodynamic consequence of PE?

8. State the two most common symptoms of PE.

   A. _____

   B. _____

9. What are the three most frequent physical findings associated with PE?

   A. _____

   B. _____

   C. _____

10. What is the incidence of hemoptysis associated with PE? _____

11. What percentage of patients with PE has an abnormal ECG? _____

12. Name the two most common ECG abnormalities associated with PE.

   A. _____

   B. _____

13. How is the chest radiograph helpful in diagnosing pulmonary embolism?

14. How helpful are arterial blood gases (ABGs) in ruling out PE? What benefit does an ABG provide in these cases?

15. One rapid blood test has been developed to help rule out embolism. Why isn't D-dimer as good for some inpatients?

16. Which test is considered the "gold standard" for the diagnosis of DVT?

_____

17. What tests might be useful in diagnosis of symptomatic proximal DVT?

Now you've got the basic idea. PE is pretty serious stuff! We'll hit the rest of the objectives as we go on. The shocking thing is that we are still pretty bad at recognizing that a patient has a clot in his or her lungs. You have to suspect and then you have to get the tests to confirm. So, whereas pneumonia is often picked up by good clinical observation, PE is not.

18. Because of the high mortality rate, it is important to make a definitive diagnosis of pulmonary embolus. What two tests are reasonably sensitive and reliable in confirming this diagnosis?

   A. _____

   B. _____

19. What is the relationship of the ventilation ($\dot{V}$) and perfusion ($\dot{Q}$) portions of scans in making a high-probability diagnosis of PE?

20. Discuss advantages and disadvantages of helical CT scans for PE.

   A. Advantages:

   B. Disadvantages:

ASSESS AND TEST

21. Prophylaxis for DVT is either pharmacologic or mechanical. Give three examples of each.

   A. Pharmacologic prophylaxis

      1. _____

      2. _____

      3. _____

B. Mechanical prophylaxis

   1. _____

   2. _____

   3. _____

22. What is the standard pharmacologic therapy for existing DVT or PE? What is the mechanism of action? What are the risks?

   A. Drug:

   _____

   B. Action:

   _____

   C. Risks:

   _____

23. How are thrombolytics different from anticoagulants? Can they be given together?

24. Give three examples of thrombolytic drugs.

   A. _____

   B. _____

   C. _____

25. List the mechanical options available for treatment of massive PE.

26. When are vena cava filters indicated?

27. Define pulmonary hypertension.

28. Describe the epidemiology of IPH in terms of age, gender, symptoms, mortality, and genetic factors.

A.   Age: _____

B.   Gender: _____

C.   Genetics: _____

D.   Symptoms: _____

E.   Mortality: _____

29. How is IPH diagnosed?

30. Why is it so important to provide oxygen as needed to keep up the sats in this condition?

31. Which drug treatment is given via inhalation? _____

32. Pulmonary hypertension is a frequent complication of COPD. What percentage of elderly patients with COPD will

develop significant pulmonary hypertension? _____

33. Explain the role of alveolar hypoxia in the development of pulmonary hypertension.

34. What other factors seen in COPD contribute to this condition?

35. What is the only treatment that improves survival in patients with COPD and pulmonary hypertension? What

treatments might help? _____

SUMMARY CHECKLIST

Identify the key points from Chapter 26. Complete the following questions by writing the correct term(s) in the blank(s) provided.

36. Venous _____ is an important cause of morbidity and _____ in hospitalized patients.

37. One third of all deaths caused by pulmonary _____ occur within _____ hour(s) of the symptoms.

38. The point of origin of pulmonary embolism is a deep venous thrombosis of the _____

    extremities or _____ in _____% of the cases.

39. Early recognition of PE and DVT is _____-_____.

40. _____ therapy reduces the risk of venous thromboembolism.

41. Treatment of venous thromboembolism includes anticoagulants such as _____ or

    _____.

42. Idiopathic pulmonary artery hypertension is a rare disease that affects _____ adult patients.

43. Drug treatment of IPAH includes _____ and vasodilators, but lung_____ is an option.

A 60-year-old man underwent total knee replacement. Two days after surgery, he complains of dyspnea and anxiety. Physical examination reveals a heart rate of 110, respiratory rate of 28, blood pressure of 115/80 mm Hg, and SpO_2 of 93% on room air. Breath sounds are clear except for faint inpiratory crackles in both bases.

44. Why is this patient at risk for PE?

45. What additional diagnostic tests would be helpful in ruling out other potential pulmonary problems?

_____

46. What treatment would you provide as a respiratory therapist?

_____

47. What medical treatment should be initiated if a diagnosis of PE is confirmed?

_____

WHAT DOES THE NBRC SAY?

Pulmonary embolism is so nonspecific in its clinical presentation that it does not have any separate category in the registry examination matrices. On the other hand, dead space–to–tidal volume ratios (D_{VD}/T_V) are definitely included. Evaluation of dyspnea, pulmonary hypertension, hypoxemia, and ventilation/perfusion scans are all mentioned. Cur pulmonale associated with COPD is a possible inclusion on the exam as well. Recommending anticoagulants is included in the pharmacology section.

You are expected to be able to make a differential diagnosis between heart attack, pneumothorax, and PE when a patient complains of sudden chest pain.

Circle the best answer.

48. A patient who is being mechanically ventilated shows an increased V_D/V_T ratio. Which of the following disorders could be responsible?
    A. atelectasis
    B. pneumonia
    C. pulmonary embolism
    D. pleural effusion

49. Which of the following is the most appropriate test to confirm the presence of a suspected PE?
    A. chest radiograph
    B. pulmonary angiography
    C. bronchogram
    D. arterial blood gas

50. A ventilation/perfusion scan reveals a defect in perfusion in the right lower lobe without a corresponding decrease in ventilation. Which of the following is the most probable diagnosis?
   A. right lower lobe atelectasis
   B. acute pulmonary embolus
   C. pneumothorax
   D. pneumonia

51. A patient presents in the ED with severe dyspnea and complains of chest pain. His respiratory rate is 24 and his minute volume is 14 L. ABG results show pH 7.44, $PaCO_2$ 37, and PaO_2 100. What is the most likely cause of a normal CO_2 when a patient has a large increase in minute ventilation?
   A. acute myocardial infarction
   B. spontaneous pneumothorax
   C. pulmonary embolus
   D. pneumonia

This topic will be covered more when we discuss hemodynamic monitoring!

FOOD FOR THOUGHT

52. What is the most common cause of pulmonary hypertension worldwide?

_____

53. Discuss the pros and cons of moving a critically ill ventilator patient to imaging for a $\dot{V}/\dot{Q}$ scan to confirm a suspected diagnosis of PE.

Chapter **26** Pulmonary Vascular Disease

27 Acute Lung Injury, Pulmonary Edema, and Multiple System Organ Failure

To be good is noble, but to teach others to be good is nobler—and less trouble.

Mark Twain

Pulmonary edema is one mean clinical problem you will encounter frequently in the emergency department and intensive care units. While the symptoms and initial goals may be similar, cardiogenic (hydrostatic) and noncardiogenic (nonhydrostatic) pulmonary edema have very different etiologies and treatments. These are complex syndromes that will challenge you to use every skill and apply all you've learned. Despite all we have learned over the years, a fairly high mortality rate still exists, especially for acute respiratory distress syndrome (ARDS).

WORD WIZARD

A helpful acronym is "SNAFU": Situation Normal, All Fouled Up. Unfortunately, most medical acronyms aren't all that much fun, but you still need to learn them. Write out the definitions of Chapter 27's alphabet soup.

1. ALI: _____

2. APRV: _____

3. ARDS: _____

4. CHF: _____

5. ECMO: _____

6. $ECCO_2R$: _____

7. GI tract: _____

8. HFV: _____

9. MODS: _____

10. PMNs: _____

11. PEEP: _____

You may hear people ask you to pass the AMBU (now a brand name) bag: the original AMBU meant Air Mask Bag Unit.

MEET THE OBJECTIVES

General Considerations

Let's talk about how to tell the various edemas apart. After all, the mortality from ARDS is 40%, so you really should try to figure this out! Start with a review of the normal physiology. When you're done, turn to Box 27-3 in your text.

12. Name two common conditions leading to hydrostatic pulmonary edema for each of the following general categories:

	CATEGORY	CONDITIONS
A.	Cardiac 1. 2.	
B.	Vascular 1. 2.	
C.	Volume overload 1. 2.	

Now let's go back to the beginning to look at the causes of ARDS or noncardiogenic edema. Check out Box 27-1 in *Egan's*.

13. List four primary and four secondary risk factors for ALI/ARDS.

A. Primary

1. _____

2. _____

3. _____

4. _____

B. Secondary

1. _____

2. _____

3. _____

4. _____

The key thing in the ICU is to take this a step further and be able to compare. This is so important; the NBRC expects you to recognize the differences between these two wet, crackly, hypoxic lungs. Refer to Box 27-2 in your text for a synopsis.

14. Compare CHF and ARDS in terms of the following criteria for diagnosis.

		CHF	ARDS
A.	Chest radiograph 1. Heart 2. Effusions 3. Infiltrates		
B.	Pulmonary capillary wedge pressure (PCWP)		
C.	Bronchoalveolar lavage fluid (BALF)		
D.	Four symptoms in common 1. 2. 3. 4.		

15. Briefly describe the pathophysiology of hydrostatic pulmonary edema.

16. Briefly describe the pathophysiology of nonhydrostatic pulmonary edema.

17. What five areas must be addressed to avoid secondary (iatrogenic) lung injury in ARDS?

A. _____

B. _____

C. _____

D. _____

E. _____

18. What two general approaches are used to maintain adequate tissue oxygen delivery (Do_2) in ARDS?

    A. _____

    B. _____

Ventilator Strategies

Most patients with ARDS will require artificial ventilatory support. Basically we're trying to avoid barotrauma, oxygen toxicity, volutrauma, sheering forces, etc. Good news for you—there are some fairly well-accepted criteria for tidal volume, PEEP, F_IO_2, and rate selection in ARDS. The following questions address the currently accepted methods for providing mechanical ventilation.

19. How does optimal PEEP differ from PEEP that delivers the best PaO_2? (The NBRC loves this one!)

20. In general, what level of PEEP is considered optimal?

    _____

21. We can avoid barotrauma by maintaining mean airway pressures at what value?

    _____

22. PEEP should be adjusted to maintain what F_IO_2 and PaO_2?

    _____

23. Compare tidal volumes delivered in conventional mechanical ventilation versus volumes delivered to ARDS patients.

    A. Conventional volume range: _____

    B. ARDS volume range: _____

24. What is meant by "permissive hypercapnia"? What is the goal of this ventilator strategy?

25. In what two conditions is permissive hypercapnia contraindicated? Why?

    A. _____

    B. _____

Innovative Strategies

When the techniques previously described are not successful, we will have to try something different. Each of these methods has had some limited success. None is foolproof for every patient. In general, innovative strategies protect patients from developing lung injury and are especially useful for patients who need high levels of support like $F_IO_2 > 60$.

26. The ARDS Net study showed that mortality is reduced when volumes are reduced to what levels? (Don't forget, it is ideal body weight, not actual body weight.)

27. One more time. A man is 6 feet tall. He has ARDS. What is the formula? The IBW? The right volume?

    A. Formula
    B. Calculate the IBW
    C. What range of tidal volume do you have to work with according to ARDSNet?

28. How does IRV differ from conventional ventilator modes?

29. What is the effect of IRV on survival of ARDS patients?

30. Pressure control ventilation (PCV) has a lot of potential since you can limit pressure trauma to the airway. Patients like the way it delivers lots of flow when they want it. What does the therapist need to monitor in PCV? What else changes when the compliance or resistance changes?

31. Now that the new ventilator valves have solved the technical problems of airway pressure release ventilation (APRV) (and bilevel, as it may be called), why do you think this is a promising mode for ARDS?

32. How does APRV compare to IRV in terms of the patient?

33. How can patient positioning be radically altered to improve gas exchange?

34. Both ECMO and $ECCO_2R$ facilitate gas exchange via what type of device?

_____

35. What is the recommendation regarding ECMO and $ECCO_2R$ in routine management of ARDS?

_____

36. Exogenous surfactant is helpful in treating infant respiratory distress syndrome and when surfactant is washed out of the adult lung. What's the story on using this with ARDS in adults?

37. Explain the role of HFOV in treating ARDS.

38. What is the last resort for viral-induced ARDS?

Pharmacologic Treatments

A variety of drugs have been used to try to turn the tide in ARDS. A few have had some limited success.

39. Surfactant is not currently recommended for ARDS. What patient group does respond to surfactant administration?

_____

40. What was the potential role of nitric oxide (NO) in treating ARDS?

41. What type of abnormal hemoglobinemia is associated with the administration of NO?

_____

42. What is the consequence of sudden discontinuation of inhaled NO?

_____

43. Like surfactant, NO didn't work out for ARDS. What group of patients does receive NO?

_____

44. What specific advice is given in regard to steroids and ARDS?

_____

SUMMARY CHECKLIST

Complete the following sentences by filling in the correct term(s) in the blank(s) provided.

45. CHF and ARDS are common causes of acute _____ failure that have similar initial

    _____ presentations.

46. CHF-associated pulmonary edema is due to elevated _____ pressures in the pulmonary

    _____.

47. ARDS-associated pulmonary edema results from _____ injury to the lungs.

48. It may be necessary to perform _____ or _____ in order to distinguish
    CHF from ARDS.

49. Recommendations regarding the treatment of ARDS have focused on supporting _____

    _____ and systemic _____ function until the patient recovers from the
    underlying illness.

Chapter **27** **Injury, Edema, and Organ Failure**

50. Ventilator strategies for patients with ARDS are designed to minimize ventilator _____ lung

_____ by using _____, low _____ volumes,

reduced airway _____, and nontoxic levels of inspired _____.

Case 1

A 5 foot 6 inch, 143-lb (65-kg) teenager did not listen (oh those teenagers . . .) when his mom told him not to pop his pimples. Now he is in the ICU with a temperature of 103° F, blood pressure of 80/50 mm Hg, heart rate of 120, and an SpO_2 of 88% on 100% oxygen. His pulmonary capillary wedge pressure is 14 mm Hg, and cardiac output is 8 L/min. Breath sounds reveal coarse crackles throughout the lungs. The patient is intubated and currently is being ventilated with a tidal volume of 800 ml, rate of 14, and PEEP of 0.

51. What is the most likely diagnosis? Why?

_____

52. With regard to the oxygenation status, what changes would you recommend?

_____

53. With regard to the volume, what changes would you recommend?

_____

54. What is the maximum recommended mean airway pressure that should be delivered to this patient to prevent alveolar damage?

_____

Case 2

A 65-year-old, 143-lb (65-kg) woman was intubated after presenting in the emergency department with pulmonary edema and severe respiratory distress. Now she is in the ICU with a temperature of 97° F, blood pressure of 80/50 mm Hg, heart rate of 120, and an SpO_2 of 90% on 60% oxygen. Her pulmonary capillary wedge pressure is 24 mm Hg and cardiac output is 3 L/min. Breath sounds reveal coarse crackles throughout the lungs. The patient is intubated and currently being ventilated with a tidal volume of 700 ml, rate of 14, and PEEP of 10.

55. What is the most likely diagnosis? What's the underlying cause?

_____

56. With regard to the oxygenation status, what changes would you recommend?

Just like it says in Chapter 27, you need to be able to differentiate CHF and ARDS based on clinical presentation and diagnostic information. You should be able to maintain oxygenation and determine optimal PEEP. Management of these patients on the ventilator is a key part of ALL THREE EXAMINATIONS! Try the following questions.

Circle the best answer.

57. Which of the following would be useful in treating an elevated shunt in a patient with ARDS who is being mechanically ventilated?

A. initiating SIMV mode

B. initiating PEEP

C. increasing the F_IO_2

D. adding expiratory retard

58. Which of the following indicates the optimal PEEP setting?

	PEEP	**PaO$_2$**	**Cardiac Output**
A.	5 cm H$_2$O	53 mm Hg	4.5 L/min
B.	10 cm H$_2$O	60 mm Hg	4.3 L/min
C.	15 cm H$_2$O	74 mm Hg	3.8 L/min
D.	20 cm H$_2$O	88 mm Hg	3.4 L/min

59. A patient is admitted to the ICU with a diagnosis of pulmonary edema. Which of the following breath sounds is consistent with this diagnosis?

A. inspiratory stridor

B. inspiratory crackles

C. expiratory rhonchi

D. pleural friction rub

60. A patient with ARDS is being ventilated with the following settings:

Mode	Assist Control
F_IO_2	0.80
Rate	10
PEEP	5 cm H$_2$O
V$_T$	600 ml
SpO$_2$	82%

Which of the following would you recommend as possible ways to improve oxygenation?

A. Increase the tidal volume.

B. Increase the PEEP.

C. Increase the F_IO_2.

D. Increase the rate.

61. Which of the following would provide necessary information regarding fluid management in a critically ill patient with cardiogenic pulmonary edema?

A. bedside pulmonary function testing

B. intake and output measurements

C. daily weights

D. pulmonary artery catheter

62. Chest radiograph changes associated with noncardiogenic pulmonary edema include _____.
    1. pleural effusion
    2. bilateral infiltrates
    3. enlarged left ventricle
       A. 1 and 2 only
       B. 2 only
       C. 2 and 3 only
       D. 1 and 3 only

63. Which of the following ventilator techniques have been suggested as useful in treating ARDS that does *not* respond to conventional therapy?
    1. high-frequency ventilation
    2. airway pressure release ventilation
    3. supine positioning
    4. pressure support ventilation
       A. 1 and 2 only
       B. 2 and 3 only
       C. 3 and 4 only
       D. 1 and 4 only
We'll come back to this subject again when we get to the chapter on hemodynamic monitoring!

FOOD FOR THOUGHT

Shock lung, Da Nang lung, adult respiratory distress syndrome, wet lung, liver lung, and *noncardiogenic pulmonary edema* are all names for ARDS. This syndrome has been recognized ever since we began to save trauma victims during modern warfare.

64. Is ARDS a homogeneous or heterogeneous lung condition? Explain.

_____

65. Lower inflection point (LIP or P_{flex}) is useful in setting appropriate PEEP and tidal volume levels. What is meant by the term LIP? How is it determined?

_____

28 Lung Cancer

I kissed my first woman and smoked my first cigarette on the same day. I have never had time for tobacco since.

Arturo Toscanini

Respiratory cancer is a popular disease of the rich and famous—John Wayne, Humphrey Bogart, Sigmund Freud, Peter Jennings, Dana Reeves; the list goes on and on. Yet there is hardly a more dreaded word in our society than *cancer*. Lung cancer is the most frequently diagnosed cancer in the world and the most difficult to treat. There is no evidence that this cancer epidemic is slowing down.

WORD WIZARD

Most people only learn the terminology of cancer when something catastrophic has happened to a loved one. You will want to be able to understand the often sad words of cancer so you can better help your patients.

Diagnosis of cancer is often made through imaging tests like _____ tomography, _____

resonance _____, and positron emission _____. Invasive tests like the transbronchial

_____ aspiration and _____ needle biopsy are used to obtain specimens. Respiratory

therapists assist the physician in performing flexible _____ to get samples directly from a

tumor or the airway. Once the tests are done the cancer is staged using the _____ _____

_____ system.

Treatment of cancer usually involves surgical _____ or _____ therapy.

MEET THE OBJECTIVES

1. How many cases of bronchogenic carcinoma were newly diagnosed in the United States in 2010? How many cases does the WHO estimate worldwide each year?

   A. _____

   B. _____

2. What percentage of cancer deaths are caused by smoking tobacco?

   _____

3. Compare lung cancer deaths of men and women in the United States.

4. What percentage of the total population in the United States smokes? Which group of smokers is the largest? (Which group are you in?)

   A. Percent of population: Men _____ Women _____

B. Most smokers: _____

C. Are we winning the war against tobacco?

5. What is another name for passive exposure to smoke? _____

6. Describe the health risks of passive exposure to smoke.

7. Besides smoking, name four other major influences linked to an increase in lung cancer.

A. _____

B. _____

C. _____

D. _____

8. What is meant by the term *apoptosis?*

_____

9. List the four major histopathologic types of lung cancer along with the epidemiology they represent and a brief description of the cells. Try Table 28-1 for help.

TYPE OF CANCER	EPIDEMIOLOGY	DESCRIPTION
A.		
B.		
C.		
D.		

CLINICAL FEATURES

10. What are the four common sites of metastasis of cancer originating in the lungs?

A. _____

B. _____

C. _____

D. _____

11. What percentage of patients with lung cancer is asymptomatic at time of presentation?

_____

12. Local tumor growth in the central airways may cause many symptoms. Name four that a respiratory therapist could easily recognize.

    A. _____

    B. _____

    C. _____

    D. _____

13. Patients with pleural or chest wall involvement will typically have what two symptoms?

    A. _____

    B. _____

14. Explain what is meant by the term "paraneoplastic syndrome."

15. Give three examples of paraneoplastic syndromes commonly associated with lung cancers. Describe briefly, please.

    A.

    B.

    C.

16. How do these imaging techniques fit into the diagnostic picture?

    A. CT:

    B. CXR:

    C. PET:

17. Two methods are used to obtain tissue for confirmation. Please describe both of the following.

    A. Flexible bronchosocopy (FB):

    B. Transthoracic needle biopsy (TNB):

18. Why is tumor staging so important?

19. Explain the meaning of the TNM staging system. Look at Figure 28-5 for this complex system.

    A. T = _____

       1 = _____

       2 = _____

       3 = _____

       4 = _____

B. N = _____

    O = _____

    1 = _____

    2 = _____

    3 = _____

C. M = _____

20. How is small cell cancer staged?

21. What's the consensus on mass screenings for people at high risk for lung cancer?

TREATMENT

22. Why is surgical resection the treatment of choice for all non–small cell lung cancers?

_____

23. What patients are *not* candidates for surgery in terms of staging?

_____

24. How are respiratory therapists involved in determining candidates for surgery?

_____

25. What test values for FEV_1 and D_{LCO} suggest a patient may (or may not!) safely undergo lobectomy or pneumonectomy?

26. Name the two nonsurgical therapy modalities.

    A. _____

    B. _____

27. What is the choice of therapy for small cell cancers?

_____

28. What is meant by *palliative* therapy? Give examples.

   A. Medications:

   B. Radiotherapy:

   C. Bronchoscopy:

ROLE OF THE RESPIRATORY THERAPIST

Respiratory therapists don't perform surgery or administer chemotherapy or radiation to patients. Still, lots of these people have preexisting lung disease or have airway problems.

29. Describe the role RTs play in

   A. Nicotine intervention:

   B. Diagnosis:

   C. Support:

Complete the following sentences by writing the correct term(s) into the blank(s) provided.

30. _____ carcinoma is the leading cause of cancer deaths in the United States.

31. Approximately _____% of all lung cancers are linked to smoking.

32. _____ represents 40% of all lung cancers and currently is the most common type.

33. The _____ classification groups patients in stages or categories that correlate with

_____.

34. Patients with _____ cancer are classified in two stages: limited or extensive.

35. The most commonly used modalities of treatment for patients with non–small cell lung cancer are surgical resection,

_____, and _____.

36. The most effective way to prevent lung cancer is to prevent _____.

CASE STUDIES

Chapter 28 has five excellent case studies in the form of Mini-Clinis. Four of these cases are particularly useful to the respiratory therapist.

Pancoast's Tumor 28-1

37. Will you be caring for patients with weakness and drooping eyelids? How is this different?

Paraneoplastic Syndrome 28-3

38. Confusion and generalized weakness are signs of what type of serious neurologic vascular accident?

Evaluating Surgical Risk 28-5

39. What therapy modalities might improve lung function prior to surgery for lung resection?

40. What methods of diagnosis might be useful for the patient with copious amounts of clear, frothy sputum?

WHAT DOES THE NBRC SAY?

For once, the NBRC is relatively silent. Obviously you need to recognize that hemoptysis is an important sign of dysfunction that may relate to cancer or tuberculosis, among other diseases. You should be familiar with the imaging techniques (see Chapter 20 for more) and of course pulmonary function tests.

FOOD FOR THOUGHT

41. Besides lung cancer, what are the other significant health risks of smoking?

42. With the high incidence and known risk factors for lung cancer, you would expect to see screening techniques. Discuss this issue.

43. What is brachytherapy? _____

44. What is the *duty* of every respiratory therapist in regard to their patients who continue to smoke?

29 Neuromuscular and Other Diseases of the Chest Wall

Expert: Someone who brings confusion to simplicity.
Gregory Nunn

Even if your lungs are normal, diseases that affect the brain, nerves, muscles, or bony thorax can lead to respiratory failure or hypoxemia. There are so many unusual conditions that produce muscular weakness that it can be difficult to keep them all straight. You will do fine if you focus on the general principles that apply to assessment and maintenance of the airway in these complex and often sad cases.

WORD WIZARD

Try matching these diseases to their definitions.

Diseases	Definitions
_____ 1. ankylosing spondylitis	A. neuromuscular conduction disorder that particularly affects the face, throat, and respiratory muscles
_____ 2. amyotrophic lateral sclerosis	B. chronic inflammatory disease that fuses the spine and affected joints
_____ 3. flail chest	C. muscle wasting disease characterized by delayed relaxation of contracted groups
_____ 4. Guillain-Barre syndrome	D. degenerative disease of motor neurons characterized by progressive atrophy
_____ 5. Lambert-Eaton syndrome	E. inflammation of muscles caused by a rheumatologic disorder
_____ 6. myasthenia gravis	F. unstable chest due to rib fractures exhibiting paradoxical movement on inspiration
_____ 7. myotonic dystrophy	G. idiopathic polyneuritis characterized by ascending weakness
_____ 8. polymyositis	H. abnormal curvature of the spine that may compromise ventilation
_____ 9. kyphoscoliosis	I. neuromuscular conduction disorder associated with underlying malignancy

MEET THE OBJECTIVES

General Principles

10. Neuromuscular abnormalities affect four major groups of muscles that may result in respiratory problems. Name these four groups.

A. _____

B. _____

C. _____

D. _____

11. The three best recognized pulmonary dysfunctions of respiratory muscle weakness are:

A. _____

B. _____

C. _____

12. What are the three common complaints of patients with respiratory muscle weakness due to neuromuscular disease?

A. _____

B. _____

C. _____

13. Give two representative diseases that affect each of the following locations in the respiratory system. Hint: check out Table 29-1.

	Location	Diseases
A.	Cortex, upper motor	_____
B.	Spinal cord	_____
C.	Lower motor neurons	_____
D.	Peripheral nerves	_____
E.	Neuromuscular junction	_____
F.	Muscle tissue	_____
G.	Interstitial lung tissue	_____

14. Pulmonary function testing of patients with neuromuscular disease and otherwise normal lung tissue will demonstrate what type of ventilatory defect?

_____

15. What three specific tests are most useful in monitoring ventilatory function in patients with neuromuscular weakness?

A. Assess volumes with _____

B. Assess muscle strength via _____

C. Assess hypoxemia and hypercapnia with _____

16. How well does pulmonary function testing assess ability to protect the airway?

_____

17. What signs and symptoms suggest performing nocturnal oximetry or formal sleep testing?

_____

18. What is the primary treatment for severe respiratory muscle weakness? What is diaphragmatic pacing?

   A. Primary treatment: _____

   B. Diaphragmatic pacing: _____

19. What problem that may require respiratory therapy is often overlooked?

_____

Specific Neuromuscular Diseases

20. What is myopathic disease? Give two examples of common myopathies.

   A. What is it? _____

   B. Example 1 _____

   C. Example 2 _____

21. Discuss the role of nocturnal ventilation in patients with myopathic diseases.

22. Most cases of myasthenia gravis arise from what abnormality at the cellular level?

_____

23. What general category of drugs is used to treat myasthenia gravis?

_____

24. What surgical treatment may be effective in some cases of myasthenia gravis?

_____

25. List four predisposing factors to Guillain-Barré syndrome (GBS).

   A. _____

   B. _____

   C. _____

   D. _____

Chapter **29** **Neuromuscular and Other Diseases of the Chest Wall**

26. What percentage of patients with GBS will have respiratory muscle compromise?

_____

27. Bilateral interruption of the phrenic nerves that results in diaphragmatic paralysis is seen in what type of injury?

_____

28. Reversible unilateral diaphragmatic paralysis occurs frequently following what commonly performed surgery?

_____

29. Describe the chest radiographic presentation of unilateral diaphragmatic paralysis.

30. How is the paralyzed diaphragm visualized during fluoroscopy?

31. What is the percentage of new spinal cord injuries in the United States each year, and what percentage of these cases results in quadriplegia?

A. _____

B. _____

32. Define the high and middle/low classification of cervical cord lesions.

A. High:

_____

B. Middle/low:

_____

33. Describe the muscle groups affected by each of the following spine injuries. See the Mini-Clini on page 653.

	Level	Muscle Groups
A.	C1-2	_____
B.	C3-5	_____
C.	C4-8	_____
D.	T1-12	_____
E.	T7-L1	_____

34. What type of breathing is the hallmark sign of significant diaphragmatic weakness?

_____

35. What percentage of patients with C3-5 injury will ultimately become liberated from mechanical ventilation?

_____

36. Both stroke and traumatic brain injuries lead to disordered breathing. What is a stroke?

_____

37. What are the two basic types of strokes?

A. _____

B. _____

38. Give examples of the effect on the respiratory system of strokes in the following locations in the brain. P.S. Breathing patterns are big on the boards. Table 29-6 is a good tool for you.

Location   **Effect on Respiration**

A. Cerebral cortex   _____

B. Bilateral hemispheric infarct   _____

C. Lateral medulla   _____

D. Mid pons   _____

39. Aside from problems similar to stroke, brain trauma can cause what respiratory "fluid" problems?

A. _____

B. _____

Disorders of the Thoracic Cage

40. Describe these two chest wall deformations that often occur together.
    A. Kyphosis:

    B. Scoliosis:

41. Describe the ventilatory defects and pulmonary function changes associated with severe kyphoscoliosis.
    A. Ventilation:

    B. Pulmonary function:

42. How is kyphoscoliosis treated in younger patients?

_____

43. Describe the role of nocturnal ventilation in treating patients with kyphoscoliosis.

44. Describe the paradoxical chest motion that is the hallmark of flail chest.

45. Name three other pulmonary injuries frequently associated with flail chest.

A. _____

B. _____

C. _____

46. Regardless of the physiologic mechanisms behind respiratory dysfunction, what are the mainstays of treatment for flail chest?

A. _____

B. _____

C. _____

SUMMARY CHECKLIST

Complete the following sentences by writing in the correct term(s) in the blank(s) provided.

47. The key components of the respiratory neuromuscular system are the _____, the nerves,

the _____ junction, and the _____ of inspiration.

48. Weakness and _____ failure are the most important respiratory dysfunctions in many neuromuscular diseases.

49. Neuromuscular diseases can also cause _____ or hypoventilation, sleep

_____ aspiration, _____, and pulmonary hypertension.

50. Signs and symptoms of muscle weakness include exertional _____, orthopnea, soft

vocalizations, and a weak _____.

51. PFTs typically show a decreased _____ lung capacity, decreased _____ capacity, and decreased _____ inspiratory pressures.

Case 1

A 27-year-old woman was admitted from her physician's office following complaints of fatigue. Upon interview, the patient reports that she becomes weak after any exertion, especially in her arms. She also complains of difficulty swallowing. She denies any recent illness. Vital signs show a normal temperature and slightly increased heart rate and respiration. Inspection reveals that she has drooping eyelids and appears to have little tone in her facial muscles.

52. Based on this information, what is the most likely diagnosis?

_____

_____

53. What drug therapy might help to confirm this diagnosis?

_____

_____

54. Why is measurement of inspiratory and expiratory pressures a more sensitive test of muscle function than measurement of vital capacity?

Case 2

A 52-year-old man was admitted from his physician's office following complaints of fatigue. Upon interview, he reports that his feet felt numb yesterday and that his legs were weak when he got up this morning. He went to the physician because he thought he might be having a stroke. He states that he had the flu about 2 weeks earlier. Vital signs show a normal temperature and slightly increased heart rate and respiration.

55. Based on this information, what neuromuscular condition is likely?

_____

_____

56. How would analysis of CSF be useful in making a diagnosis?

Chapter **29** **Neuromuscular and Other Diseases of the Chest Wall**

57. What two treatment strategies have improved outcome in this syndrome?

A. _____

B. _____

_____

WHAT DOES THE NBRC SAY?

One or two cases on the Clinical Simulation Examination will be devoted to adult patients with neuromuscular or neurologic conditions. Myasthenia gravis, Guillain-Barré, tetanus, muscular dystrophy, and drug overdose are listed as examples in the matrix. You should be able to recommend or interpret the results of bedside tests such as vital capacity and maximum inspiratory pressure. So while there won't be too many multiple-choice questions on neuromuscular pathophysiology, this is an important part of the testing process. Questions on the chest and spinal trauma are also included on your boards. In particular, you should pay attention to the subject of flail chest. Here are a few questions for practice.

Circle the best answer.

58. A 23-year-old patient with flail chest is transferred to the ICU for observation following a motor vehicle accident. After 2 hours, the patient complains of increasing dyspnea and arterial blood gas analysis is performed.

pH	7.27
$PaCO_2$	55 mm Hg
PaO_2	61 mm Hg

What action should the respiratory therapist recommend at this time?
A. Place the patient on oxygen therapy.
B. Initiate mask CPAP.
C. Administer a bronchodilator drug.
D. Initiate mechanical ventilation.

59. A patient with Guillain-Barré syndrome has had serial vital capacity measurements.

0900	3.1 L
1100	2.6 L
1300	2.1 L
1500	1.6 L

In regard to these data, what should the respiratory therapist recommend?
A. Increase the monitoring to every hour.
B. Administer Tensilon.
C. Provide intubation and mechanical ventilation.
D. Continue to monitor the patient every 2 hours.

60. A vital capacity below what value indicates the need for intubation and ventilation in a patient with acute neuromuscular disease?
A. 30 ml/kg
B. 20 ml/kg
C. 15 ml/kg
D. 10 ml/kg

61. A patient with myasthenia gravis presents in the emergency department with profound muscle weakness. Administration of which of the following will improve ventilation?
    A. pancuronium
    B. neostigmine
    C. epinephrine
    D. atropine

62. The presence of paradoxical chest motion on inspiration following a motor vehicle accident most likely indicates
    _____.
    A. flail chest
    B. pulmonary contusion
    C. pneumothorax
    D. hypoxemia

FOOD FOR THOUGHT

63. ALS is the disease that strikes down heroes in the prime of life. Prognosis is poor. Two new ideas for ALS include riluzole and NSIF. Please discuss.
    A. Riluzole:

    B. NSIF:

30 Disorders of Sleep

Most people spend their lives going to bed when they're not sleepy and getting up when they are.
Cindy Adams

Does someone you know snore excessively? Does that mean the snorer has sleep apnea? Have you ever wondered just exactly what you do while you're sleeping? The polysomnography lab is just the place to find out. Many respiratory therapists (RTs) have found rewarding careers in the sleep or neurodiagnostic lab setting.

Another reason RTs are interested in disorders of sleep is the cardiopulmonary consequences of sleep apnea. Finally, even in the acute care setting, you will be called on to deal with patients who utilize CPAP or bilevel airway pressure devices to control their apnea. Once again, you will find yourself in the position of being the expert on the assessment and equipment involved in treating this not-so-unusual condition.

WORD WIZARD

Acronyms can be fun if they sound cool, like SCUBA (Self-Contained Underwater Breathing Apparatus). Too bad most of the medical acronyms are dull. Give the full name of the following acronyms from Chapter 30. (You're probably already familiar with some of these by now.)

1. BiPAP: _____

2. CSA: _____

3. CPAP: _____

4. RDI: _____

5. EEG: _____

6. EPAP: _____

7. IPAP: _____

8. OSA: _____

9. PSG: _____

10. UPPP: _____

11. AHI: _____

MEET THE OBJECTIVES

12. What is the definition of sleep apnea? What about hypopnea?

13. How does OSA differ from CSA?

14. What is the estimated incidence of OSA in the adult population?

_____

15. Why does airway closure occur during sleep?

16. Name five adverse cardiopulmonary consequences of untreated OSA.

A. _____

B. _____

C. _____

D. _____

E. _____

17. Name two neurobehavioral and two metabolic consequences of untreated OSA.

Neurobehavioral

A. _____

B. _____

Metabolic

C. _____

D. _____

18. List three factors that predispose a patient to OSA.

A. _____

B. _____

C. _____

19. Describe the six common clinical features seen in many cases of OSA.

A. _____

B. _____

C. _____

D. _____

E. _____

F. _____

20. What is the current gold standard for making a diagnosis of OSA?

_____

21. An apnea-hypopnea index of what value is consistent with moderate to severe sleep apnea? What is considered

normal? _____

22. What are the three goals of treatment for OSA?

A. _____

B. _____

C. _____

23. Discuss the behavioral options that should be pursued in all patients with sleep-disordered breathing.

24. Why do you think nocturnal CPAP has become the first-line medical therapy for OSA?

25. How does CPAP work to relieve OSA?

26. What is auto-titrating CPAP?

27. Identify the indications and explain how the titration of bilevel positive airway pressure therapy differs from that of CPAP.

28. Describe five of the common minor side effects of positive-pressure therapy. Identify what you can do to help the patient solve these annoying problems.

A. _____

B. _____

C. _____

D. _____

E. _____

29. What is the role of tracheostomy in treating sleep apnea?

30. What is the success rate of UPPP, and what is the current recommendation regarding this procedure as a treatment for OSA?

Identify the key points from Chapter 30. Complete the following questions by writing the correct term(s) in the blank(s) provided.

31. The three types of sleep apnea are obstructive, _____, and _____.

32. The predominant risk factor for airway narrowing or closure during sleep is a _____ or _____ upper airway.

33. The long-term adverse consequences of OSA include poor _____ functioning as well as increased risk of _____ morbidity and mortality.

34. Risk factors for OSA include _____ gender, age greater than _____ years, upper body _____, and habitual _____.

35. The first-line medical therapy for OSA is _____.

36. _____ positive airway pressure therapy may be useful in salvaging patients who have difficulty complying with CPAP.

37. _____ therapy may be an option for a select group of patients who have undergone extensive upper airway analysis and do comply with medical therapy.

38. In mild to moderate OSA, _____ _____ can be an effective alternative therapy.

WHAT DOES THE NBRC SAY?

The NBRC usually considers CPAP to be a ventilator mode or freestanding strategy to improve oxygenation, but that is changing. Nasal CPAP (and BiPAP, which by the way, is a trademark of a particular company, not a generic term) is included. To be specific, CPAP devices (mask, nasal, or bilevel) are mentioned, and you need to know about the equipment and the therapy. You may even see a simple tracing like you see on Figure 30-1, A of your text.

Circle the best answer.

39. An RT notes in the medical record that a patient is receiving BiPAP therapy with a machine he brought from home. Which of the following is the most likely diagnosis for the patient?
    A. pulmonary emphysema
    B. congestive heart failure
    C. obstructive sleep apnea
    D. atrial fibrillation

40. A sleep study shows simultaneous cessation of airflow and respiratory muscle effort. These findings are consistent with _____.
    A. pulmonary hypertension
    B. obstructive sleep apnea
    C. congestive heart failure
    D. central sleep apnea

271

41. Which of the following is *true* regarding BiPAP therapy?
    1. Expiratory pressure is always set above inspiratory pressure.
    2. BiPAP units are pneumatically powered.
    3. IPAP should be increased until snoring ceases.
        A. 1 and 3
        B. 2 only
        C. 2 and 3
        D. 3 only

FOOD FOR THOUGHT

If you want to gain more professional expertise on this subject, look no further than the journal *Respiratory Care*, which has editions devoted only to sleep-disordered breathing!

31 Neonatal and Pediatric Respiratory Disorders

Any man who hates dogs and babies can't be all bad.
Leo Rosten

There's hardly a more joyous event than bringing new life into the world—unless you look at it from the perspective of the respiratory therapist. We don't see the healthy babies, just the sick ones!

WORD WIZARD

Try this matching exercise to test your ability to understand the new terms and acronyms found in Chapter 31.

Terms	Definitions
_____ 1. RDS	A. poor clearance of lung fluids (type II RDS)
	B. aspiration of fetal feces
_____ 2. croup	C. chronic problem from alveolar trauma and oxygen toxicity
_____ 3. GERD	D. life-threatening upper airway infection
_____ 4. PPHN	E. virus-induced subglottic swelling
	F. acute infection of the lower airways
_____ 5. MAS	G. leading cause of death in infants <1 year old
_____ 6. TTN	H. complex syndrome of newborn hypertension
_____ 7. SIDS	I. stomach problem associated with asthma
	J. surfactant deficiency in preemies
_____ 8. epiglottitis	
_____ 9. BPD	
_____ 10. bronchiolitis	

BABY BLUES

11. How many babies in the United States have RDS?

_____

12. What is the primary pathophysiology in infants with RDS?

_____

_____

13. Describe the four clinical signs of RDS that are listed below.

A. Respiratory rate: _____

B. Breathing pattern: _____

C. Auscultation: _____

D. Audible sounds: _____

14. How is the definitive diagnosis usually made?

15. Discuss the four main therapies for treating RDS.
    A. CPAP: starting values? Device?

    B. Ventilator: when do you start? What is the goal of PEEP for this baby?

    C. Surfactant: when to give? Positioning?

    D. HFV: what does this acronym mean?

16. How does the chest radiograph of a baby with transient tachypnea of the newborn (TTN) (type II RDS) differ from that of primary RDS?

17. List two typical respiratory treatments for TTN.

A. _____

B. _____

18. Meconium aspiration is usually associated with what fetal event?

_____

19. What age baby usually has MAS?

_____

20. Name the three primary problems in MAS.

A. _____

B. _____

C. _____

21. Immediate treatment of the MAS baby is vital! What should you do?

A. Upon delivery: _____

B. Repeat until: _____

C. If the condition worsens: _____

D. What case of meconium aspiration does not require suctioning with immediate intubation?

_____

22. In some ways, bronchopulmonary dysplasia is a result of our efforts to save preterm infants. What are the five events implicated in causing BPD?

A. _____

B. _____

C. _____

D. _____

E. _____

23. What is the "best management" of BPD, and how and where does this begin?

A. Best: _____

B. How: _____

C. Where: _____

24. Please define "periodic breathing," and compare that to "abnormal apneic spells."
   A. Periodic breathing:

   B. Abnormal apneic spells:

25. Describe how the following strategies work to alleviate infant apneic events. (Check Table 31-3 if you get lost!)
   A. Tactile stimulation:

   B. CPAP:

   C. Caffeine (xanthines):

   D. Doxapram (Dopram):

   E. Transfusion:

26. Persistent fetal circulation may result in hypertension in the newborn. Name the three types of PPHN and at least one factor that might have caused the problem.

	TYPES	FACTORS
A.		
B.		
C.		

27. What's the basic idea behind each of these treatments for PPHN?
A. Oxygen

B. Glucose

C. Inotropes

D. Sedation

E. HFV

F. Inhaled NO

G. ECMO

28. An infant with profound cyanosis at birth most likely has one of two conditions. Name them.

A. _____

B. _____

29. What are the four defects seen in tetralogy of Fallot?

A. _____

B. _____

C. _____

D. _____

30. Acyanotic heart diseases are also seen in newborns. PDA is of special interest to RTs. Describe PDA. Name two treatments.

   A. Description:

   B. Treatments:

   C. Explain the use of two pulse oximeters in this situation. You'll need to look back at PPHN to find the answer.

NEONATAL RESUSCITATION

There is nothing more exciting than neonatal resuscitation; except flying in the back of a small plane and doing neonatal resuscitation. RTs are always key members of the transport team. Refer to the American Academy of Pediatrics Neonatal Resuscitation Protocol and you'll find out the scoop.

PEDIATRIC PROBLEMS

Kids get sick a lot and they have little airways. The combination of infection and airway problems like reactive airways and cystic fibrosis makes for a lot of visits to the emergency department (ED).

Sudden infant death syndrome (SIDS) is the leading cause of death in infants less than 1 year of age in the United States, with about 7000 deaths each year! Diagnosis isn't made until a previously healthy baby dies unexpectedly. That's pretty sad, don't you think?

31. What is the cause of SIDS? _____

_____

32. Describe the typical profile of a baby who dies of SIDS.

_____

_____

33. What sleeping position is strongly linked with SIDS?

_____

34. Identify the six infant characteristics often seen near the time of death.

   A. _____

   B. _____

   C. _____

D. _____

E. _____

F. _____

35. Once an at-risk infant is identified, what can be done to try to prevent a SIDS death?

36. What is gastroesophageal reflux disease (GERD)? Name a few of the many respiratory problems this condition can trigger.

37. What group of kids usually gets bronchiolitis?

_____

38. RSV is one particularly nasty virus that's the culprit in many cases of bronchiolitis. Discuss:

A. Immunization. Who gets it?

_____

B. What does RSV stand for?

_____

C. How is the diagnosis made?

_____

39. Dyspnea, tachypnea, wheezing, and cough are common in these kids. If they have to be hospitalized, what respiratory treatments are indicated?

A. Bronchodilators, what's the controversy? _____

B. Why give antibiotics for a virus? _____

C. Hygiene? _____

D. What's ribavirin? _____

Bronchiolitis, croup, epiglottitis, and cystic fibrosis are all serious and relatively common pediatric respiratory disorders that you should be able to recognize and differentiate from each other. So is asthma, but we covered most of that in Chapter 23.

Case 1

A mother brings her previously healthy 1-year-old to the ED. She states that her baby had a cold 2 days ago, but he still has a slight fever and has been coughing. Mom became concerned when she heard audible wheezing. A treatment with albuterol in the ED has had no effect. Vital signs are essentially normal, except for a slight elevation in respiratory rate. The chest radiograph shows mild hyperinflation with no signs of consolidation. Pulse oximetry shows a saturation of 94%.

40. What diagnosis is most likely?

_____

41. How can a diagnosis of RSV be ruled out?

_____

42. The physician decides to send mom and baby home. What treatment would you recommend?

Case 2

A 3-year-old is brought to the ED with respiratory distress and a barking cough (like a seal!). The child has been sick for several days with a low-grade fever and stuffy nose. Examination reveals moderate inspiratory stridor and retractions. The pulse oximeter shows a saturation of 88% on room air. A lateral neck film identifies subglottic narrowing with a "steeple sign."

43. What is the most likely diagnosis?

_____

44. What aerosolized medication is traditionally delivered?

45. When should you add nebulized budesonide?

280

46. How would you deliver oxygen to this child?

_____

Case 3

A 5-year-old is brought to the Emergency Department with labored breathing and a high fever. Examination reveals marked inspiratory stridor. The child is listless, and dad says he has had a sore throat. When you talk to the boy, he responds very quietly with short answers. A lateral neck radiograph identifies a "thumb sign."

47. What is the most likely diagnosis?

_____

48. What organism is usually responsible for this condition? How could you confirm?

_____

49. What is the immediate treatment for this condition? Who should perform the intervention and where?

_____

50. What should not be done? _____

Case 4

A grandmother brings her son's 2-year-old in to the clinic because "his breathing just isn't right." She states, "This boy is coughing all the time. Besides, he isn't growing very well, and when I kiss him his skin tastes salty!"

51. How would your diagnosis be confirmed? What values indicate CF (this is NBRC stuff!)?

_____

Mayo Clinic has a good Web site for CF. They state that diagnosis begins with blood screening in most states for all newborns. The traditional test is used to confirm. If it is still not clear, genetic testing is performed.
If genetic testing is the best method, why do you think we don't do this first?

52. What dietary modifications are needed in cystic fibrosis?

_____

53. Name four respiratory treatments aimed at decreasing airway obstruction.

A. _____

B. _____

281

C. _____

D. _____

54. Nebulizing drugs here is one of the key treatments. Tell me more about:
   A. Mucolytic drugs:

   B. 7% solution:

   C. Who's this Tobi?

If you want to get serious about this disease, look up the Cystic Fibrosis Foundation.

WHAT DOES THE NBRC SAY?

The Entry-Level Examination may ask you a couple of questions related to pediatrics, usually recall questions, but this is not the primary proving ground for this area of knowledge. The Registry tests make detailed references to the material in Chapter 31. Neonates are on the Registry tests. The Examination Matrices (all of them!) contain these items (just a partial list!):

Perinatal data
- Maternal history
- Perinatal history
- Apgar scores
- Gestational age
- L/S ratio
- Preductal and postductal studies

Recommend procedures
- Umbilical line
- Transcutaneous monitoring

Inspect the patient
- Apgar score
- Gestational age
- Retractions
- Transillumination of the chest

Inspect lateral neck and chest radiographs

Equipment
- Oxygen hoods and tents
- Specialized ventilators-oscillators, high frequency

The Clinical Simulation Examination Matrix makes it clear that you will have one pediatric and one neonatal problem. Basically, you can't be an RT without specialized, in-depth neonatal and pediatric knowledge. That's why most schools have a separate course and text for this topic. BUT *Egan's* contains much of the information you need to pass your boards. These cases are typical examples from the clinical simulations:
- Neonatal

Delivery room management, resuscitation, infant apnea, meconium aspiration, respiratory distress syndrome, congenital heart defect

■ Pediatric

Epiglottitis, croup, bronchiolitis, asthma, cystic fibrosis, foreign body aspiration, toxic substance ingestion, bronchopulmonary dysplasia

Try these multiple-choice questions. Circle the best answer.

55. A premature infant is experiencing episodes of apnea and cyanosis. The respiratory therapist should recommend which of the following?
    A. albuterol
    B. Narcan
    C. Exosurf
    D. theophylline

56. A 5-year-old child presents in the ED with complaints of a severe sore throat. The child has inspiratory stridor and muffled phonation. He has a fever of 40° C. His mother states he will not drink anything, so she brought him in. The most likely diagnosis is _____.
    A. croup
    B. bronchiolitis
    C. foreign body aspiration
    D. epiglottitis

57. Which of the following tests is helpful in establishing a diagnosis of cystic fibrosis?
    A. sweat chloride
    B. L/S ratio
    C. Apgar score
    D. pneumogram

58. Which of the following is the most appropriate imaging technique to help confirm a diagnosis of croup?
    A. computed tomogram
    B. PA chest film
    C. lateral neck film
    D. bronchogram

59. A 4-year-old child with LTB presents in the ED with moderate stridor and harsh breath sounds. The RT should recommend which of the following?
    A. albuterol
    B. racemic epinephrine
    C. immediate intubation
    D. aminophylline

FOOD FOR THOUGHT

Many students ask, "What's the difference between an infant, baby, child...?" Here are some definitions for you that are not in *Egan's:*

■ **Fetus:** The unborn offspring from the end of the eighth week after conception (when the major structures have formed) until birth. Up until the eighth week, the developing offspring is called an embryo.

■ **Premature baby:** A baby born before 37 weeks of gestation have passed. Historically, the definition of prematurity was 2500 grams (about $5^1/_2$ pounds) or less at birth. The current World Health Organization definition of prematurity is a baby born before 37 weeks of gestation.

■ **Neonate:** This is a newborn baby. If the baby leaves the newborn nursery, goes home, and comes back to the hospital, he or she may be put into the pediatric unit.

■ **Post-term baby:** A post-term baby is born 2 weeks (14 days) or more after the usual 9 months (280 days) of gestation.

■ **Child:** This is a person 6 to 12 years of age. An individual 2 to 5 years old is a preschool-aged child. Sometimes we use the following criteria: Ages 1 to 8 for a child. Obviously size is important when you're talking about ET tubes and drug dosages, because some children are quite large. When a child is the physical size of an adult, you would use adult dosages.

32 Airway Pharmacology

All things are poison and poison is in all things. Whether it is a medication or a poison…depends on the dose.

Paracelsus

When the first edition of *Egan's* came out in 1969, only a limited number of drugs were available by inhalation. Most of those medications are no longer used, due to the advent of newer, more specific agents with longer action and fewer side effects. New categories of inhaled medicines require the respiratory therapist (RT) to have a strong grasp of pharmacologic principles and the specific indications and actions for these newer tools for managing the airway. You'll need to stay on top of things; for example, a new dry powder drug, Arcapta (indacaterol), has been approved by the FDA for COPD and Cayston (aztreonam), an inhalation solution, was recently approved for cystic fibrosis. You will be the one who can advise physicians, nurses, and patients on methods and options for producing bronchodilation, reducing the inflammatory response, clearing secretions, and treating infection.

This chapter is long and can be difficult. However, delivering medications can occupy as much as 30-50% of our time on a daily basis in some hospital settings! Your hard work will pay off with an excellent grasp of the meds you give to your patients.

WORD WIZARD

Try this matching exercise to test your ability to understand the new terms found in Chapter 32. (You may have to really dig for some of these—use the chapter, the glossary, and a medical dictionary if necessary!)

Terms	Definitions
1. _____ indication	A. time it takes to metabolize 1/2 drug dosage
2. _____ tolerance	B. drug may not be given for any reason
3. _____ adrenergic	C. effect of acetylcholine on smooth muscle
4. _____ vasopressor	D. reason for giving a drug to a patient
5. _____ prodrug	E. undesired effect of a drug
6. _____ muscarinic	F. drugs that mimic the effect of epinephrine
7. _____ pharmacodynamic	G. has receptor affinity and exerts an effect
8. _____ side effect	H. mimics the effect of acetylcholine
9. _____ absolute contraindication	I. drug that exerts a constricting effect on blood vessels
10. _____ leukotriene	J. given in an inactive form that converts to active in the body
11. _____ mydriasis	K. dilation of the pupil of the eye
12. _____ agonist	L. phase related to mechanism of action
13. _____ pharmacokinetic	M. maximum effect from a drug dosage
14. _____ cholinergic	N. time it takes a drug to start working
15. _____ antagonist	O. how long the drug's effect lasts
16. _____ tachyphylaxis	P. increasing dose needed for effect
	Q. has receptor affinity but produces no effect
	R. rapidly developing tolerance
	S. compounds that produce allergic or inflammatory responses
	T. phase related to metabolism of a drug

17. _____ onset

18. _____ peak effect

19. _____ duration

20. _____ half-life

MEET THE OBJECTIVES

Chapter 32 has six broad objectives that cover more than 20 medications. You will need to focus on the five main classes of drugs used for management of respiratory disease. Respiratory therapists both administer and recommend these medications. Bronchodilators, mucolytics, and glucocorticoids are all commonly administered by RTs. We'll cover the objectives by classes in this chapter following the text.

JUST SAY YES

21. What is the most common route of administration that is used by RTs?

_____

22. Name four advantages of this route.

A. _____

B. _____

C. _____

D. _____

23. Name two disadvantages of this route.

A. _____

B. _____

24. How do medications delivered by this route usually end up in the systemic circulation?

_____

25. Describe the two primary divisions of the autonomic nervous system in terms of name, main neurotransmitter, and effect on bronchial smooth muscle.

	DIVISION	OTHER NAME	NEUROTRANSMITTER	AIRWAY MUSCLE EFFECT
A.	Sympathetic			
B.	Parasympathetic			

ADRENERGIC BRONCHODILATORS

Adrenergic bronchodilators come in two basic types: short and long acting. LABAs, or long-acting beta agonists are used to control asthma and COPD. Special warnings exist for the use of these drugs.

26. State the three receptors of the sympathetic nervous system and their basic effects.

	RECEPTOR	PRIMARY EFFECT
A.		
B.		
C.		

27. Give the generic name, brand name, strength, and dose for the following commonly used beta-adrenergic bronchodilators.

	GENERIC NAME	BRAND NAME	STRENGTH	DOSE
A.	Racemic epinephrine SVN			
B.	Epinephrine SVN			
	Epinephrine MDI			
C.	Albuterol SVN			
	Albuterol MDI			
D.	Levalbuterol SVN			
	Levalbuterol MDI			
E.	Pirbuterol MDI			
F.	Salmeterol DPI			
G.	Formoterol DPI			
H.	Arformoterol SVN			

28. Epinephrine and racemic epinephrine are bronchodilators, but these drugs are usually administered to:

A. Stimulate what receptor? _____

B. Produce what effect? _____

C. Accomplish what clinical goals? _____

29. What would you recommend if a patient experienced bronchospasm from a CFC inhaler?

_____

30. It is especially important that you know how long it takes for a drug to start working and reach its maximum effect and how long the drug will last. Fill in the information for the drugs listed below.

	DRUG	ONSET	PEAK EFFECT	DURATION
A.	Xopenex			
B.	Micronefrin			
C.	Proventil			
D.	Serevent			
E.	Formoterol			
F.	Arformoterol			

31. List the most common side effects of bronchodilator drugs. Which one is number 1?

A. _____

B. _____

C. _____

D. _____

32. Adverse reactions are more serious, but less frequently seen. List six potential adverse effects you must watch for in patients receiving adrenergic bronchodilators.

A. _____

B. _____

C. _____

D. _____

E. _____

F. _____

33. What should you monitor when administering any drugs via the aerosol route?

A. _____

B. _____

C. _____

D. _____

And the fifth vital sign?

E. _____

34. What specific tests or data can be obtained to monitor the effects of bronchodilator therapy?

A. _____

B. _____

C. _____

D. _____

35. How would you assess long-term bronchodilator use?

A. _____

B. _____

C. _____

D. _____

E. _____

36. Long-acting beta agonists have some risks that can be addressed by new FDA regs. List three of these safety precautions.

A. _____

B. _____

C. _____

ANTICHOLINERGIC BRONCHODILATORS

37. Generally, ipratropium is indicated for use in what types of patients?

_____

38. Fill in the blanks to complete your knowledge of ipratropium.

NAME	BRAND NAME	STRENGTH	DOSE
Ipratropium bromide			
MDI (HFA)			
SVN			
Nasal			
Tiotropium			

39. Now try this one.

DRUG	ONSET	PEAK EFFECT	DURATION
Ipratropium			
Tiotropium			

40. What medication is available by MDI or SVN with both ipratropium and albuterol? What are the possible advantages and disadvantages of this medication?

41. Describe the side effects to watch for when administering this class of drugs.

Common side effects

A. _____

B. _____

MDI occasional side effects

A. _____

B. _____

SVN occasional side effects

A. _____

B. _____

42. Why does *Egan's* talk about the eyes of patients who get treatments? How do we protect them (and yourself!)?

MUCUS CONTROLLING AGENTS

43. Describe the mucoactive agents available for nebulization.

	AGENT	BRAND NAME	DOSE	INDICATION
A.				
B.				
C.				
D.				

44. Bronchospasm is a common side effect of the administration of mucolytic agents. How would you recommend modifying the therapy to prevent or treat this problem?

45. What types of short- and long-term assessments should you make to monitor the effectiveness of these drugs?

46. When is mucoactive therapy a potential danger to a patient? Your book discusses three potential scenarios where you could make things worse.

INHALED GLUCOCORTICOIDS

Like bronchodilators, there are a lot of inhaled steroids out on the market. You can expect many of your patients to be receiving these medications. Physicians, patients, and family members have many misconceptions about steroids, including "steroid phobia." Again, it's up to you to be the expert and to be able to clearly explain the use of these very important tools in the fight against asthma.

47. How long will it take for inhaled steroids to have a noticeable effect on the symptoms of asthma?

48. What significance does this have in terms of patient education?

49. The most common side effects of inhaled steroids are local ones (as opposed to systemic). Name the four most common problems.

A. _____

B. _____

C. _____

D. _____

50. Besides a reservoir device, what two additional recommendations are made by GOLD and NAEPP in regard to corticosteroid inhalers?

51. What would you assess to determine if the steroids were working in the long run?

The National Institutes of Health Asthma Education and Prevention Program guidelines were first issued in 1997 and contain definitive information on the use of drug therapy for the treatment of asthma. You can get a copy of these guidelines from the American Lung Association or your instructors or you can download the information from the NIH Web site.

NONSTEROIDAL ANTIASTHMA DRUGS

Drugs that prevent the release of histamine or block the release or effects of other mediators of inflammation are hot items right now. These drugs, whether oral, inhaled, or injected, hold tremendous promise for treating asthma and preventing the long-term pulmonary consequences of this increasingly serious condition. They fall into the category of "controllers" rather than "rescue" drugs like albuterol.

52. What is believed to be the mode of action of cromolyn sodium?

_____

53. Which two mediator antagonists are recommended for use in young children? Hint: Look at Table 32-6.

_____

54. Which of these mediator antagonists is available by inhalation?

_____

55. List the number one side effect for each of the following:

   A. Cromolyn sodium (Intal): _____

   B. Nedocromil (Tilade): _____

   C. Zafirlukast (Accolate): _____

   D. Zileuton (Zyflo): _____

   E. Montelukast (Singulair): _____

56. No one can pronounce it, but omalizumab, or Xolair (easier, "zo-lair"), can make a dramatic difference for severe asthma that is caused by what type of response? Based on the time between shots, how long do you think this might take to start working? (The answer doesn't have to be exact; just check Table 32-6 and give your best guess.)

TREATING INFECTION BY THE AEROSOL ROUTE

It should make sense to you that lung infections can be treated by aerosolizing medications. This technique for delivery is limited to very specific situations.

57. What agent may be nebulized to treat *P. jiroveci* (formerly called PCP or *Pneumocystis carinii* pneumonia) seen in severely immunocompromised patients?

_____

58. Why isn't the drug used much anymore?

_____

_____

59. What are the common undesired respiratory side effects of administration? What modification of therapy would you recommend if they occur?

60. While *P. jiroveci* (PCP) is not a hazard to healthy people, patients with AIDS often have what other disease that is transmitted via the airborne route?

_____

61. Describe the use of ribavirin in terms of indication, patient population, and special equipment needed for administration.

A. Indication: _____

B. Type of patient: _____

C. Nebulizer: _____

D. Organism: _____

62. What about TOBI?

A. Drug: _____

B. Type of patient: _____

C. Nebulizer: _____

D. Organism: _____

63. Describe the new antimicrobial aztreonam™

A. Drug: _____

B. Type of patient: _____

C. Nebulizer: _____

D. Organism: _____

INFLUENZA

Influenza can be fatal to the elderly and those with heart or lung problems. While vaccination is still the best protection, there is an inhaled drug that shortens the course and alleviates symptoms.

64. What's the drug? What's the problem with giving it to asthma and COPD patients?

A. Drug: _____

B. Problem: _____

C. Delivery system: _____

D. What is the "off-label use?"

A FUNGUS AMONG US

No FDA-approved drugs are available specifically for inhalation right now. Invasive pulmonary fungal infections like aspergillosis love the lungs of the immunocompromised. Intravenous amphotericin B is the drug of choice but does not always penetrate the lung effectively. In the past, RTs nebulized amphotericin B to administer to patients with fungus in their lungs on many occasions. A lot more science has been developed since then and there will soon be a dry powder amphotericin for the treatment of pulmonary aspergillosis.

INHALED VASODILATORS

People have been inhaling vasodilators for recreation for years, and now we have medications like nitric oxide for newborns. Iloprost and treprostenil can be nebulized to administer to adults with pulmonary hypertension.

65. Specifically, when is nitric oxide used for newborns? When is it contraindicated?

66. What is the most common adverse reaction during weaning from nitric oxide? What type of hemoglobin disorder could be monitored?

67. What is the brand name of iloprost? What is the class of drugs? (Be specific.)

    A. _____

    B. _____

68. What nebulizer is used to deliver the drug?

69. Describe trepostinil.

    A. Indications and goal: _____

    B. Delivery system: _____

    C. Mode of action: _____

Case 1

A patient who has asthma is admitted to the hospital for the second time in 2 months. She has not been able to get relief and is using her albuterol inhaler frequently.

70. In addition to inhaled beta agonists, steroids are commonly administered to *reduce* inflammation associated with asthma. Name one inhaled steroid and recommend a dose.

   _____

71. What device is important to use along with MDIs to prevent deposition of these drugs in the mouth?

   _____

72. Why should this patient rinse her mouth after use of her inhaled steroid?

   _____

73. Recommend another drug that can be delivered by MDI as a long-term controller to *prevent release* of inflammatory mediators.

   _____

74. What long-acting bronchodilator may help this patient sleep through the night without being awakened by dyspnea and wheezing?

   _____

Case 2

Cystic fibrosis is diagnosed in a 7-year-old. This patient has extremely thick mucus (like glue!). Auscultation reveals scattered wheezing and rhonchi.

75. What drug would you recommend aerosolizing for treatment of the thick mucus?

   _____

76. What other drug should be given to treat the wheezing?

   _____

77. He has *Pseudomonas* in his sputum. What could you nebulize to treat gram-negative bad boys in CF?

   _____

Case 3

A 67-year-old man with long-standing COPD characterized by chronic bronchitis is coughing up copious amounts of very thick white sputum. He complains that his chest feels tight, and he cannot catch his breath. His albuterol inhaler is not providing relief.

78. What bronchodilator is appropriate to add to the therapeutic regimen?

   _____

79. What alternative delivery methods might be useful?

80. What mucolytic may be considered if other means of sputum clearance are ineffective? Why might this drug be counterproductive?

A respiratory care student is administering a standard dose of albuterol via SVN to a 65-year-old male admitted for pneumonia and COPD. Five minutes into the treatment the patient's heart rate increases from 92 to 156 on the monitor. The instructor walks in at this moment.

81. What action should the student do first? What other actions might be taken right away at the bedside?

82. What diagnostic test should be ordered?

83. What change in medication could provide bronchodilation with fewer side effects?

WHAT DOES THE NBRC SAY?

Sure enough, the NBRC has scattered a number of drug questions strategically throughout the tests. In fact, pharmacology appears in at least six different parts of the matrix. You need to administer aerosol therapy to remove secretions. Administer aerosol, dry powder, and endotracheal meds. The biggest one area is IIIG, "Recommend modifications in the respiratory care plan based on patient response." Section 4 includes: Recommending pharmacologic interventions such as bronchodilators, leukotriene modifiers, corticosteroids, cromolyn, hypertonic saline, acetylcysteine, rHDNAse, antimicrobials, and surfactant. It is pretty specific, so you will know what to study. There is more on the delivery of medications in Chapter 36, so this is just the introduction.

296

84. A patient with *P. jiroveci* pneumonia is unable to tolerate oral antibiotics due to gastrointestinal side effects. Which of the following would you recommend?
    A. aerosolized acetylcysteine (Mucomyst)
    B. aerosolized albuterol (Proventil)
    C. aerosolized dornase alfa (Pulmozyme)
    D. aerosolized pentamidine iethionate (NebuPent)

85. An asthmatic patient presents in the emergency department with dyspnea, hypoxemia, and wheezing. All of the following are appropriate at this time *except* _____.
    A. administration of oxygen
    B. nebulized cromolyn sodium (Intal)
    C. nebulized albuterol (Ventolin)
    D. measurement of peak expiratory flow rates

86. Following extubation, a patient has mild stridor. Which of the following would you recommend at this time?
    A. administration of oxygen
    B. aerosolized albuterol (Proventil)
    C. aerosolized virazole (Ribavirin)
    D. aerosolized racemic epinephrine (Vaponefrin)

87. After administering a corticosteroid via MDI, the RT should ask the patient to perform which of the following actions?
    A. Rinse and gargle with water.
    B. Deep breathe and cough.
    C. Inhale an adrenergic bronchodilator.
    D. Inhale via a spacer device.

88. The heart rate of a patient receiving an adrenergic bronchodilator rises from 80 to 94 per minute during the treatment. Which of the following actions is most appropriate?
    A. The RT should discontinue the therapy.
    B. Let the patient rest for 5 minutes.
    C. Continue the treatment.
    D. Reduce the dosage of the bronchodilator.

89. A physician calls in an order for bronchodilator therapy for a patient with COPD. The order states "0.05 ml of albuterol in 3 ml of normal saline via SVN four times per day." The RT should _____.
    A. deliver the treatment as ordered
    B. recommend substituting Atrovent
    C. carefully monitor heart rate during the treatment
    D. call the physician to verify the order

90. When administering nebulized ipratropium (Atrovent), the respiratory therapist must take care to avoid
    A. contamination of the nebulizer
    B. mixing albuterol with the atrovent in the nebulizer
    C. nebulized solution contact with the eye
    D. nebulized solution contact with oral mucosa

91. Which of the following is the most commonly used rescue medication for acute episodes of bronchospasm?
    A. Albuterol
    B. Atrovent
    C. Advair
    D. Primatene

92. A patient's asthma is poorly controlled with bronchodilators and inhaled steroids. This individual has multiple allergies that trigger her asthma. What additional medication could the respiratory therapist recommend to achieve better control?
   A. Methylxanthines
   B. Leukotriene modifiers
   C. Oral steroids
   D. Nonsteroidal antiinflammatory agents

FOOD FOR THOUGHT

You might be wondering how you can retain all this drug information. It's not easy! Especially when you might not use many of these medications on a regular basis. One suggestion is a time-honored technique: make drug cards. All you need is some 3 × 5 or 4 × 6 index cards. Write out the following on each card:
   • Generic and brand names of the drug
   • Routes (like MDI, oral, SVN)
   • Dose
   • Strength
   • Adverse reactions and side effects
   • Contraindications
   • Patient teaching points
   Another trick is to make a memory matrix. You can use a spreadsheet program to do this or any paper. Make rows down the left with the drug names and columns across the top with headings such as indication, dose, etc. You can put most of this chapter on one page!

93. Besides treatment of excessively thick mucous, what can Mucomyst be used for?

_____

33 Airway Management

When you can't breathe, nothing else matters.
American Lung Association Motto

Airway management is a rewarding subject. It is very satisfying to help patients breathe better in such a dramatic fashion. While there is no substitute for experience, Chapter 33 will help you learn how to use equipment, tubes, and techniques to deal with airway emergencies. You will want to become an expert in every aspect of this subject so that you can become a skilled, knowledgeable provider and a resource for other health care professionals.

MEET THE OBJECTIVES

This chapter has a ton of material but it all falls into three basic areas:
- Airway clearance devices and techniques
- Insertion and maintenance of artificial airways
- Special airway management procedures

There are specific sections on your board examinations for each of these three areas which we will examine at the end of the chapter. The workbook will follow along with the chapter outline in the text and meet the 13 objectives. Let's start with the three important areas under the suctioning procedure.

"THE HALLS ARE ALIVE WITH THE SOUND OF MUCUS..."

Patients who can't clear their own secretions are at risk for all kinds of problems like increased work of breathing, atelectasis, and lung infections. It's your job to get in there and clean out those airways. Respiratory therapists (RTs) suction both the upper and lower airways.

---

10 Commandments for Endotracheal Suctioning

    I. Thou shall assess thy patient.
   II. Thou shall use the correct vacuum setting.
  III. Thou shall use the right catheter size.
  IV. Thou shall preoxygenate and hyperinflate thy patient.
   V. Thou shall suction shallow or withdraw prior to suctioning.
  VI. Thou shall suction on withdrawal only.
 VII. Thou shall limit the duration to 10 to 15 seconds.
VIII. Thou shall reoxygenate and reinflate after each attempt.
  IX. Thou shall only irrigate when indicated.
   X. Thou shall monitor thy patient.

---

1. Oral suctioning alone is usually accomplished with a rigid plastic tube called a tonsil tip. What's the other common name for this device?

_____

2. Why do you need to be careful when you're putting a device in someone's mouth? Hint: Did you ever stick your toothbrush too far into the back of your mouth?

_____

_____

ENDOTRACHEAL SUCTIONING

Endotracheal suctioning is a vital, but potentially risky procedure. Closely following the rules will greatly reduce your chances of causing an adverse reaction. The AARC Clinical Practice Guidelines in your textbook give a good overview of this subject.

3. Describe the cause of and how to prevent each of the following complications.

	COMPLICATION	CAUSE	PREVENTION
A.	Hypoxemia		
B.	Cardiac arrhythmia		
C.	Hypotension		
D.	Atelectasis		
E.	Mucosal trauma		
F.	Increased ICP		

4. Discuss the advantages and disadvantages of closed-system multiuse catheters.
    A. Advantages:

    B. Disadvantages

5. What special catheter is used to facilitate entry into the left mainstem bronchus?

_____

6. How should you position a patient for nasotracheal suctioning?

_____

7. How is the catheter prepared to prevent trauma during this procedure?

_____

8. What specialized airway is used to facilitate repeated nasal suctioning?

_____

9. What device do you need to include when you want to collect a sputum specimen during suctioning?

_____

ESTABLISHING THE ARTIFICIAL AIRWAY

Start off by learning the parts of the two most important artificial airways used to maintain adequate ventilation.

WORD WIZARD

Establishing the Artificial Airway

Complete the following paragraph by writing in the correct term(s) in the blank(s) provided.

_____ tubes are long, semirigid tubes, usually made of _____ chloride or some other type of plastic. A typical ET tube has nine basic parts. The proximal end (sticking out of the mouth) has a standard

_____-mm adapter. The body of the tube has _____ markings in centimeters. The tube ends

in a _____ tip. There is a port, or slot, cut in the side of the tip called a _____ eye. This slot

helps ensure gas flow if the tip is obstructed. Just above the tip, a _____ that can be inflated to seal the

airway to prevent aspiration or provide for _____ pressure ventilation is bonded to the tube. A small filling

tube leads to a _____ balloon. This small balloon has a spring-loaded _____ with a connector

where a syringe can be attached to allow inflation or deflation. A _____ indicator, or line, is embedded in the wall of the tube body to make it easier to see the tube position on a chest x-ray.

   Another commonly used tube, inserted through a surgical opening in the trachea, is called a _____ tube.

These tubes are also made of plastic, or occasionally of metal such as _____. The _____ cannula

forms the primary structural unit of the tube. Like the ET tube, a _____ may be attached near the end to

seal the airway. A _____ is attached to the proximal end to prevent slippage and provides a means to secure

the tube to the neck. Many tubes have a removable _____ cannula with a standard _____-mm

adapter. This cannula can be removed for cleaning. A special device called an _____ has a rounded blunt end and is used to facilitate insertion.

ET TUBES

There are three specialized endotracheal tubes you should know about: double-lumen tubes, jet ventilation tubes, and CASS tubes. Pay attention, this is board material!

10. What type of lung disease requires the use of a double-lumen ET tube?

   _____

   These are also called Carlen's, or endobronchial, tubes. What is the name of the special type of ventilation used

   with this tube? _____

11. High-frequency jet ventilation tubes look like standard tubes with two additional lines. What are they?

   A. _____

   B. _____

12. Continuous aspiration of subglottic secretions is the generic name for the Hi-Lo Evac Tube. What is the reported benefit of the subglottic suction (i.e., CASS or Hi-Lo Evac Tube) tube?

_____

_____

INTUBATION PROCEDURES

13. What is the preferred route for establishing an emergency tracheal airway?

_____

_____

14. Name the four types of practitioners who most commonly perform endotracheal intubation.

A. _____

B. _____

C. _____

D. _____

15. Why is suction equipment needed for intubation?

_____

_____

16. Describe two common troubleshooting procedures used when the laryngoscope does not light up properly.

_____

_____

17. How are tube sizes selected for infants?

_____

_____

18. How are tube sizes selected for adults? How does size differ for men and women? Do you agree with the sizes for men and women in Table 33-2 (if you have clinical experience for comparison, what do you see in your ICU)?

_____

_____

_____

_____

_____

19. Prior to insertion, how should the RT test the tube?

_____

_____

20. How is the head positioned to align the mouth, pharynx, and larynx?

_____

_____

21. What other actions *must be taken* before making any attempt to intubate?

_____

_____

22. How long may you attempt intubation? Why do you think we have a rule like this one?

_____

23. Name at least two anatomic landmarks *besides the glottis* to be visualized prior to intubation.

A. _____

B. _____

24. Compare the use of the Miller and Macintosh laryngoscope blades during the intubation procedure (Figure 33-17!).

25. Your textbook describes nine methods for bedside assessment of correct tube position. While none of these methods absolutely confirms position, they are essential assessments to make right after the tube is placed. Fill in the information from Box 33-4 in your textbook.

A. _____

B. _____

C. _____

D. _____

E. _____

F. _____

G. _____

H. _____

I. _____

26. The hottest thing in intubation right now is the video laryngoscope. When should you use it, and what are some advantages?

27. What is the disadvantage of using capnographic or colorimetric analysis of carbon dioxide to assess intubation in a cardiac arrest victim?

Chapter **33** **Airway Management**

28. What is the final step of confirmation?

    _____

29. Give two examples of clinical situations where nasotracheal intubation might be preferred over oral intubation.

    A. _____

    B. _____

30. Describe the two techniques used for nasal intubation.

    A. _____

    B. _____

31. Let's compare oral and nasal intubation. Each has advantages and disadvantages. Place a letter "O" by items that match oral intubation and a letter "N" by items that go with nasal intubation. Check out Table 33-1 for help.

    A.   avoids epistaxis and sinusitis   _____

    B.   greater comfort for long-term use   _____

    C.   easier to suction   _____

    D.   larger   _____

    E.   greater risk of extubation   _____

    F.   improved oral hygiene   _____

    G.   bronchoscopy more difficult   _____

    H.   increased salivation   _____

    I.   reduced risk of kinking   _____

    J.   decreased laryngeal ulceration   _____

    K.   increased risk of sinusitis   _____

32. Now might be a good time to talk about medications we didn't cover in Chapter 32. You may need to use meds to have a successful intubation, whether it is oral or nasal. What drugs would you use to:
    A. Numb the airway and reflexes

    B. Sedate the patient

C. Vasoconstrict/prevent bleeding

TRACHEOTOMY

33. What is the primary indication for performing a tracheotomy?

_____

34. When is tracheotomy the preferred primary route of airway management?

_____

35. Describe the sequence for removing an ET during the tracheotomy procedure. You might want to remember this procedure!

PERC ME UP!

The percutaneous, or bedside, tracheal tube insertion is the most common method for ICU patients.

36. Compare the location of placement in percutaneous and traditional surgical tracheotomy.

37. Name at least three advantages of the percutaneous technique compared with traditional surgical tracheotomy.

A. _____

B. _____

C. _____

AIRWAY TRAUMA

38. Compare the following laryngeal injuries associated with intubation in terms of symptoms and treatment.

	INJURY	SYMPTOMS	TREATMENT
A.	Glottic edema		
B.	Vocal cord inflammation		
C.	Laryngeal ulceration		
D.	Polyp/granuloma		
E.	Vocal cord paralysis		
F.	Laryngeal stenosis		

305

39. Name the three most common tracheal lesions.

A. _____

B. _____

C. _____

40. Compare tracheal malacia and tracheal stenosis in terms of cause, pathology, and treatment.

	INJURY	CAUSE	PATHOLOGY	TREATMENT
A.	Malacia			
B.	Stenosis			

41. Describe the tracheoesophageal fistula in terms of cause, complications, and treatment.

42. Tracheoinnominate fistula is a rare, but serious, complication. What are the clues, and what are the immediate and corrective actions taken?

What is the survival rate?

CARE OF YOUR NEW ARTIFICIAL AIRWAY

Once placement of an artificial airway is successfully completed, the real fun begins. As an RT, you will be expected to secure the airway, maintain adequate humidification, manage secretions, care for that cuff, and troubleshoot problems that arise—some of which are life threatening.

43. What is the most common material used to secure endotracheal tubes? Tracheostomy tubes?

_____

What's the alternative?

_____

44. How do flexion and extension of the neck affect tube motion? What is the average distance the tube will move (in cm)?

45. People with endotracheal tubes can't talk, and they shouldn't try. What device is used to help with communication?

_____

46. What is a "talking" trach? What are some of the problems with these gadgets?

47. A trach can be temporarily closed with a finger (the patient's finger or yours, with a glove of course!). A more effective solution in the long run is the Passy-Muir Valve. What do you need to do with the cuff? How about the ventilator?

HUMIDIFICATION

48. What is the worst problem that results from inadequate humidification of the artificial airway?

_____

49. What temperature range must be maintained in a heated humidification system to provide adequate inspired moisture?

_____

50. What device can be used as an alternative to heated humidifiers for short-term humidification of the intubated patient?

_____

Look into Chapter 35 for more details on this subject.

51. State at least four reasons why tracheal airways always increase the risk of infection.

A. _____

B. _____

C. _____

D. _____

52. Describe three techniques that can be used to decrease the risk of infection.

A. _____

B. _____

C. _____

53. What is the most common cause of airway obstruction in the critically ill patient?

_____

CUFF CARE

54. Describe the shape of a modern tube cuff.

_____

55. What is the recommended safe cuff pressure? What is the consequence of elevated cuff pressures?

A pressure of 25 cm H$_2$O is considered the top number for the board exams!

56. Why are minimum leak and minimum occluding volume no longer recommended?

The NBRC still includes "cuff volume" in the examination matrices. Cuff volume is the volume of air or water in milliliters that it takes to achieve an adequate seal or pressure on the airway.

57. What happens to cuff pressures when the tube is too small for the patient's trachea?

_____

58. How is food coloring used to test for aspiration?

RTs and nursing personnel may share some of the tracheotomy care duties. These tubes require daily care to keep the wound clean and the tube functioning properly.

Your textbook makes changing a trach tube sound simple, but it can be a harrowing experience. The first change is most often performed by the surgeon. Always have intubation and emergency airway equipment handy. Be especially careful when:

- The neck is thick.
- The site is inflamed or infected.
- The trach is fresh.

59. What protective gear do you need to use when performing trach care?

_____

60. Briefly describe the eight basic steps of tracheotomy care.

A. _____

B. _____

C. _____

D. _____

E. _____

F. _____

G. _____

H. _____

AIRWAY EMERGENCIES

61. State three airway emergencies.

A. _____

B. _____

C. _____

62. Give four reasons why a tube may become obstructed.

A. _____

B. _____

C. _____

D. _____

63. What simple technique is used to assess tube obstructions that are not relieved by repositioning the head or deflating the cuff?

_____

64. If you cannot clear the obstruction, what action should you be prepared to take?

_____

65. What additional troubleshooting step can often be performed on patients with tracheostomies?

_____

66. What effects will occur with a cuff leak when a patient is being mechanically ventilated?

_____

67. What action should you be prepared to take if the cuff is blown?

EXTUBATION AND DECANNULATION

Extubation is a procedure commonly performed by the RT. You will need to be familiar with the indications for extubation and techniques used to minimize risk during this procedure.

68. The decision to remove the airway and to remove the ventilator are NOT THE SAME! What kind of patients might need to remain intubated even after the ventilator is removed?

_____

69. Describe the method for performing a "cuff-leak test."

What does *Egan's* suggest as a good percentage of leak for considering extubation?

70. List five types of equipment you will want to assemble *prior* to extubation.

A. _____

B. _____

C. _____

D. _____

E. _____

71. You will need to suction which two places before extubating? Name them, and describe the correct sequencing for this important step. _____

_____

72. Describe the two different strategies for removing the tube itself.

   A. _____

   B. _____

73. What therapeutic modality is usually applied immediately after extubation?

_____

74. List two or three of the most common problems that occur after extubation.

75. The worst complication of extubation is laryngospasm. What can you do if this persists for longer than a few seconds?

76. A common complication of extubation is glottic edema. How will you recognize *and* treat this problem?

77. Oral feeding should be withheld for how long following extubation? Why?

_____

78. State the three methods for weaning from a tracheostomy tube. Give one advantage and one disadvantage for each technique. This is national exam material.

	TECHNIQUE	ADVANTAGE	DISADVANTAGE
A.			
B.			
C.			

AIRWAY ALTERNATIVES

You might need to have a few more airway tricks up your sleeve. LMAs are increasingly popular devices, especially in the operating room and the EMS settings. Combitubes are also a part of the prehospital setting. Both of these tubes are now a part of Advanced Cardiac Life Support (ACLS) training. Emergency cricothyroidotomy may be needed if the upper airway is obstructed. Paramedics may put in cricothyrotomy tubes but RTs usually do not.

79. Give three advantages of the LMA.

A. _____

B. _____

C. _____

80. Give two disadvantages of the LMA.

A. _____

B. _____

81. Why is the Combitube potentially useful in the field?

_____

_____

BRONCHOSCOPY

While rigid scopes are usually used in the operating room, flexible bronchoscopy is often done at the bedside with the RT playing a key role in patient preparation and monitoring during the procedure.

82. State one advantage and three disadvantages of the metal rigid bronchoscope.

83. Give an example of a specific drug and the general goal for each of the following classes of premedication used in bronchoscopy.

	DRUG CLASS	EXAMPLE	GOAL
A.	Tranquilizer		
B.	Drying agent		
C.	Narcotic-analgesic		
D.	Anesthetic		

84. What drugs would RTs nebulize prior to the procedure on a nonintubated patient? What about after the procedure?

A. Before: _____

B. After: _____

85. What three types of cardiopulmonary monitoring devices are considered essential for this procedure?

A. _____

B. _____

C. _____

86. What are some of the activities we RTs might perform while assisting with the procedure?

A. _____

B. _____

C. _____

CASE STUDIES

Case 1

During your first day of clinical training in the ICU, a patient sustains a cardiac arrest. Your clinical instructor asks you to assist in preparing the equipment needed for endotracheal intubation. The patient is a small 56-year-old female.

87. What size endotracheal tube should you select?

_____

88. How should you test the tube prior to insertion?

_____

89. How will you test the laryngoscope and blade for proper function?

_____

90. Once the tube is inserted, how can you quickly assess placement?

91. A colorimetric CO_2 detector is attached to the ET tube. The end-tidal CO_2 is 2% on exhalation and 0% on inhalation as the chest rises with bagging. What does this suggest regarding the effectiveness of the chest compressions?

_____

Case 2

After your heart-pounding initiation into resuscitation, it is time to check the other ventilator patients in the unit. A 19-year-old woman with a head injury is receiving mechanical ventilation via a cuffed No. 8 tracheostomy tube with an inner cannula. As you enter the room, the high-pressure alarm is sounding.

Chapter **33** **Airway Management**

92. How will you determine the need for suctioning in this situation?

_____

93. What vacuum pressure should be set prior to suctioning?

_____

94. What size suction catheter is suggested using the Rule of Thumb found in *Egan's?*

_____

95. How long, and with what F_IO_2, should you preoxygenate this patient?

_____

96. After suctioning, you will need to check the cuff pressure. What is a safe cuff pressure?

_____

WHAT DOES THE NBRC SAY?

Chapter 33 is the longest one we've had so far! That must mean this is extremely important material. The NBRC agrees! The Examination Matrix says you must perform procedures to achieve maintenance of the airway including artificial airway care, adequate humidification, cuff monitoring, positioning, and removal of secretions. They go on to include modification of the management of artificial airways including changing the type of humidification, inflating or deflating the cuff, and initiating suctioning. You should be able to assemble and check the function of the airways and the intubation equipment. Finally, you need to assist the physician in performing bronchoscopy, tracheostomy, and, of course, intubation. The actual number of airway questions varies from exam to exam, but you should be prepared for at least six to eight questions on any given test.

Circle the best answer.

97. Which of the following will decrease the risk of damage to the trachea from the endotracheal tube cuff?
   1. inflating the cuff with less than 10 ml air
   2. maintaining cuff pressures of 25 cm H_2O
   3. utilizing a high-volume low-pressure cuff
   4. inflating the cuff to 25-35 mm Hg
      A. 1 and 2
      B. 1 and 3
      C. 2 and 3
      D. 3 and 4

98. The diameter of the suction catheter for an adult should be no larger than
   A. one-tenth the inner diameter of the ET tube.
   B. one-third the inner diameter of the ET tube.
   C. one-half the inner diameter of the ET tube.
   D. three-fourths the inner diameter of the ET tube.

99. A patient with a tracheostomy tube no longer requires mechanical ventilation. All of the following would facilitate weaning from the tracheostomy tube *except* a(n) _____.
   A. fenestrated tracheostomy tube
   B. cuffed tracheostomy tube
   C. tracheostomy button
   D. uncuffed tracheostomy tube

100. Extubation is performed on a patient with an endotracheal tube. Presence of which of the following suggests the presence of upper airway edema?
    A. rhonchi
    B. crackles
    C. wheezes
    D. stridor

101. All of the following are useful in nasotracheal intubation *except* a _____.
    A. laryngoscope handle
    B. stylette
    C. Miller blade
    D. Magill forceps

102. While performing endotracheal suctioning, an RT notes that flow-through is minimal and secretion clearance is sluggish. Which of the following are possible causes of this problem?
    1. The vacuum setting is greater than 120 mm Hg.
    2. The suction canister is full of secretions.
    3. There is a leak in the system.
    4. The tube cuff is overinflated.
        A. 1 and 2
        B. 1 and 4
        C. 2 and 3
        D. 3 and 4

103. Rapid, initial determination of endotracheal tube placement can be achieved by _____.
    1. auscultation
    2. arterial blood gas analysis
    3. measurement of end-tidal CO_2
    4. measurement of SpO_2
        A. 1 and 2
        B. 1 and 3
        C. 2 and 4
        D. 3 and 4

104. A patient with a tracheostomy tube shows signs of severe airway obstruction. A suction catheter will only pass a short distance into the tube. The RT should _____.
    A. remove the tracheostomy tube
    B. inflate the cuff of the tube
    C. ventilate the tube with positive pressure
    D. remove the inner cannula

105. Which of the following can be used to assess pulmonary circulation during closed-chest cardiac compressions?
    A. capnometry
    B. arterial blood gas analysis
    C. pulse oximetry
    D. blood pressure monitoring

106. Prior to performing bronchoscopy, an RT is asked to administer a nebulized anesthetic to the patient. What medication is most appropriate to place in the nebulizer?
    A. Versed
    B. atropine
    C. morphine
    D. lidocaine

Here's an idea that could help you learn a topic as huge, complex, and important as this one: digital flashcards. Take photographs of equipment, scan pictures from books, and download from the Internet to create a pile of pictures. Set up a slide show and you've got digital flashcards. Many students find this a fun and effective way to learn, and they help each other out on the project.

107. What is a King™ airway, and why should you be excited about it?

34 Emergency Cardiovascular Life Support

We're in the resuscitation business, not the resurrection business.

Anonymous RT

Nothing is more satisfying than being a part of the team that helps save someone's life! A successful resuscitation is an exciting event that you will remember forever. Of course, a poorly managed effort is completely frustrating, and attempting to save someone who should never have cardiopulmonary resuscitation (CPR) in the first place is about as depressing as it gets. Because respiratory therapists play an integral role in hospital resuscitations, you will want to know both the basic and advanced life support techniques. Chapter 34 summarizes the important concepts of these two activities and provides you with knowledge and skills you will be expected to demonstrate on your boards. **There is no substitute for formal training and certification in basic and advanced life support!**

WORD WIZARD

Acres of Acronyms

You must have noticed by now that medicine loves acronyms. There are 14 in Chapter 34 that will enable you to talk the talk. (Walking the walk is another story altogether!)

Write out the full definition of each acronym below.

1. CABD: _____

2. ACLS: _____

3. AED: _____

4. AHA: _____

5. ARC: _____

6. BLS: _____

7. SCA: _____

8. CDC: _____

9. CNS: _____

10. CPR: _____

11. FBAO: _____

12. EMS: _____

13. NRP: _____

14. PALS: _____

CAUSES AND PREVENTION OF SUDDEN DEATH

15. What is the primary cause of sudden death among adults in the United States?

_____

16. What is the most common rhythm immediately after cardiac arrest? What are the two basic treatments?

A. Rhythm: _____

B. Treatments: _____

_____

BASIC LIFE SUPPORT

17. Compare adult, child, and infant resuscitation for the following categories for two rescuers (see Table 34-1).

	CATEGORY	ADULT	CHILD	INFANT
A.	Compression 1. Hand placement 2. Depth 3. Rate 4. Check pulse			
B.	Obstructed 1. Mild 2. Unresponsive			
C.	Ventilation 1. Rate 2. Ratio			

18. You wouldn't want to do CPR on someone who is just sedated. Once you carefully assess unresponsiveness, you need HELP! What should you do in each of these situations?

A. Collapsed outside hospital:

_____

B. In the hospital:

_____

C. How do you quickly check for "signs of life?"

_____

_____

19. When is the jaw-thrust maneuver indicated?

_____

20. How can you determine if a victim is breathing?

_____

21. Describe the technique for mouth-to-mouth breaths for adults and children. What is the hazard to the *victim* in this procedure?

    A. Adults:
       1. Technique

       2. Hazard or problem

    B. Children:
       1. Technique

       2. Hazard or problem

    C. Infants:
       1. Technique

       2. Hazard or problem

22. When is mouth-to-nose indicated in adults?

_____

23. Mouth-to-tube or stoma? Seriously, folks, you might be able to bring yourself to do this on a loved one, but in the hospital, you will want to modify this technique. What would you do?

_____

24. How is assessment of pulselessness different in adults and infants?

When can you just "go by the monitor" and not assess the patient's pulse?

25. How is hand positioning for chest compression different in adults, children, and infants?

A. Adults:

B. Children:

C. Infants:

26. Describe the modifications to CPR that you need to consider under these special circumstances:

A. Near drowning:

B. Electrocution:

C. Implanted pacemakers, etc.:

27. Once CPR is begun, it is normally only stopped for what three reasons?

    A. _____

    B. _____

    C. _____

28. Health care providers and lay providers might do CPR a little differently. Please explain the differences.

WHO PUT THE "D" IN DEFIBRILLATION?

The American Heart Association (AHA) added defibrillation (D) to the ABCs because it is lifesaving in many cases of sudden cardiac arrest.

29. A person with sudden cardiac arrest is probably in what rhythm? What is the treatment for this rhythm?

    _____

30. Why is early defibrillation so important?

    _____

31. Describe the AED briefly. Is the shock really automatic? After hooking up the electrodes, what else is the operator supposed to do?

YES, BUT IS IT GOOD CPR?

32. How can you easily and quickly determine the effectiveness of ventilations and compressions delivered during CPR?

    A. Ventilation:_____

    B. Compression:_____

33. CPR can have complications. Give a way to avoid these classics.

A. Neck injury: _____

B. Gastric inflation: _____

C. Vomiting: _____

D. Internal trauma (liver laceration): _____

E. FBAO removal: _____

34. CPR is contraindicated under what two circumstances?

A. _____

B. _____

35. What barriers does the CDC suggest to protect us during CPR?

_____

FOREIGN BODIES

36. What is the universal distress signal for foreign body obstruction of the airway?

_____

37. When should back blows be used on an adult victim?

_____

38. Give another name for the abdominal thrust maneuver.

_____

When should you avoid this maneuver in an adult?

_____

What should you do if you cannot or should not perform the abdominal thrust on a choking victim?

39. Describe four ways you can tell that you have effectively removed a foreign body from the airway.

A. _____

B. _____

C. _____

D. _____

RTs are often called on to perform oxygenation, assessment, and airway management techniques during resuscitation. It is recommended that you take the AHA course in ACLS. Besides making you a smarter member of the code team, it will enhance your marketability to employers. Many hospitals now use "precode" medical emergency teams of an RT and RN to get the jump on an impending crisis. You'll need to follow protocols like ACLS to assess and treat.

40. What concentration of oxygen should be administered during a life-threatening emergency?

_____

41. What is the technique to select the best-sized oropharyngeal airway (OPA)?

42. Name and describe the two basic types of oral airways.

A. _____

B. _____

43. What could go wrong if you insert an oral airway in a conscious victim?

_____

44. What airway would you choose for the patient who cannot tolerate an oral airway?

_____

45. Describe two ways to insert an oral airway without pushing the tongue back.

A. _____

B. _____

46. How would you lubricate the following airways prior to insertion?

A. Oral: _____

B. Nasal: _____

47. Why is an endotracheal tube the preferred method for securing the airway during CPR?

48. Describe characteristics of the ideal mask.

49. Describe the proper way to ventilate during resuscitation. Include volumes, rates, ratios—all methods to avoid hyperinflation and other problems. The Mini-Clini on page 803 reviews this material nicely.

50. When should the endotracheal route of drug administration be used? Hint: Check out the Mini-Clini.

51. What is the primary treatment for pulseless ventricular tachycardia and ventricular fibrillation?

_____

52. Give three examples of drugs that can be delivered via the ET route.

A. _____

B. _____

C. _____

D. What is the acronym for these ET drugs? _____

53. What modification to dosage and technique must be made for endotracheal instillation of emergency drugs?

_____

54. What initial energy level is recommended for electrical countershock during ventricular fibrillation using a biphasic defibrillator? What about monophasic? How about any subsequent shocks?

55. Explain the difference between cardioversion and defibrillation.

56. When is electrical pacing indicated?

_____

57. What are the two primary types of pacing mentioned in *Egan's*?

A. _____

B. _____

You can also use the defibrillator to pace via the pads on the chest with many models used in the ED and ICU.

DRUG THERAPY

58. Identify the drug indicated to treat each of the following. (Check out Table 34-2 in your text.)

	EVENT	DRUG THERAPY
A.	Ventricular tachycardia	
B.	Pulseless electrical activity	
C.	Asystole	
D.	Poor cardiac contractility	
E.	Hypotension	
F.	Hypertension	
G.	Ventricular fibrillation	
H.	SVT	
I.	Coronary artery occlusion	
J.	CHF/pulmonary edema (fluid overload)	

CASE STUDIES

Let's review some of the basics via cases.
You enter the local coffeehouse to get some java before facing a tough shift in the ICU. The place is packed. While you wait for your venti mocha cappuccino with an extra shot...

Case 1

A man at the corner table is eating and having coffee. Suddenly he puts his hands to his throat and tries to stand. He is unable to cough or speak.

59. What is your first action?

60. How would you relieve the FBAO?

61. If the victim becomes unconscious, how will you modify your technique?

Case 2

Your coffee is ready, but before you can drink one sweet sip, a red-faced executive-type in a suit collapses to the floor, splashing you with dairy-free latte . . .

62. According to "Basic Life Support" guidelines, you need to perform 6 steps in the right order.

   A. First determine unresponsiveness. What would you check? What would you do?

   B. Step two is check the _____.

   C. Now you need to call for help. Be specific for this setting.

   D. This victim has become unresponsive and basically dead on the spot. What device do you need right now to assess the heart and treat the most likely rhythm for sudden cardiac arrest?

   E. No devices are available. You need to start _____ at a rate of

   _____.

   F. Open the _____ and check for _____.

   G. He's still dead. You should give two _____.

Case 3

You are dreaming of your coffee, but the paramedics arrive. They defibrillate the victim and his pulse returns but not his breathing. The paramedics ask for your help with airway management.

63. Select an initial device to manage the airway in an unconscious victim.

64. You must begin ventilation with bag and mask. Of course you use oxygen, but what rate is needed in this case and how long is inhalation?

65. What is the biggest hazard to the patient during bag-mask ventilation?

WHAT DOES THE NBRC SAY?

The Examination Matrix no longer makes it clear what you need to know in regard to resuscitation. They do tell you there are eight questions in the category between the Certified Respiratory Therapist (CRT) and Written Registry Examination (WRE). Be familiar with the following concepts for treating cardiopulmonary collapse:
   A. BCLS

   B. ACLS

   C. PALS

   D. NRP

   Questions are mostly simple recall and application of facts. The matrix also mentions laryngoscopes, all the tubes, and CO_2 detectors. If you pay attention to this one chapter, you'll get those eight questions right! Admittedly, there is a lot to know. I don't think there is any substitute for an ACLS or PALS course to complete your knowledge in preparation for work in the ICU or the examinations. In fact, the examination matrices are clear that you must know ACLS, BLS, PALS, and NRP information even if you are not certified in these techniques! Finally, the Clinical Simulation Examination may present you with a case on resuscitation as well.

Here are a few sample questions. Circle the correct answer.

66. When is the jaw-thrust technique indicated to help maintain an open airway?
   A. only when foreign body obstruction is suspected

   B. only following trauma to the head

   C. only in cases of suspected neck injury

   D. only during most CPR efforts

67. While attempting mask-to-mouth ventilation, an RT notes that the chest does not rise with each breath. The most appropriate action to take at this time is to _____.
   A. intubate the patient
   B. switch to bag-mask ventilation
   C. use an oxygen-powered breathing device
   D. give another breath after repositioning the head

68. Where should you check the pulse of an unresponsive infant?
   A. brachial artery
   B. carotid artery
   C. femoral artery
   D. radial artery

Chapter **34** **Emergency Cardiovascular Life Support**

69. Upon entering a hospital room, you see a physical therapist administering CPR to a patient who is lying on the floor. Your first action would be to _____.
   A. move the patient onto the bed
   B. call for help
   C. take over chest compressions
   D. deliver two slow breaths to the airway

70. What is the correct number of rescue breaths to deliver per minute during mouth-to-mouth ventilation of an adult victim with one lay rescuer performing CPR?
   A. No breaths are delivered
   B. 5 breaths per minute
   C. 10 breaths per minute
   D. 12 breaths per minute

71. An unconscious patient begins gagging during your attempt to insert an oropharyngeal airway. The correct action to take at this time would be to _____.
   A. insert a smaller oral airway
   B. intubate the patient
   C. perform the jaw-thrust maneuver
   D. insert a nasal airway

72. The correct ratio of compressions to ventilations during two-rescuer CPR of an adult is _____.
   A. 3 : 1
   B. 30 : 2
   C. 1 : 3
   D. 1 : 30

73. The ideal airway to use during a resuscitation effort is a(n) _____.
   A. oropharyngeal airway
   B. nasopharyngeal airway
   C. fenestrated tracheostomy tube
   D. oral endotracheal tube

74. A patient is coughing and wheezing after accidentally aspirating a piece of meat. At this time, the RT should _____.
   A. allow the patient to clear his airway
   B. perform the Heimlich maneuver
   C. deliver five back blows
   D. call for help

75. Upon entering an ICU room, an RT observes ventricular fibrillation on the cardiac monitor. The most appropriate treatment for this rhythm is _____.
   A. CPR
   B. administration of lidocaine
   C. administration of epinephrine
   D. defibrillation

76. During an adult resuscitation effort, no IV line can be established. The RT should recommend _____.
   A. intraosseous infusion of the medications
   B. endotracheal instillation of the medications
   C. insertion of a central line
   D. aerosol administration of the medications

77. The effectiveness of chest compressions in producing circulation can be measured by _____.
    1. pulse oximetry
    2. capnography
    3. transcutaneous monitoring
    4. arterial blood gases
       A. 1 and 2 only
       B. 2 and 3 only
       C. 2 and 4 only
       D. 1 and 4 only

78. A patient has atrial fibrillation with serious signs and symptoms that do not respond to medications. The treatment of choice would be _____.
    A. vagal stimulation
    B. defibrillation
    C. oxygen administration
    D. cardioversion

Get the picture? Any question on the subject of resuscitation is fair game. Start by learning the basic rates, depths, and management techniques. Then move on to the advanced material.

FOOD FOR THOUGHT

79. How can we improve the quality of care given during codes?

80. Who provides emotional support to the family of a resuscitation victim? Support for the health care providers?

Humidity and Bland Aerosol Therapy

Water, taken in moderation, cannot hurt anyone.
Mark Twain

Have you ever travelled to a low-humidity environment and experienced a humidity deficit? The dry air in winter? Even your hair is unhappy without humidity. Imagine what happens to patients when we give them dry gases to breathe. Or worse, when we bypass the upper airway's natural humidification system. Humidification is a simple thing, really, but then it's often the simple things in life that matter most.

WORD WIZARD

Complete the following paragraph by writing in the correct term(s) in the blank(s) provided.

The amount of relative humidity in gas can be measured by a device called a _____. When air

does not have enough moisture to meet the normal _____ humidity of 44 mg/L, a humidity deficit
is present. This problem may occur when the normal upper airway is bypassed by an endotracheal tube. Secretions may

become very thick or _____, resulting in airway obstruction. A _____
is a device that adds gaseous water to inspired air. When you heat a humidifier it can deliver more water to the lungs. An

artificial nose, or _____ and _____ exchanger, is a simple device that

does not require a water-filled chamber. _____—devices that produce particles of water—are

also useful for adding moisture to inspired air. An electrically powered device called an _____

nebulizer, utilizes a _____ crystal, and produces a large output of small particles of water for
deposition in the lung.

MEET THE OBJECTIVES

Humidity Therapy

1. How are heat and moisture normally exchanged in your body?

   _____

2. List at least four consequences of prolonged inspiration of improperly conditioned gases.

   A. _____

   B. _____

   C. _____

   D. _____

3. Liter flows exceeding what value require humidification?

_____

4. Give one other situation where you would **ALWAYS** provide humidification.

_____

5. List the two primary and two secondary indications for humidification (see Box 35-1).

Primary   **Secondary**

A. _____   A. _____

B. _____   B. _____

6. What are the three variables that determine how well a humidifier works?

A. _____

B. _____

C. _____

Which is most important?

_____

7. Bubble humidifiers are added to what type of oxygen delivery system?

_____

8. What is the typical range for absolute humidity delivered by a bubble humidifier? What does this amount convert to in terms of relative body humidity?

A. Output _____ to _____ mg/L

B. Relative body humidity = _____ %

9. What safety device is incorporated into the design of a bubble humidifier?

_____

10. Discuss the three primary advantages of passover humidifiers compared with bubble humidifiers.

A. _____

B. _____

C. _____

11. Describe the principle of operation of each of the following artificial noses.

    A. Condenser humidifier:

    B. Hygroscopic condenser humidifier:

    C. Hydrophobic condenser humidifier:

12. What are the five contraindications to using heat-moisture exchangers (HMEs), according to the AARC Clinical Practice Guideline on humidification during mechanical ventilation?

    A. _____

    B. _____

    C. _____

    D. _____

    E. _____

13. Where does research suggest placing the HME in the breathing circuit?

14. What is an "active HME"?

15. Both Pari Hydrate and Vapotherm offer unique humidification devices with wide-ranging clinical applications. Please briefly describe these popular new humidifiers.

    A. Pari Hydrate _____

    B. Vapotherm _____

16. Identify three possible risks of using heated humidifiers. Hint: See Box 35-2 and the Clinical Practice Guideline!

    A. _____

    B. _____

    C. _____

17. Identify three hazards associated with water that "rains out," or condenses, in humidified breathing circuits.

    A. _____

    B. _____

    C. _____

18. How should you protect yourself from condensate?

19. What specialized breathing circuit circumvents (usually) the condensation problem?

20. The AARC recommends what range of alarm settings for electronically controlled heated humidifiers?

    _____

21. What is the most reliable and scientific method used to determine the effectiveness of a humidification system? What do secretions tell you about effectiveness of humidification?

    A. Scientific method:

    B. Secretions:

22. Your textbook describes what really simple way to estimate the performance of an HME or heated-wire circuit without using a hygrometer?

    _____

Chapter **35** **Humidity and Bland Aerosol Therapy**

Bland Aerosols

Bland doesn't mean boring or dull in this case. Bland aerosols simply don't have medications in them.

23. List the seven indications given in the AARC Clinical Practice Guidelines for bland aerosol administration.

A. _____

B. _____

C. _____

D. _____

E. _____

F. _____

G. _____

24. Give three examples of solutions used to make bland aerosols.

A. _____

B. _____

C. _____

25. Identify the parts of the ultrasonic nebulizer (USN) shown here.

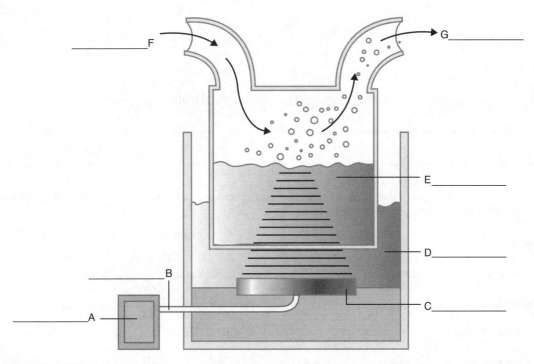

Functional schematic of a typical large-volume ultrasonic nebulizer. (Modified from Barnes TA: *Core Textbook of Respiratory Care Practice*, ed 2, St. Louis, 1994, Mosby.)

26. What preset variable determines the size of the aerosol particles generated by a USN?

_____

27. What adjustable control determines the actual amount of aerosol produced?

_____

28. USNs are primarily used to accomplish what specific clinical goal/procedure?

_____

29. When performing this procedure, what type of water is placed in the nebulizer cup?

_____

30. Large volume jet nebulizers are often used to provide moisture to the airway of patients with tracheostomy tubes. When would you use this on a patient who is not intubated?

31. What provides the power to operate a jet nebulizer?

_____

32. Jet nebulizers are also useful in controlling F_IO_2. How is this accomplished?

33. Identify the two primary clinical problems associated with tents and body enclosures?

A. _____

B. _____

34. Your text identifies six important problems associated with bland aerosol therapy. For each of these problems, give a possible solution or means of prevention.

Problem	Solution
A. Cross-contamination/infection	_____
B. Environmental safety	_____
C. Inadequate mist	_____
D. Overhydration	_____
E. Bronchospasm	_____
F. Noise	_____

MATHEMAGIC

Concepts like relative humidity were covered in Chapter 6. Here is a review of these questions since they may be on your board examinations!

35. At body temperature, gas has a saturated capacity of about 44 mg of water vapor per liter. If a gas has an absolute humidity of 22 mg/L, what is the relative humidity?

Formula _____

Solution _____

Answer _____

36. What is the humidity deficit in Question 35?

Formula _____

Solution _____

Answer _____

SUMMARY CHECKLIST

Let's review some basic concepts from Chapter 35. Complete the following sentences by writing in the correct term(s) in the blank(s) provided.

37. Conditioning of _____ gases is done primarily by the _____.

38. Gases delivered to the trachea should be warmed to _____ to _____°C.

39. A _____ is a device that adds invisible molecular water to a gas.

40. A _____ generates and disperses particles into the gas stream.

41. _____ is the most important factor affecting humidifier output.

42. At high flows, some bubble humidifiers may produce _____, which can carry infectious bacteria.

43. Breathing circuit _____ must always be treated as _____ waste.

44. Bland aerosol therapy with sterile _____ is often used to treat _____

airway _____, overcome humidity _____ in patients with tracheal

airways, and help obtain _____ specimens.

CASE STUDIES

Use the algorithm in Figure 35-17 to choose the right humidity or bland aerosol system.

Case 1

A man is brought to the emergency department with a core temperature of 30° C after falling into a lake while ice fishing. The patient is intubated with a No. 8 endotracheal tube. The patient is unconscious and requires mechanical ventilation.

45. Why can't you use an HME on this patient?

_____

46. What humidification system would you recommend?

_____

Case 2

A 32-year-old man is admitted to the medical floor with a diagnosis of *Mycoplasma pneumoniae*. He is receiving oxygen via nasal cannula at 5 L/min. He complains of a stuffy, dry nose a few hours after admission.

47. What humidification system would you recommend for this patient?

_____

48. Why is this patient unable to benefit from an HME?

_____

Case 3

A 57-year-old man who has undergone coronary artery bypass graft surgery (CABG) is being mechanically ventilated with a No. 8 ET tube pending recovery from the procedure. He has no secretion problems or history of lung problems. Body temperature is normal.

49. What humidification system would you recommend?

_____

50. What signs would you see on chest exam that would tell you that you need to switch this patient to a different device?

WHAT DOES THE NBRC SAY?

You should be able to recommend and administer bland aerosol and humidity therapy. You should know when to change to another system. Selecting, assembling, cleaning, and troubleshooting are in there, too. Expect three to five questions, and especially expect something on HMEs and USNs.

Here are a few sample questions. Circle the best answer.

51. A respiratory therapist hears a loud whistling sound as she enters the room of a patient receiving oxygen via cannula at 6 L/min. In reference to the humidifier, what is the most likely cause of the problem?
    A. The top of the humidifier is cross-threaded.
    B. The humidifier has run out of water.
    C. The flow rate is set at less than the ordered amount.
    D. There is a kink in the oxygen supply tubing.

52. A USN is ordered for sputum induction. Which of the following solutions should be placed in the medication cup to accomplish this goal?
   A. sterile distilled water
   B. 0.45% NaCl solution
   C. 0.9% NaCl solution
   D. 3% NaCl solution

53. A large-volume all-purpose nebulizer is set at an F_IO_2 of 40% and a flow rate of 10 L/min to deliver humidified oxygen to a patient with a tracheostomy. The nebulizer is producing very little mist. Which of the following could be done to improve the aerosol output?
   1. Check the water level in the nebulizer.
   2. Increase the flow rate to the nebulizer.
   3. Drain condensate from the supply tubing.
   4. Turn off the nebulizer's heating system.
      A. 1 only
      B. 1 and 2 only
      C. 1 and 3 only
      D. 1, 3, and 4 only

54. While performing a ventilator check, the respiratory therapist observes a large amount of thin, white mucus in the tubing connected to the HME. Which of the following actions should be taken at this time?
   A. Rinse out the HME with sterile water.
   B. Suction the mucus from the tubing.
   C. Place the patient on a heated humidification system.
   D. Replace the HME.

55. Sputum induction via USN is ordered. The nebulizer will produce a 5 ml of water per minute output on the maximum amplitude setting. The treatment is to last for 15 minutes. How much solution should the RCP respiratory therapist place in the nebulizer?
   A. 5 ml
   B. 15 ml
   C. 50 ml
   D. 75 ml

FOOD FOR THOUGHT

56. The industry standard for adding simple humidification to an oxygen delivery system is a flow rate of greater than 4 L/min. Can you think of any situations where you might add humidification when the flow rate is lower than 4?

57. Why wouldn't you use Vapotherm or another similar system for every patient?

■ Just for fun (respiratory fun), place yourself on a nasal cannula at 6 L/min (be sure to use a clean one!) or a simple mask at 10 L/min in the laboratory setting. Breathe through your nose for 10 or 15 minutes. How does it feel?

36 Aerosol Drug Therapy

The pen is mightier than the sword! The case for prescriptions rather than surgery.

Marvin Kitman

Now that you have the drugs, what do you do with them? In the past, RTs gave almost all their medications via intermittent positive-pressure breathing (IPPB). It was expensive, complicated and time and labor intensive and was not exactly customized to the customer! You, however, are expected to learn a wide variety of ways to deliver aerosolized drugs and find the most cost-effective and therapeutic method of delivery. Chapter 36 will get you off to a good start on this quest.

WORD WIZARD

By now you must have noticed that respiratory care has a language all its own. You won't go far without the passwords. Drug administration is no different, so you need to start by matching the following terms to their definitions.

Terms	Definitions
1. _____ aerosol	A. suspension of solid or liquid particles in a gas
2. _____ atomizer	B. difference between therapeutic and toxic drug concentrations
3. _____ baffle	C. device that produces uniformly sized aerosol particles
4. _____ deposition	D. device that removes large particles
5. _____ hygroscopic	E. device that produces non–uniformly sized aerosol particles
6. _____ inertial impaction	F. deposition of particles by collision
7. _____ MMAD	G. testimony of a witness (or, particles being retained in the respiratory tract!)
8. _____ nebulizer	H. absorbs moisture from the air
9. _____ propellant	I. measurement of average particle size
10. _____ therapeutic index	J. amount of drug left in the SVN
11. _____ residual drug volume	K. something that provides thrust

CHARACTERISTICS OF THERAPEUTIC AEROSOLS

12. Why is particle size so important in aerosol therapy?

_____

13. What is the primary method of deposition for large, high-mass particles?

_____

14. Particles of 10 microns or larger tend to deposit in what part of the respiratory tract?

What about particles between 5 and 10 microns?

A. ≥10: _____

B. 5 to 10: _____

15. In what part of the lung would you like to deposit beta-adrenergic bronchodilator drugs? What particle size is needed to accomplish this goal?

A. Where: _____

B. Particle size: _____

16. Sedimentation is an important factor in lung deposition that RTs can influence.

A. How long is an ideal breath hold maneuver? _____

B. How much will you increase drug deposition? _____

C. What about drug distribution? _____

17. Respiratory therapists influence diffusion by choosing the right delivery device for the particle size needed for the objective and by what other important method?

_____

18. Deposition increases with proper breathing patterns influenced by the practitioner delivering the medications (proper coaching matters!). Increases in what three breath variables will result in increased drug deposition?

A. _____

B. _____

C. _____

19. It is extremely difficult to predict exactly what happens to particles once they enter the lung. What is the most practical way to determine how well you are delivering a drug?

_____

HAZARDS OF AEROSOL THERAPY

What is the number one hazard of aerosol drug therapy? Why, the drugs themselves, of course! (But you knew that....)
20. Nebulizers are a great source for nosocomial infections. Describe three of the CDC's recommendations for preventing this serious problem.

A. _____

B. _____

C. _____

21. List five aerosolized substances associated with increased airway resistance.

    A. _____

    B. _____

    C. _____

    D. _____

    E. _____

22. What can you do to prevent bronchospasm from happening when you nebulize reactive substances?

    _____

23. Aerosolizing drugs **always** has the potential for inducing bronchospasm. Describe at least four ways you can monitor this potential problem.

    A. _____

    B. _____

    C. _____

    D. _____

24. What group(s) of patients is most prone to harm from bland aerosols?

    _____

25. What is meant by the term "drug concentration?" When is this most likely to occur?

26. Eye irritation or drug reactions are most likely to occur under what circumstances?

27. What could happen to a therapist who inhales bronchodilator exhaust from the nebulizers (…and you thought second-hand smoke was bad!)?

Chapter **36** **Aerosol Drug Therapy**

As mentioned earlier, there are a lot of different delivery options available. Naturally, every company claims their system is the best. Let's see if we can figure out the best using the information in *Egan's*.

Metered Dose Inhalers

Metered dose inhalers (MDIs) are the most widely prescribed aerosol drug delivery system, even though they are not completely socially accepted. It's OK to pop your antacids in the boardroom, but most executives will hide their inhalers!

28. What is meant by priming the MDI?

29. What propellant was used in most MDIs, and why was it a problem? What new propellant is safer for patients and

    the environment? _____

30. What other substances are found in MDIs that may produce clinical problems?

    _____

31. What percentage of the drug in an MDI is actually deposited in the lung? Why is there so much variability?

    _____

32. What is a "serious limitation" of pMDIs? How can you solve the problem?

    _____

33. Put the following steps of optimal open-mouth MDI delivery in order.

    A. Hold your breath for 10 seconds   _____

    B. Breathe out normally   _____

    C. Wait 30-60 seconds   _____

    D. Actuate cannister (dose)   _____

    E. Hold the MDI two fingers from mouth   _____

    F. Slowly inhale as deeply as you can   _____

    G. Warm and shake the canister   _____

    H. Actuate the canister (prime)   _____

    I. Take off the cap   _____

34. What is the difference between a spacer and a holding chamber? Does it matter?

35. Holding chambers and spacers are especially useful for what class of inhaled medications?

_____

36. How does the recommended breathing pattern differ with a holding chamber from that with a spacer or unassisted

MDI? _____

37. Describe the Turbo or the Easihaler. How will these devices help patients get their medications?

Dry Powder

Dry powder makes sense, because wet powder never did work. You'll want to get familiar with the four or five different types of devices in common use.

38. What is a DPI? What's the big deal?

39. How does DPI breathing technique differ from that recommended with an MDI?

_____

40. What patients cannot use DPIs?

_____

41. Name an example of an active DPI delivery system.

_____

42. In general, what is the role of the DPI in management of acute bronchospasm?

Small Volume Nebulizers

Small volume nebulizers (SVNs) have been around a long time and are still widely used. They have an amazing number of aliases: mini-neb, acorn neb, hand-held neb, updraft neb, micro-neb, med neb...the list seems to go on forever. These devices are indicated when a patient is unable to physically use an MDI or cannot generate sufficient inspiratory flow rates for an MDI or DPI. Some drugs are only available for nebulization.

43. List three potential power sources to drive the small medication nebulizer.

    A. _____

    B. _____

    C. _____

44. How does an atomizer differ from an SVN? When would you want to use one?

45. What is the ideal flow rate and amount of solution to put in an SVN for a typical albuterol treatment?

    A. Flow rate: _____

    B. Amount of solution: _____

46. Why is it so important to match nebulizer and compressor systems for home use?

    _____

47. Several nebulizers on the market are designed to reduce the amount of drug expelled into the atmosphere and wasted. Describe the following in terms of physical design, class of nebulizer, and key features.

    A. Circulaire:

    B. Pari LC Sprint:

    C. Aeroclipse:

48. What is meant by nebulizer "sputter," and why is it important to RTs?

49. What potential problem exists when you deliver an SVN via mask? How can you deal with this problem?

50. Explain what is meant by the "blow-by" technique used with infants, and discuss the effectiveness of this technique.

51. You really can't nebulize all of the solution. Explain the idea of residual volume. How broad is the range?

Large Volume Nebulizers

Large volume nebulizers are usually used to deliver bland aerosols (see Chapter 35). Special large volume nebulizers, like the HEART and HOPE nebulizers, are used to deliver continuous bronchodilator therapy. You may want to try one to deliver drugs when a severely obstructed patient does not respond to SVN treatments and needs a repeated series over time.

52. What potential clinical problem may exist with continuous bronchodilator therapy?

_____

53. Why is the SPAG generator unique? When is it indicated?

_____

Small Ultrasonic Nebulizers

Small ultrasonic nebulizers (USNs) have a lot of advantages: small uniform particles, high output, and they can be used with ventilators.

54. List three advantages and three disadvantages of USNs to deliver medications (see Table 36-3 in your text).

	ADVANTAGES	DISADVANTAGES
A.		
B.		
C.		

Use the algorithms in Figure 36-33 or 36-29 in *Egan's* to answer the following questions about selection of aerosol drug delivery devices and doses.

Case 1

An alert, cooperative 52-year-old man has recently been diagnosed with chronic bronchitis. He quit smoking (60-pack-year history) 6 months ago, but still has respiratory symptoms. He is in your pulmonary clinic today to receive his pulmonary function test (PFT) results and medications. The physician has ordered Atrovent and Flovent.

55. What method of delivery would you recommend for this patient?

_____

56. What other equipment is indicated?

_____

57. What general considerations for patient education would you stress for this patient?

_____

58. How will you know that he is able to perform the therapy correctly?

_____

Case 2

A 27-year-old man presents in the emergency department with acute respiratory distress. He is diagnosed with status asthmaticus. He has high-pitched diffuse wheezes, a respiratory rate of 24, heart rate of 106, and SpO$_2$ of 92%. His PEFR is 150 after 4 puffs of albuterol via MDI.

59. What are the possible options for treating this patient at this point?

_____

60. What method of bronchodilator delivery would you recommend?

_____

61. What is meant by "dose-response" assessment?

_____

Case 3

You are asked to deliver a bronchodilator to a patient in the neuro unit. When you arrive to assess the patient, you note that she is obtunded. Breath sounds reveal scattered rhonchi and wheezing in the upper lobes.

62. What method of bronchodilator delivery would you recommend in this situation?

_____

348

63. What modification will you need to make?

_____

64. Because peak flow is unlikely to be performed, how will you assess the effectiveness of therapy?

_____

INTUBATED PATIENTS

Delivering bronchodilators to intubated patients has always been difficult. Much of the drug ends up in the circuit or the endotracheal tube. Assessment of effectiveness can be difficult as well. Both SVNs and MDIs can be used to achieve good results if you follow some guidelines and use the right equipment.

65. What is the starting dose for albuterol via SVN for an intubated patient?

_____

66. What standard starting dosage is recommended for albuterol by MDI to a ventilator patient?

_____

67. Where should you place the SVN in the ventilator circuit?

_____

68. When should an MDI be activated for a ventilator patient?

_____

69. What adjustments to dilution need to be made with the SVN for ventilator delivery?

_____

70. Describe the method for giving a bronchodilator to a patient on noninvasive mask ventilation.

71. Describe the method for giving a bronchodilator to a patient who is on an oscillator.

72. What changes do you need to make to ensure delivery? (Look at Box 36-9 for clues.)

A. HME: _____

B. Flow-by: _____

C. Alarms, limits: _____

It will come as no surprise that this information is on your boards. What *is* unusual is how little of this material is on the test considering the importance and frequency of aerosol drug administration in the clinical setting. One reason is that only recently have good studies been done to provide more scientific conclusions about how best to deliver medications. The matrix specifically mentions MDIs, spacers, DPIs, and pneumatic-powered nebulizers. Of course, peak flows and assessment are included. Continuous nebulization is now included as well.

Try the following questions. The following information pertains to questions 73 and 74. Circle the best answer.

Asthma has been recently diagnosed in a 16-year-old patient. The respiratory therapist is asked to teach the patient how to self-administer QVAR via MDI.

73. In addition to the inhaler, what other equipment would be needed to teach the patient?
    1. spacer device
    2. pulse oximeter
    3. peak flowmeter
        A. 1 only
        B. 1 and 2 only
        C. 1 and 3 only
        D. 2 and 3 only

74. After performing the inhalation, the RT instructs the patient to perform a breath holding maneuver. The purpose of this maneuver is to _____.
    A. promote a strong cough
    B. improve venous return
    C. improve inertial impaction
    D. increase medication delivery

75. While attempting to administer albuterol via SVN to a patient who has had a recent CVA, the RT notes that the patient is unable to hold the nebulizer or keep her lips sealed on the mouthpiece. The RT should recommend _____.
    A. switching to an MDI
    B. utilizing an aerosol mask for delivery
    C. discontinuing the medication
    D. subcutaneous administration of the medication

76. An MDI is ordered for a patient who is intubated and being mechanically ventilated and humidified with a heat-moisture exchanger (HME). Which of the following is the most appropriate way to administer the bronchodilator?
    A. Place the MDI in the expiratory limb of the ventilator circuit.
    B. Place the MDI between the HME and the endotracheal tube.
    C. Recommend changing the delivery method to a small volume nebulizer.
    D. Remove the HME during delivery of the drug.

77. An alert adult patient with asthma is receiving bronchodilator therapy via small volume nebulizer during a hospitalization. What recommendations should the RT make in regard to this therapy when the patient is ready for discharge?
    A. Recommend MDI instruction.
    B. Recommend oral administration of the medication.
    C. Recommend training in home use of the SVN.
    D. Recommend administration of the drug via IPPB.

78. Which of the following devices is most suitable for delivery of Virazole (ribavirin)?
    A. continuous large volume nebulizer
    B. small particle aerosol generator
    C. ultrasonic nebulizer
    D. atomizer

Chapter 36 ends with some important material about protecting the practitioner from continuous exposure to a wide variety of inhaled agents.

79. What two inhalational drugs have proved to be an occupational risk for RTs?

A. _____

B. _____

80. Describe some of the physical ways to control environmental contamination when delivering medications that have potential side effects for the provider.

81. What do the terms HEPA and PAPR refer to?

_____

37 Storage and Delivery of Medical Gases

O Lord, help me to be pure, but not yet.
St. Augustine

RTs have to learn more about medical gases than any other mortals on this planet! This information will come in handy many times in the clinical setting, and it is good to be an expert when the delivery systems malfunction and no one knows quite what to do but the respiratory therapist!

WORD WIZARD

You will learn about the safety systems in this chapter. Listed here are some other terms that might come in handy. Look up these nine terms and give a brief description.

Characteristics
Flammable
Nonflammable
Oxidizing

Equipment
Bourdon gauge
Thorpe tube
Reducing valve
Regulator
Flowmeter
Zone valves

CHARACTERISTICS OF MEDICAL GASES

1. Name three gases categorized as nonflammable.

    A. _____

    B. _____

    C. _____

2. Most therapeutic gases will oxidize or support combustion. Name three gases in this category.

    A. _____

    B. _____

    C. _____

3. Describe the four basic steps of the fractional distillation process.

   A. _____

   B. _____

   C. _____

   D. _____

4. What purity level is required for medical grade oxygen?

   _____

5. Describe the two methods used to separate oxygen from air. What concentration is produced by each method?

   A. _____

   B. _____

6. Describe the devices used to produce medical grade air for hospital systems and for home use.

   A. Hospital:

   B. Home:

7. To this day, medical carbon dioxide is occasionally used in neonatal and adult medicine. State the primary use of CO_2 for respiratory labs. Give one clinical example.

   _____

8. What is heliox? What is it used for?

   _____

9. What is the primary medical use for nitrous oxide? What are some of the hazards of nitrous oxide administration?

10. What is the only type of patient who receives nitric oxide in current clinical practice?

   _____

11. Describe two possible hazards of using nitric oxide.

    A.

    B.

12. Give the chemical symbol for each of the following medical gases.

Gas	Symbol
A. Oxygen	_____
B. Air	_____
C. Carbon dioxide	_____
D. Helium	_____
E. Nitrous oxide	_____
F. Nitric oxide	_____

STORING MEDICAL GASES

High-pressure medical gas cylinders have been around for over 100 years. The modern cylinder is the subject of numerous regulations and rules that control manufacturing, storage, and transportation of these potentially dangerous steel bottles. Naturally, you will be expected to have considerable knowledge on this subject even if you don't use it on a daily basis!

13. Identify the cylinder markings on the diagram shown here.

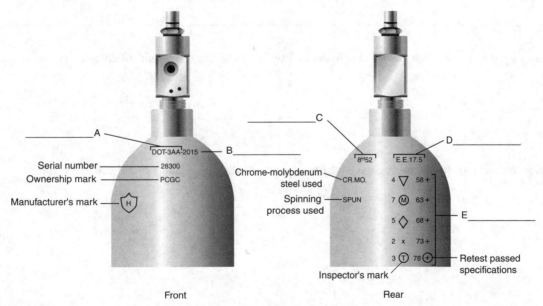

Typical markings of cylinders containing medical gases. Front and back views are for illustration purposes only. Exact location and order of markings vary.

14. What do the symbols * and + mean when stamped on a cylinder?

A. * _____

B. + _____

15. Identify the proper color for these gas cylinders (in the United States).

A. Oxygen _____

B. Carbon dioxide _____

C. Nitrous oxide _____

D. Helium _____

E. Nitrogen _____

F. Air _____

16. Because cylinder color is only a guideline, how do you actually determine what gas is in a tank?

_____

17. What is the best way to determine the actual oxygen concentration in a cylinder?

_____

FILL 'ER UP

Cylinders are filled with either gas or liquid. The liquid will either be at room temperature or in a cryogenic state.

18. Name two gases that can be stored in the liquid state at room temperature.

A. _____

B. _____

19. Explain why the pressure in a gas-filled cylinder is different from that of a liquid-filled cylinder.

20. Describe the methods for measuring the contents of a gas-filled cylinder and a liquid-filled cylinder.
A.

B.

21. Write the formula for calculating the cylinder factor for a gas-filled cylinder.

22. What are the factors for the "E" and "H" oxygen cylinders?

A. _____

B. _____

23. Now write the formula for calculating duration of flow in minutes.

_____

We'll practice these calculations later in this chapter. They are important for clinical practice and for your board exams!

BULK OXYGEN

Try to imagine how much oxygen a large hospital needs every day. If you had 100 patients wearing oxygen at 6 L/min, you would need over 800,000 L for 1 day! Ventilators draw much more gas! You could do this with individual cylinders in each room, but think how much work that would involve. A bulk system, by definition, has at least 20,000 cubic feet of gas. Check out the cool picture in Figure 37-9. Better yet, go on a field trip and look at the bulk system with a hospital engineer.

24. Describe a gaseous bulk system. Be sure to discuss the manifold, the primary, and reserve banks.

25. Why do most hospitals use a liquid bulk oxygen system?

_____

26. Where are small liquid oxygen cylinders usually used?

_____

27. What is the critical temperature of oxygen? How is the bulk liquid oxygen maintained at this temperature?

28. What is the normal working pressure for a hospital oxygen piping system?

_____

29. What are zone valves? Give two reasons you might need to use these valves.

SAFETY SYSTEMS

Ah, the fabled safety systems. They come in two general types: those built into the cylinder valve stem to prevent rupture from high pressures, and indexed systems designed to keep you from giving the wrong gas to a patient.

30. Remember the gas laws? If a cylinder overheats, the pressure will rise. Describe the type of pressure release valve usually found in these cylinder stems.

    A. Small cylinder: _____

    B. Large cylinder: _____

31. Name the three basic indexed safety systems for medical gases. Both names!

Abbreviated name	Full name
A. _____	_____
B. _____	_____
C. _____	_____

32. A large cylinder of oxygen is described as follows: CGA-540 0.903-14NGO-RH-Ext. Explain what this means.

33. What type of cylinder uses pins and holes for the safety connection system?

_____

34. What system was established to prevent accidental interchange of low-pressure medical gas connectors? What do they mean by "low-pressure?"

_____

35. What is the purpose of the quick-connect system?

_____

358

Because a large cylinder of oxygen may have a pressure as high as 2400 psi, we need to have a way to lower this pressure and control it or our equipment (or the patient) could be harmed.

36. Describe the action of the following devices.

   A. Reducing valve: _____

   B. Flowmeter: _____

   C. Regulator: _____

37. Describe the normal way each of the following is used in respiratory care.

   A. Preset reducing valve:

   B. Adjustable reducing valve:

   C. Multiple-stage reducing valve:

38. What two hazards can be created when you open a cylinder attached to a high-pressure reducing valve?

Three categories of flowmeters are used in respiratory care. The next set of questions will test your knowledge of these commonly used devices.

39. What are two advantages and two disadvantages of flow restrictors?

	ADVANTAGES	DISADVANTAGES
A.		
B.		

359

40. Describe the Bourdon flowmeter.

_____

41. What is the chief advantage of the Bourdon-type flowmeter?

_____

_____

42. How will indicated flow compare to actual flow when a Bourdon flowmeter meets up with downstream resistance?

_____

_____

43. What do Bourdon gauges actually measure? Thorpe tubes?

    A. Bourdon: _____

    B. Thorpe: _____

44. Compare indicated flow and actual flow in a compensated Thorpe flowmeter when downstream resistance occurs.

45. What happens to the float in a compensated Thorpe tube when you connect it to a 50 psi gas source?

_____

_____

CASE STUDY

Case 1

A patient is to be transported from the ICU to the imaging department for a CT scan. The patient requires continuous supplemental oxygen at 10 L/min by mask. You will need to provide portable oxygen for the transport. An E cylinder is available.

46. What type of regulator is most appropriate for transport?

_____

47. How long will the cylinder last at the given flow rate if the pressure is 1000 psi?

    Formula: _____

    Calculation: _____

48. When you turn on the cylinder valve, a hissing noise is heard from the regulator. The flowmeter is off, so there must be a leak. What should you check to try to correct the leak?

    A. _____

    B. _____

Now, back to the problem of cylinder duration calculations. Obviously, this is important—not just because it is on tests! Let's say you have to transport a patient by airplane, or send someone home with oxygen, or just go from the emergency department to the ICU. Will you have enough gas? Running out in the elevator is not really acceptable!

There are two ways to do this: the board-exam, precise way and the Rule of Thumb quick and dirty way.

Precise way first.

The two most common cylinders you will be using are the small E type and the larger H or K type. Factors are 0.28 and 3.14.

Example: You are sending a patient home by car. The E cylinder is full (2200 psi) and the patient is wearing a cannula at 2 L/min. How long will the O_2 last?

Start by writing out the formula. (You have to know this one.)

$$\text{Duration} = \text{psi} \times \text{Factor/Flow}$$

Now plug in the numbers.

$$\text{Calculation: } 2200 \times 0.28/2 = 616/2 = 308 \text{ minutes}$$

OK, how many hours is that?

$$308/60 = 5.1 \text{ hours}$$

49. Calculate duration of an E cylinder with 1500 psi running at 2 L/min.

Formula: _____

Calculation:

Answer: Minutes _____   Hours _____

50. Calculate the duration of an H cylinder with 1500 psi running at 2 L/min.

Formula: _____

Calculation:

Answer: Minutes _____   Hours _____

Now for the quick and dirty way.

0.28 is roughly $1/3$. One third of 2200 is 700.

700 divided by 2 = 350 minutes, divided by 60 minutes in an hour = 5+ hours

You can see how you could get into trouble with this. Of course if the patient is taking a 30-minute trip home, it would hardly matter. Be sensible when you take shortcuts! A safer shortcut is to use $1/4$. One fourth of 2200 is about 550. Divided by 2, that is only 275 minutes, but you have a little cushion of extra gas.

P.S. If you use this on the boards, you could check your work pretty easily, or you might be able to skip the mathematics and just use the shortcut.

P.P.S. When transporting a patient who needs oxygen, it's a good idea to start with a full cylinder if it is at all possible.

P.P.P.S. Remember that a full E cylinder will last 10 hours at 1 L or 1 hour at 10 L. This rule is easy to remember and can be useful.

361

You won't see too many questions on the material in Chapter 37. Cylinder duration is one common question and usually involves duration of an E or H cylinder. Here are some typical problems for you to try.

Circle the best answer.

51. An H cylinder of oxygen is being used to deliver oxygen to a patient in a subacute care facility where no piped-in oxygen is available. The cylinder gauge shows a pressure of 1000 psi. The patient is receiving oxygen at 5 L/min by cannula. Approximately how long will the cylinder gas last at this flow rate?
    A. 1 hour
    B. 8 hours
    C. 10 hours
    D. 628 hours

52. A respiratory therapist notices that a flowmeter plugged into the wall outlet continues to read 1 L/min even though it is not turned on. What is the most appropriate action at this time?
    A. Replace the flowmeter.
    B. Include the extra liter in any calculations.
    C. Disassemble the flowmeter and replace the "O-rings."
    D. Do nothing; this is not an unusual situation.

53. A respiratory therapist has to transport a patient via air from the island of Maui to Honolulu. The patient is being manually ventilated with an oxygen flow set at 10 L/min using an E cylinder of gas. The cylinder gauge reads 2000 psi. How long will the cylinder last?
    A. 42 minutes
    B. 56 minutes
    C. 60 minutes
    D. 10 hours

54. When a respiratory therapist unplugs a Thorpe-type flowmeter, a huge leak occurs from the wall outlet. What action should the RT take at this time?
    A. Shut off the gas to the room with the zone valve.
    B. Shut off the bulk oxygen system.
    C. Plug the flowmeter back into the outlet.
    D. Call maintenance to fix the outlet.

55. A fire breaks out in the pediatrics unit due to a faulty electrical cord. One respiratory therapist has ensured that patients with oxygen are safe. Your responsibility in this situation would be to:
    A. Prepare to shut off the zone valves to the unit.
    B. Obtain an additional crash cart for emergencies.
    C. Obtain additional E cylinders of oxygen.
    D. Prepare to document the incident in the record.

FOOD FOR THOUGHT

56. What would happen if nitrous oxide leaked into the room in the emergency department or operating room setting?

57. Your text describes the catastrophic consequences of bulk-system failures. Describe what some of your actions might be in this type of emergency.

58. What protective gear is appropriate when opening a valve on a high-pressure cylinder?

_____

Chapter **37** **Storage and Delivery of Medical Gases**

38 Medical Gas Therapy

Smile, breathe and go slowly.
Thich Nhat Hanh

The respiratory care profession has come a long way, but medical gas therapy is still a cornerstone of respiratory care. Of course we think of oxygen as a drug now, and things have changed a lot in our understanding of administering this powerful medication. The modern respiratory therapist must have a much firmer grasp of the goals and objective of medical gas therapy. You will be expected to assess and make recommendations for modifications. Protocols will allow you to change liter flow, F_IO_2, and delivery devices as required to meet specific clinical outcomes for the patient.

WORD WIZARD

Let's try something different in the war of the words. Many students have a hard time with the spelling of medical terms. Check your ability by circling the correct spelling for this gas jargon.

1. canulla   cannula
2. reservore   reservoir
3. lasitude   lassitude
4. diaphramatic   diaphragmatic
5. retanopathy   retinopathy
6. hypoxemia   hypoxemea
7. toxicity   toxisity
8. infarction   infraction
9. displasia   dysplasia
10. pendent   pendant
11. concentration   concintration
12. entranement   entrainment
13. wye   why

TANK JOCKEYS AND GAS PASSERS

Let's start by reviewing the reasons for giving oxygen and how to clinically recognize those needs.

14. What is acute hypoxemia? _____

15. What are the threshold criteria for defining hypoxemia in adults according to the AARC Clinical Practice Guidelines?

     1. PaO_2 _____

     2. SaO_2 _____

16. Specifically, what beneficial effect does oxygen have on the symptoms of patients with COPD and chronic hypoxemia (besides treating hypoxemia!)?

     A. COPD (and interstitial disease) _____

     B. Chronic hypoxemia _____

17. Describe the two compensatory mechanisms of the cardiopulmonary system when faced with hypoxemia.

A. Lungs: _____

B. Heart: _____

18. In what acute cardiac condition is oxygen therapy especially important?

_____

19. What effect does hypoxemia have on the pulmonary blood vessels? What are the long-term consequences of this effect?

20. State the three basic ways to determine if a patient needs oxygen.

A. _____

B. _____

C. _____

21. List six common acute clinical situations where hypoxemia is so common that oxygen therapy is usually provided.

A. _____

B. _____

C. _____

D. _____

E. _____

F. _____

22. Give two signs of mild and severe hypoxia for each of the following systems. (Table 38-1)

	SYSTEM	MILD	SEVERE
A.	Respiratory		
B.	Cardiovascular		
C.	Neurologic		

There are four great big problems associated with oxygen therapy (besides burning down the hospital!). Naturally, you need to know them.

Toxic Talk

23. Oxygen toxicity affects what two organ systems?

    A. _____

    B. _____

24. The harm caused by oxygen is influenced by what two factors?

    A. _____

    B. _____

25. Describe the effects on the lung tissue of breathing excessive oxygen.

26. What is meant by a "vicious circle" in reference to oxygen toxicity?

27. While every patient is unique, what general rule of thumb can be applied to prevent oxygen toxicity?

28. When should oxygen be withheld from a hypoxic patient to avoid the consequences of toxicity?

    _____

I Feel Depressed

29. What specific type of COPD patient is likely to experience depression of ventilatory drive while breathing oxygen?

    _____

30. Give two explanations for this effect.

    A. _____

    B. _____

31. When should oxygen be withheld from a hypoxic COPD patient to avoid depressing ventilation?

_____

RLF or ROP?

32. Describe the pathophysiology of how excessive blood oxygen causes blindness in premature newborns.

33. During what time period after birth is a preemie likely to develop ROP?

_____

34. How can you reduce the risk of ROP?

_____

Absorbing Information

35. Describe how oxygen can cause atelectasis.

36. What groups of patients are at increased risk for absorption atelectasis?

_____

37. How can you reduce the risk of absorption atelectasis?

_____

Fire!

38. What is the fire triangle?

39. What type of regulator has been associated with fires?

40. What is the biggest hazard in the home setting?

Now that you know why to give a patient oxygen and some of the hazards of administration, it's time to learn how to make tasty selections from the complex choices offered on the medical gas menu.

41. The three basic categories are low flow, high flow, and reservoir. Match the category to the description below.

	CATEGORY	DESCRIPTION
A.	Low flow	1. Always exceeds patient's inspiratory needs
B.	Reservoir	2. Provides some of patient's inspiratory needs
C.	High flow	3. May meet needs if no leaks occur

LOW FLOW

42. Why do you think the nasal cannula is the most commonly used low-flow system?

_____

43. When should you attach the cannula to a bubble humidifier?

_____

44. What maximum flow does the text suggest for newborns?

_____

45. How does the patient's breathing pattern affect the F_IO_2 delivered to the lung when wearing a low-flow device like a cannula? Hint: What happens to the delivered oxygen if the patient gets in trouble or exercises and breathes faster and deeper?

Low-Flow Experiment

If you have access to a cannula, humidifier, and some medical oxygen, find out what it feels like to be a patient!
1. Attach the cannula to a flowmeter with the nipple adaptor (or "Christmas tree" if you like that term better).
2. Insert the prongs in your nose and set the flow to 1 L/min.
3. Try that for one minute.
4. Increase the flow by 1 L/min.
5. Continue this until you get to the 8 L/min maximum suggested by the text.
6. Try again with a humidifier.

Questions
- How well could you feel the gas at 1 L? What implication does this have for patient care?
- When did the flow start to become noticeable? Uncomfortable?
- What happened to the humidifier as the flow rates exceeded 5 L/min?

---

46. Give me one good reason to use the ancient nasal catheter.

47. What is the primary advantage of using a transtracheal oxygen catheter?

_____

48. What is the primary disadvantage of the transtracheal catheter?

49. What range of F_IO_2 is usually delivered by low-flow devices?

_____

50. Because you can't tell exactly how much oxygen the patient is receiving at any given moment from a cannula or any low-flow device, how can you assess the effects of administering the drug?

_____

51. What are the advantages and disadvantages of reservoir cannulas?

   A. Advantages _____

   B. Disadvantages _____

52. In what setting are reservoir cannulas usually used?

_____

RESERVOIR

53. Use Table 38-3 to help you find the information about oxygen masks.

	MASK	F_IO_2 RANGE	ADVANTAGE	DISADVANTAGE
A.	Simple			
B.	Partial rebreathing			
C.	Nonrebreathing			

54. What is the primary difference between the partial rebreathing and nonrebreathing masks?

_____

55. How can you tell if a nonrebreathing mask has an adequate flow rate?

_____

56. Give a solution for each of these common problems with reservoir masks. See Table 38-6 for clues!

Problem   **Solution**

  A. Confused patient removes mask   _____

  B. Humidifier pop-off activated   _____

  C. Mask causes claustrophobia   _____

  D. Bag collapses on inspiration   _____

  E. Bag fully inflated on inspiration   _____

Reservoir Experiment

Get a nonrebreather (NRB), a simple mask, a bubble humidifier, a nipple adaptor, and a flowmeter. Try to use a non-rebreather with two valves on the mask if you can find one.

1. **First,** try the simple mask without a humidifier. Set the flowmeter at 2 L/min and breathe from the simple mask for a few breaths. Now take deep breaths. Set the flowmeter at 10 L/min and try again.
2. **Next,** set up the NRB. Repeat the experiment. Breathe as deeply as you can and adjust the flowmeter until the bag doesn't collapse. **Try** the mask with one expiratory flap valve in place and with two (if possible).
3. **Finally,** attach the bubble humidifier, set the flow at 10, and put on the mask. Now increase the flow rate to 15, then flush.

Questions

- How did it feel to breathe on the simple mask at a low flow rate?
- What happened when you tried the NRB at a low flow?
- How did mask performance vary when you used two valves?
- What difference did the humidifier make?
- What happened to the humidifier when you increased the flow?

Remember, lab experiments should be done under lab conditions with appropriate supervision!

HIGH-FLOW

Air-entrainment systems are commonly used to provide high-flow oxygen because they are simple and inexpensive to operate. Oxygen is directed through a small tube, or jet, which creates a very high forward velocity. Room air is entrained or mixed into the system, which dilutes the oxygen and increases the total flow rate delivered to meet the patient's needs.

57. Describe the effects of varying the jet size or entrainment port opening on F_IO_2 and total flow rate.

	FACTOR	INCREASED SIZE	DECREASED SIZE
A.	Jet 1. F_IO_2 2. Flow		
B.	Port 1. F_IO_2 2. Flow		

58. Fill in the air-to-oxygen ratios for the following oxygen concentrations. (See Table 38-7.)

A. 100% _____

B. 60% _____

C. 40% _____

D. 35% _____

E. 30% _____

F. 24% _____

59. What is the common name for an air entrainment mask (AEM)?

_____

60. Why does the AEM have larger openings on the side of the mask than a simple oxygen mask?

_____

61. What effect does raising the delivered flow from the flowmeter have on the F_IO_2 delivered by an AEM?

_____

62. Air-entrainment devices are classified as high-flow. For what F_IO_2 settings is this usually true?

_____

63. How do you boost the total flow when using an AEM?

_____

64. Why is this not possible with an air-entrainment nebulizer?

_____

65. There are four devices used to deliver gas from an air-entrainment nebulizer to the patient. Choose the device(s) that fits each of the following patients. (See Figure 38-16 in your text.)

Patient   **Aerosol Delivery Device**

A. Tracheostomy tube   _____

B. Endotracheal tube   _____

C. Intact upper airway _____

D. After nasal surgery _____

66. Describe an easy way to tell if an air-entrainment nebulizer is providing sufficient gas to meet the patient's needs.

67. Give one example of a specialized flow generator that produces an aerosol, and one example that produces dry gas. These devices produce high flow and high F_IO_2, thus solving the problem created with nebulizers and AEMs! (See Figure 38-19 for an example.)

   A. Aerosol: _____

   B. Dry: _____

68. What effect does downstream resistance to flow have on F_IO_2 and total flow delivered by a typical AEM or nebulizer entrainment system?

High-Flow Experiment

You will need an AEM, oxygen analyzer, and an air-entrainment jet nebulizer with a length of corrugated tubing.
   1. First, set the AEM at 40% with a flow of 5 L/min of oxygen. Analyze the F_IO_2 (detach the mask and put the analyzer tee on). Increase the flow to 8 L/min. Analyze again.
   2. Next, set up the nebulizer. Use 40% and a flow of 10. Analyze the output. Increase the flow to 12 and analyze again.
   3. Now pour enough water into the corrugated tubing to partially occlude it. Analyze. Add enough water to completely occlude the tubing. Analyze.
   4. Finally, drain out the water. Try to increase the flowmeter setting past 15.

Concentration Questions
   - What is the effect of altering flow rate on the AEM?
   - What is the effect of water (resistance) in the tubing of a jet neb?
   - What happened when you tried to increase the flow with the neb? Why?

MATHEMAGIC

Oxygen–to–air entrainment ratios and total flow from air-entrainment devices is another one of the universal clinical and board exam expectations that has driven countless students to the brink of insanity. Take a slow, deep breath; exhale. Straighten shoulders. Engage.... You have three choices.
   - Memorize the ratios for each F_IO_2.
   - Learn the algebraic formula.
   - Learn the magic box.

You must learn and master this information!
   If you like the first method, you must memorize every detail in Table 38-7. READ the fine print.
   Or
   Look at the Mini-Clini "Computing the Total Flow Output of an Air-Entrainment Device." A three-step method is provided for calculating the ratio and the subsequent total flow. Let's try one.

A patient is receiving oxygen at 40% via a Venti-mask with the flowmeter set at 8 L/min. What is the ratio of oxygen to air? What is the total flow?

Step 1: Compute the ratio

$$\frac{\text{Liters of Air}}{\text{Liters of O}_2} \qquad \frac{(100 - 40)}{(40 - 21)}$$

$$\frac{\text{Liters of Air}}{\text{Liters of O}_2} \qquad \frac{(60)}{(19)}$$

$$\frac{\text{Liters of Air}}{\text{Liters of O}_2} \qquad \frac{3}{1}$$

Step 2: Add the numerator and denominator parts

$$3 + 1 = 4$$

Step 3: Multiply the sum of the parts by the oxygen flow rate

$$4 \times 8 = 32 \text{ L/min total flow}$$

Now you try.

69. What is the oxygen–to–air entrainment ratio and total flow for a patient who is receiving 60% oxygen via an entrainment nebulizer with the flowmeter set at 10 L/min?

    A. Step 1: Compute the ratio

       Formula: _____

       Calculation: _____

       Reduce answer to get ratio: _____

    B. Step 2: Add the parts

    C. Step 3: Multiply the sum of the parts by the O_2 flow rate

The "magic box" is a favorite of many RTs. (See Figure 38-14 for an example.) Retry the sample problem above for the patient on 40%. Pretty nifty! The only problem with this method is that you substitute 20 (instead of 21) to make the math easy. At percentages below 40, your answers will start to vary from the algebraic method. You can solve this by using "21" for low percentages and "20" for 40% or more.

Practice with your chosen method until you can solve for every F_iO_2. There is no way out of this!

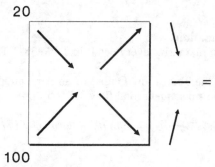

The magic box used to estimate air–to–oxygen ratio.

BLENDERS

Oxygen blenders are another kind of "magic box." The blender requires a 50 psi input of air and oxygen. When you twirl the knob to set the F_IO_2, you are actually adjusting a proportioning valve. Turning toward a high percentage of oxygen makes the opening for oxygen larger and the opening for air smaller. Use of 100% closes the air side and only lets oxygen out. Vice versa for turning the knob toward 21%. The blender is a very handy device. It gives you high flow rates or 50 psi to power equipment at any F_IO_2 you desire.

70. Describe the three-step process for confirming the proper operation of a blender (see Box 38-3).

    A. _____

    B. _____

    C. _____

PUT THOSE KIDS IN A TENT!

The opening scene of the venerable *Marcus Welby, MD* television show depicted a man in an oxygen tent. Wearing a nasal cannula! You may see this being done on soap operas as well. Nowadays, enclosures are a simple way to deliver oxygen to infants and children.

71. What is the major problem with oxygen tents?

72. What is the highest F_IO_2 you can expect to deliver with a tent?

73. Why is a hood the best method for delivering oxygen to an infant?

74. What minimum flow must be set for a hood? Why?

75. What harmful consequence occurs when flow rates into the hood are too high?

76. What effect will cold air flowing into the hood have on a premature infant?

_____

77. What is the best way to control oxygen delivery to an infant inside an incubator?

_____

78. What is the primary benefit of the infant incubator?

_____

HIGH-FLOW SYSTEMS AND HYPOXEMIA

High-flow oxygen systems are a valuable new tool for managing serious hypoxemia.

79. Compare the Vapotherm™ and Salter high-flow systems.

80. What are the major limitations of these devices?

81. What device could you use during resuscitation or in the emergency setting to administer 100% oxygen?

82. What are the 3 "P's" of delivery?

HYPERBARIC OXYGEN

Life under pressure: that's hyperbaric oxygen, or HBO. We can administer oxygen to the patient at 2 or 3 atmospheres (ATA) to treat several acute and chronic problems. Originally designed for decompression sickness in divers, HBO operates according to Boyle's law. RTs often work with patients who require this mode of oxygen administration, and it is also common for RTs to work in hyperbaric units. So pick up your pencils and let's get on with the show!

83. Compare the monoplace and multiplace hyperbaric chambers.

	CHAMBER	O₂ DELIVERY	PATIENT	STAFF
A.	Monoplace			
B.	Multiplace			

84. List three acute and three chronic conditions where HBO is indicated. (Try Box 38-6.)

Acute   **Chronic**

A. _____   _____

B. _____   _____

C. _____   _____

85. Under what circumstances is HBO indicated in cases of carbon monoxide poisoning? (See Box 38-7.)

OTHER GASES

86. Two other therapeutic gases are commonly administered by RTs. Give indications for each.

Gas   **Indications**

A. NO   _____

                _____

B. Helium   _____

                _____

87. What other gas is always mixed with helium? What is the most common combination?

_____

88. What physical property of helium results in decreased work of breathing?

_____

89. Helium is so diffusible that special balloons are used to hold it! What type of gas delivery device is used to administer helium to patients who are not intubated?

_____

CASE STUDIES

Case 1

A 52-year-old college professor is admitted for chest pain and possible myocardial infarction (MI). Electrocardiogram (ECG) monitoring reveals sinus tachycardia. The chest pain has been decreased by the administration of nitroglycerin. Respirations are 20 per minute, and SpO_2 on room air is 92%.

90. What is your assessment of this patient's oxygenation status?

91. What is your recommendation in regard to administration of supplemental oxygen?

Case 2

A man has been admitted for exacerbation of his COPD. The patient is wearing oxygen at 2 L/min via nasal cannula. The pulse oximeter shows a saturation of 94% while at rest. The nurse calls you to ask for your assistance in evaluation of the patient's dyspnea during ambulation.

92. What changes occur in breathing pattern during exercise?

_____

93. How are low-flow oxygen devices affected by changes in breathing pattern?

_____

94. How would you assess dyspnea on ambulation for a patient wearing oxygen?

Case 3

A patient is recovering from surgery following a head injury. The patient is trached and requires supplemental oxygen at 60% via T-piece. The flowmeter is set at 12 L/min. Each time the patient inhales, the mist exiting the T-piece disappears.

95. Air-entrainment nebulizers are considered high-flow delivery systems. Discuss this in terms of the disappearing mist.

_____

96. What should be added to the T-piece to help deal with this problem?

_____

97. Describe a common method of increasing the delivered flow when administering high F_IO_2

via air-entrainment nebulizers. _____

98. What is the oxygen–to–air entrainment ratio for 60%?

_____

99. What is the total flow in the system described in this case?

_____

There must be some reason why this chapter is so long. The NBRC will expect you to know about all types of delivery systems and when to use them. You should know when oxygen is indicated and recognize and minimize potential hazards and complications. The Entry-Level Exam and Registry Exams will expect you to know most of the material in this chapter! Specialty gases, blenders, and oxygen devices are all included in addition to changing flow, mode, F_IO_2, and assessing the patient. Answer the following questions. Circle the best answer.

100. During a suctioning procedure a patient experiences tachycardia with PVCs. Which of the following could be responsible for this response?
    A. inadequate vacuum pressure
    B. lack of sterile technique during the procedure
    C. fear of the suctioning procedure
    D. inadequate preoxygenation

101. A patient with a history of carbon dioxide retention is receiving oxygen at 6 L/min via nasal cannula. He is becoming lethargic and difficult to arouse. In regard to the oxygen delivery, what change would you recommend?
    A. Change to a 40% Venturi mask.
    B. Maintain the present therapy.
    C. Change to a partial rebreathing mask.
    D. Reduce the flow to 2 L/min and obtain an ABG.

102. A newborn requires oxygen therapy. Which of the following methods of delivery would you select?
    A. partial rebreathing mask
    B. oxygen hood
    C. Venturi mask
    D. oxygen tent

103. A patient is receiving oxygen therapy from a nonrebreathing mask with a flow rate of 10 L/min. The respiratory therapist observes the bag deflating with each inspiration. What action is indicated in this situation?
    A. Replace the mask with a cannula.
    B. Immediately perform pulse oximetry.
    C. Increase the flow to the mask.
    D. Change to a Venturi mask.

104. A patient is to receive a mixture of helium and oxygen. Which of the following delivery devices would be appropriate?
    A. nasal cannula
    B. oxygen tent
    C. Venturi mask
    D. nonrebreathing mask

105. An 80/20 mixture of helium and oxygen is administered. An oxygen flowmeter is set at 10 L/min. What is the actual flow delivered to the patient?
    A. 10 L
    B. 14 L
    C. 16 L
    D. 18 L

106. A patient is receiving 40% oxygen via an air-entrainment mask with the flowmeter set at 8 L/min. What is the total flow delivered to the patient?
    A. 24 L/min
    B. 32 L/min
    C. 40 L/min
    D. 48 L/min

107. Water has accumulated in the delivery tubing of an aerosol system. This will result in all of the following *except*
_____.
   A. increased F_IO_2
   B. decreased aerosol output
   C. increased total flow
   D. increased back-pressure in the system

108. A patient requires a flow rate of 40 L/min to meet his inspiratory demand for gas. He is to receive oxygen via a Venturi mask set at 24%. What is the minimum setting on the flowmeter to produce the appropriate flow?
   A. 1 L/min
   B. 2 L/min
   C. 3 L/min
   D. 4 L/min

FOOD FOR THOUGHT

109. Why does common use of the term "100% nonrebreather" create a clinical problem?

110. Why would an AEM be preferred over an air-entrainment nebulizer for a patient who has asthma or COPD?

Chapter **38** **Medical Gas Therapy**

39 Lung Expansion Therapy

Cheer the patient up by having someone tell him jokes.
(Postoperative instruction to surgical residents in medieval text.)
A. De Mondeville, 1260-1320

Postoperative complications are dreaded by everyone involved: surgeons, nurses, third-party payers, and, yes, even patients. Postoperative pulmonary complications have been recognized as a problem for as long as surgery has been around, and respiratory therapists have been at the forefront of the battle against atelectasis (incomplete expansion) and retained secretions for many years. Anesthesia, pain, medications, and preexisting lung disease are the enemy. Fortunately, we have a powerful arsenal of lung expansion devices and treatments on our side. (In addition to telling jokes to the patient.)

WORD WIZARD

One of the problems associated with lung expansion therapy is explaining the goals, procedures, and equipment so the patient can understand. For each of the following terms or treatments, give a simple, short explanation in lay terms that even your kid brother could understand.

1. Atelectasis: "When you don't take deep breaths…"

   _____

2. Incentive spirometer (IS):

   A. "The purpose of this treatment is to…"

   _____

   B. "This device will…" _____

3. Sustained maximal inspiration (SMI): "I want you to take…"

   _____

4. Intermittent positive-pressure breathing (IPPB)

   A. "Your doctor has ordered a breathing treatment that will help you…"

   _____

   B. "This machine will…" _____

5. Continuous positive airway pressure (CPAP)

   A. "This treatment will…" _____

   B. "I am going to put a mask on your face…"

   _____

   In fact, maybe you should try out your explanations on friends or family members to see if they make sense! Think of it as a play and act your part.

Answer the following questions to test your understanding of this chapter's objectives.

6. What is the definition of atelectasis?

   _____

7. What is resorption atelectasis, and when is it likely to occur?

8. What causes passive atelectasis?

9. Why are postoperative patients at highest risk for development of atelectasis?

10. What specific group of postoperative patients are at highest risk?

    _____

11. Name two other types of patients who have increased likelihood of developing atelectasis. Explain why.

    A. _____

    B. _____

12. Explain how each of the following may help provide clues that atelectasis is present or likely. (You can use the exact same indicators to tell if the atelectasis is improving after lung expansion therapy, except for the history, of course.)

    A. History

    B. Breath sounds

C. Respiratory rate

D. Heart rate

E. Chest film

13. All modes of lung expansion therapy increase lung volume by increasing the transpulmonary pressure gradient. What are the two methods for increasing the gradient?

A. _____

B. _____

INCENTIVE SPIROMETRY

14. List three indications, two contraindications, and two hazards of incentive spirometry. (See Boxes 39-1, 39-2, and 39-3.)
   A. Indications

   1. _____

   2. _____

   3. _____

   B. Contraindications

   1. _____

   2. _____

   3. _____

   C. Hazards

   1. _____

   2. _____

15. Consider the top two complications. What are your ideas about dealing with these problems?

A.

B.

IPPY-BIPPY

Seriously, it was called ippy-bippy. Intermittent positive pressure breathing (IPPB) is a time-honored way to pump someone up. That means ancient. Still, for the right patient this machine works well. It is also expensive, complicated, and intimidating to students! IPPB was first described by Motley in 1947 following its use in aviation medicine during the war.

16. Give a brief general idea of how it works to inflate the lung when the patient cannot take a deep breath.

_____

17. Like IS, IPPB is used to treat atelectasis. Specifically, when would IPPB be indicated compared with IS?

18. What is the one absolute contraindication to IPPB?

19. List at least five additional partial contraindications.

A. _____

B. _____

C. _____

D. _____

E. _____

20. Name two common complications of IPPB administration.

    A. _____

    B. _____

21. What outcomes will tell you that your IPPB therapy has been effective? Name at least four. Try Box 39-8 if you get lost.

    A. _____

    B. _____

    C. _____

    D. _____

PUMP 'EM UP WITH POSITIVE AIRWAY PRESSURE

22. Name the three current PAP therapies. Which one is the best?

    A. _____

    B. _____

    C. _____

    D. The best one is... _____

23. Physiologic effects of CPAP are poorly understood but probably include:

    A. _____

    B. _____

    C. _____

    D. _____

24. Name two contraindications to CPAP therapy.

    A. _____

    B. _____

25. The text suggests the major complications of this therapy. Discuss each of the following problems.

    A. Hypoventilation:

B. Barotrauma:

C. Gastric distention:

26. What alarm system is essential for monitoring patients receiving continuous mask CPAP?

27. Adequate flow is important to maintain CPAP levels. How does the author suggest you determine the initial setting?

Look at Figure 39-7 in *Egan's*.

To operate this simple PAP generator, you use flows of 5 to 15 L/min and the patient breathes as coached. Whether you use commercial CPAP/flow generators or your institution makes a continuous flow system, the methodology is sound and the patients breathe *spontaneously*.

SUMMARY CHECKLIST

Complete the following sentences by writing in the correct term(s) in the blank(s) provided.

28. Atelectasis is caused by persistent _____ with _____ tidal volumes.

29. Patients who have undergone upper _____ or _____ surgery are at the greatest risk for atelectasis.

30. A history of _____ disease or _____ are additional risk factors.

31. The chest _____ is often used to confirm the presence of atelectasis.

32. Patients with atelectasis usually demonstrate _____ _____ breathing.

33. The most common problem associated with lung expansion therapy is the onset of respiratory _____, which occurs when the patient breathes _____.

Use the protocol found in Figure 39-8 and the section on "selecting an approach" to help answer the following questions.

Case 1

An alert, 34-year-old man is admitted for a hernia repair. He smokes 2 packs of cigarettes per day. Following surgery, the physician asks for your recommendation for therapy to prevent lung complications. The patient's vital capacity is 1.4 L and he weighs 80 kg with ideal body weight. He complains of cough but produces no sputum.

34. Discuss potential risk factors for atelectasis in this case.

_____

35. What therapy would you recommend for prevention of atelectasis for this patient?

_____

Case 2

A 70-year-old 5 foot 2 inch female patient is immobilized following hip replacement. Her predicted inspiratory capacity is 1.8 L. She is performing incentive spirometry at 500 ml per breath. Breath sounds reveal bilateral basilar crackles, and she is coughing up lots of thick mucus.

36. What is the minimum acceptable volume for incentive spirometry for this patient according to her predicted IC and her measured volume?

_____

37. What treatment would you recommend adding to the therapeutic regimen at this time?

_____

Case 3

An obese, mildly confused 59-year-old woman is recovering from CABG (open-heart surgery). The patient has persistent atelectasis with mild hypoxemia. Her radiograph shows an elevated left hemidiaphragm with air bronchograms in the left base. Vital capacity is 10 ml/kg ideal body weight. She has no prior lung disease, and is not coughing up any mucus.

38. What is the significance of the elevated diaphragm and air bronchograms seen on the chest film?

39. What treatment would you recommend? Why? What's the minimum goal for this therapy?

Lung expansion techniques like IS, IPPB, and CPAP are important parts of your board examinations. PEP is usually discussed under secretion management. The main difference between the CRT and RRT exams is the difficulty level of the questions. For example, the CRT exam is more likely to ask you to recall facts or apply them. The RRT exam asks more difficult questions that ask you to analyze information. Lung inflation is a very rich topic for the boards:

- Assessment items: crackles, air bronchograms, elevated diaphragm
- Diagnostic studies: chest radiographs, oxygenation
- Equipment: spirometer, IPPB, circuit, disinfection
- Mathematics, communication, instructing the patient, and more!

Here are a few practice questions. Circle the best answer.

40. A patient complains of a "tingling" feeling in her lips during an incentive spirometry treatment. The RT should instruct the patient to _____.
    A. breathe more slowly
    B. take smaller breaths
    C. continue with the treatment as ordered
    D. exhale through pursed lips after each breath

41. Which of the following alarms are a vital part of the system when setting up CPAP therapy for treatment of atelectasis?
    A. exhaled volume
    B. high respiratory rate
    C. pulse oximetry
    D. low pressure

42. During administration of IPPB therapy, the practitioner observes the system pressure rise up suddenly at the end of inspiration. The RT should instruct the patient to _____.
    A. "Help the machine give you a deep breath."
    B. "Inhale slowly along with the machine."
    C. "Exhale gently and normally."
    D. "Exhale through pursed lips after each breath."

43. A patient is having difficulty initiating each breath with an IPPB machine. The practitioner should adjust the _____.
    A. pressure limit
    B. peak flow
    C. F_IO_2
    D. sensitivity

44. Which control is used to increase the volume delivered by an IPPB machine?
    A. pressure limit
    B. peak flow
    C. F_IO_2
    D. sensitivity

45. Continuous positive airway pressure is used to increase which of the following?
    A. functional residual capacity
    B. peak expiratory flow rate
    C. FEV_1
    D. arterial carbon dioxide levels

46. An IPPB machine cycles on with the patient effort but does not shut off. The most likely cause of this problem is _____.
    A. The pressure is set too low.
    B. The sensitivity is set incorrectly.
    C. There is a leak in the system.
    D. The patient is not blowing out hard enough.

47. How should you instruct a patient to breathe during incentive spirometry?
   A. "Exhale gently, then inhale rapidly through the spirometer."
   B. "Inhale deeply and rapidly through the spirometer."
   C. "Exhale until your lungs are empty, then inhale and hold your breath."
   D. "Exhale normally, then inhale slowly and deeply and hold your breath."

48. How often should a patient be instructed to use the incentive spirometer after being taught to perform the procedure correctly?
   A. 10 breaths, four times per day
   B. 6 to 10 breaths every hour
   C. 10 to 20 breaths every 2 hours
   D. 6 to 8 breaths three times daily

49. A patient who has had surgery for an abdominal aortic aneurysm suffers from arrhythmias and hypotension after surgery. The physician asks for your recommendation for lung expansion therapy. The best choice in this situation would be _____.
   A. IS
   B. IPPB
   C. PEP
   D. CPAP

50. When adjusting the flow rate control on an IPPB machine, the RT would be altering the _____.
   A. maximum pressure delivered by the device
   B. effort required to initiate a breath
   C. volume delivered by the machine
   D. inspiratory time for a given breath

To get good at lung expansion therapy you will need to get out the equipment and practice in the lab. All of these treatments can be delivered to classmates in practice sessions until you are skilled with the devices, the coaching, and the breathing circuits. Some students say the hardest part is learning to explain and coach therapy, not the equipment!

FOOD FOR THOUGHT

51. A really interesting topic in critical care is how best to reinflate the acutely restricted or atelectatic lung. "Lung recruitment maneuvers" is the correct name. Why don't you search out that one and explain briefly, in your own terms, how a lung recruitment maneuver is done.

40 Airway Clearance Therapy

Sputum is *our bread and butter.*
Anonymous Respiratory Therapist

After medical gas administration, playing with sputum is what makes our profession famous (or infamous). (Picture asking a man to "cough it up" while turning your head away to gag.) Eventually you will get used to that lovely rattling sound. The halls are alive with the sound of mucus, and secretion management awaits!

WORD WIZARD

Acronyms Again?

After you've read Chapter 40 (You have read it, right?), you will have noticed an awful lot of acronyms (check out Table 40-3). Let's get those out of the way before we dive into bronchial hygiene. Write the definition for each of these mystic medical markings.

1. ACBT _____

2. PEP _____

3. AD _____

4. PDPV _____

5. CPT _____

6. CPAP _____

7. EPAP _____

8. FET _____

9. HFCWC _____

10. HZ _____

11. ICP _____

12. IPV _____

13. MI-E _____

MEET THE OBJECTIVES

The objectives for this chapter fall into two basic parts: the rationale for secretion clearance and the techniques. We'll start with the fundamentals.

Normal lungs generate a modest amount of mucus from the goblet cells, glands, and Clara cells. The mucociliary escalator whips that stuff up and out in no time. You hardly even notice. Of course, things go wrong. That's where RTs come in.

14. Name the four phases of the normal cough. Give examples of impairments for each (Table 40-1).

Phase   **Impairments**

A. _____   _____

B. _____   _____

C. _____   _____

D. _____   _____

15. Compare the effects of full and partial airway obstruction caused by retained secretions.

A. Full obstruction, or _____ plugging, results in _____.

B. Partial obstruction increases _____ of breathing and leads to air _____.

16. Just for fun, state the airflow velocities and rise in lung pressures created by a good strong cough.

A. Expiratory velocity: _____ miles per hour!

B. Pleural/alveolar pressure: _____ mm Hg

DISEASE AND BAD CLEARANCE

17. Name at least three conditions that may cause internal obstruction or external compression of the airway lumen (opening).

A. _____

B. _____

C. _____

18. Name two obstructive lung diseases that result in excessive secretion of mucus and impairment of normal clearance.

A. _____

B. _____

19. List four neurologic or musculoskeletal conditions that impair cough.

A. _____

B. _____

C. _____

D. _____

SECRETION MANAGEMENT: GOALS AND INDICATIONS

Obviously getting the gunk out of the lungs is the main idea, but there's more to it, of course! The big picture is made up of acute conditions, chronic disorders, prevention, and assessment.

20. Name four acute conditions in which bronchial hygiene is indicated.

A. _____

B. _____

C. _____

D. _____

21. Explain why you think bronchial hygiene is not useful in treating most cases of pneumonia or uncomplicated asthma.

22. Discuss bronchial hygiene therapy for chronic lung conditions. How much sputum needs to be produced daily for the therapy to be useful? What are three typical diseases that we treat?

23. Describe the two well-documented preventive, or prophylactic, uses of this type of therapy.

A.

B.

24. In order to determine the need for bronchial hygiene therapy, you would assess the patient and the medical record. Give a brief explanation of the significance of each factor listed below (see Box 40-3).

Factor	Significance
A. History	_____
B. Airway	_____
C. Chest radiograph	_____
D. Breath sounds	_____
E. Vital signs	_____

BRONCHIAL HYGIENE METHODS

There are five general noninvasive approaches to managing secretion problems. Within each general approach are several choices. You will need to customize therapy for each patient based on cost, effectiveness, clinical condition, and ability to participate in therapy.

Postural Drainage

25. Kinetic therapy has many pulmonary benefits. Name two *non*pulmonary benefits.

A. _____

B. _____

26. Postural drainage therapy includes up to four components, not counting cough. What are they?

A. _____

B. _____

C. _____

D. _____

Exercise: Learn Those Pesky Positions!

Here are some suggestions for ways to learn the positions for chest drainage:

- Photocopy Figure 40-2, *Patient Positions for Postural Drainage*. Cut out each position, and cut off the heading that names the position. Tape the picture to the front of a 3 × 5 index card and the title (lung segment) to the back. Flash cards are a good visual learning tool.
- Get a partner (two partners works better) and a hospital bed (can be in the lab or the medical center).
  1. One person should name a lung segment.
  2. Position your partner in what you think is the correct position.
  3. Check the position to see if you got it right or have a third person check. This way you will physically learn the positions and have to move someone around, add pillows, etc.

Since there are about 12 different positions for the 18 lung segments, you will need to spend 30 to 45 minutes on this exercise. You will need to repeat this at least two or three times before you have the positioning and related segments rock solid in your memory. It will pay off when you get tested…

P.S. If you don't have a partner, use a mannequin.

---

27. List two absolute and two relative contraindications to turning.

A. Absolute

1. _____

2. _____

B. Relative

1. _____

2. _____

28. How long should you wait to schedule postural drainage after a patient eats? Why?

_____

29. What is the minimum range of time for effective application of postural drainage therapy?

_____

30. Give two recommended interventions for each of the complications of postural drainage listed below (check out Table 40-2).

Complication	Interventions
A. Hypoxemia	_____
B. Increased ICP	_____
C. Acute hypotension	_____
D. Pulmonary bleeding	_____
E. Vomiting	_____
F. Bronchospasm	_____
G. Cardiac dysrhythmias	_____

31. Discuss vigorous cough efforts in relationship to position and postural drainage.

32. How long does it take to determine the effectiveness of postural drainage? If therapy is effective, how often should you reevaluate in the hospital? In the home?

A. How long? _____

B. Reevaluate hospital patients? _____

C. Reevaluate home patients? _____

33. Describe at least five factors that must be documented after each postural drainage treatment:

A. _____

B. _____

C. _____

D. _____

E. _____

34. Describe percussion and vibration as techniques to loosen secretions. Are they really effective?

35. Compare manual and machine methods of percussion and vibration.

Cough It Up

Bronchial hygiene therapy is frustrating and sometimes useless if you can't get the patient to make an effective cough. Directed cough, cough staging, huff coughing, autogenic drainage, and active cycle of breathing are all really good tools you'll want to have in your bag of tricks. Each patient may require a combination of hygiene and coughing techniques. The latest research suggests that cough and other clearance techniques are the most important part of bronchial hygiene.

36. How would you position a patient (ideally) for an effective cough? (Don't forget the part about the legs—try it!)

37. Standard directed cough must frequently be modified. Give three examples of types of patients who may need modified cough techniques.

A. _____

B. _____

C. _____

38. What is splinting? _____

39. What special form of cough assistance is used with patients who have neuromuscular conditions?

_____

40. Describe the forced expiratory technique (FET).

41. Describe the three repeated cycles of the ACB technique.

A. _____

B. _____

C. _____

42. What is the primary problem with autogenic drainage?

_____

43. Describe the two cycles of MI-E in terms of time and pressure.

A. Inspiratory:

B. Expiratory:

Positive Airway Pressure

44. Positive airway pressure is a popular way to help mobilize secretions. What are the four indications for PAP adjuncts according to the AARC Clinical Practice Guidelines?

    A. _____

    B. _____

    C. _____

    D. _____

45. What type of monitoring is essential regardless of the equipment used to deliver positive airway pressure to help mobilize secretions?

High-Frequency Compression/Oscillation of the Chest Wall

46. Describe the two general approaches to oscillation.

    A. _____

    B. _____

47. What do you think are the primary problems with vests and shells? What group of patients most commonly uses the vest?

    _____

48. Describe the way IPV delivers gas to the airway.

49. Describe at least four of the benefits or advantages of the flutter valve as a secretion management tool.

    A. _____

    B. _____

    C. _____

    D. _____

Mobilization and Exercise

Early mobilization and frequent position changes are standards of care in preventing pulmonary complications after surgery or trauma.

50. Describe the benefits of adding exercise as a mobilization technique.

51. What should you specifically monitor when exercising patients with lung problems?

CASE STUDIES

Case 1

Refer to Figure 40-12 for some clues.

A 60-year-old professor who has had a colon resection for an intestinal tumor is receiving incentive spirometry to help expand his lungs. You are asked to assess the patient for retained secretions. Auscultation reveals coarse rhonchi bilaterally in the upper lobes. A few scattered crackles are heard in the bases. SpO_2 on room air is 94%. The patient states he is unable to cough up anything "because it hurts too much."

52. What technique could you use to decrease the pain associated with cough in a postoperative patient?

_____

53. What type of cough would you teach him?

_____

Case 2

A 75-year-old woman with bronchiectasis states she coughs up "cups of awful mucus every day." She is admitted with a diagnosis of pneumonia.

54. What therapy is indicated while this patient is in the hospital?

_____

As you provide the therapy, you find out that the patient is a widow who lives alone. She takes albuterol treatments via SVN when she has difficulty breathing.

55. What therapy alternatives could you recommend for home use?

_____

399

Remove Bronchopulmonary Secretions

- Conduct therapeutic procedures to remove bronchopulmonary secretions.
- Instruct and encourage proper coughing, AD, PEP, IPV, HFCWO and flutter.
- Perform postural drainage, percussion, and/or vibration (use vibrators, percussors).

The only real difference between CRT and RRT is the difficulty level of the questions, not the actual content.

Here's a sample of what you can expect. Circle the best answer.

56. During the initial treatment, a PEP device is set to deliver a pressure of 15 cm H_2O. The patient complains of dyspnea and can only maintain exhalation for a short period of time. Which of the following should the RT recommend?
    A. Decrease the PEP level to 10 cm H_2O.
    B. Increase the PEP level to 20 cm H_2O.
    C. Discontinue the PEP therapy.
    D. Add a bronchodilator to the PEP therapy.

57. A patient is lying on her left side, one-quarter turn toward her back, with the head of the bed down. What division of the lung is being drained?
    A. lateral segments of the right lower lobe
    B. right middle lobe
    C. left upper lobe, lingular segments
    D. posterior segment of the right upper lobe

58. A patient is receiving postural drainage in the Trendelenburg position. The patient begins to cough uncontrollably. What action should the RT take at this time?
    A. Encourage the patient to use a huff cough.
    B. Administer oxygen therapy.
    C. Administer a bronchodilator.
    D. Raise the head of the bed.

59. In explaining the therapeutic goal of PEP therapy to a patient, it would be most appropriate to say _____.
    A. "This will help prevent pneumonia."
    B. "This will increase your intrathoracic pressure."
    C. "This will help you cough more effectively."
    D. "This will prevent atelectasis."

60. A COPD patient with left lower lobe infiltrates is unable to tolerate a head-down position for postural drainage. What action would you recommend?
    A. Perform the drainage with the head of the bed raised.
    B. Do not perform the therapy until 2 hours after the last meal.
    C. Administer a bronchodilator prior to the postural drainage.
    D. Notify the physician and suggest a different secretion management technique.

61. Active patient participation is an important part of which of the following procedures?
    1. postural drainage
    2. directed cough techniques
    3. airway suctioning
    4. positive expiratory pressure (PEP)
        A. 1 and 2
        B. 2 and 4
        C. 1 and 3
        D. 3 and 4

62. An RT is preparing a patient with bronchiectasis for discharge. Which of the following techniques would be most appropriate for self-administered therapy in the home?
    A. IPPB
    B. flutter
    C. suctioning
    D. percussion and postural drainage

FOOD FOR THOUGHT

63. How does hydration affect secretion clearance? What respiratory therapy modality can augment hydration of the airway?

64. Your text mentions never clapping directly over the spine or clavicles. Can you think of other places you should not clap? Use your imagination! (Could you get fired for clapping on certain parts of the anatomy?) So where *exactly* should you clap?

One more thing! When a patient has lung disease in only one lung, or "unilateral lung disease," positioning is very important. The rule of thumb is **down with the good lung.** When you put the good lung down, gravity takes the blood flow to the best ventilation. IF you put the bad lung down, perfusion goes to the bad lung and oxygenation can significantly worsen. There are some exceptions: lung abscess, PIE, and internal bleeding may require you to put the bad lung down. Otherwise, watch your patients for signs of distress if you turn them so the diseased lung is down!

41 Respiratory Failure and the Need for Ventilatory Support

There's no success like failure, and failure's no success at all.
Bob Dylan

Chapter 41 is short, sweet, and essential to your understanding of why patients need mechanical ventilation. Remember, 35% of all the patients diagnosed with acute respiratory failure die in the hospital! When you understand the material in this chapter, you will be ready to tackle the very complex and difficult subject of mechanical ventilation and critical care. Chapter 41 is really the gateway to becoming a registered respiratory therapist (RRT). The National Board for Respiratory Care (NBRC) places a special emphasis on the material in Section VI. Work hard on this chapter and it will help you pass your boards, and perhaps that 35% will have a better chance at survival.

WORD WIZARD

Here is a brief exercise to help with the new terms you need to know. Match the definitions to these seven concepts.

_____ Auto-PEEP

_____ Barotrauma

_____ Dynamic hyperinflation

_____ Type I respiratory failure

_____ Type II respiratory failure

_____ Respiratory alternans

_____ Work of breathing

A. Switching from abdominal to ribcage breathing
B. Another term for dynamic hyperinflation
C. The oxygen is too low
D. The carbon dioxide is too high
E. The physiologic cost of increased dead space and resistance
F. Hyperinflation, elevated airway pressures, and procedures lead to this harmful outcome
G. Low rates, high flows, and moderate volumes avoid this harmful outcome

SO, WHAT COULD GO WRONG?

1. Complete this sentence: "Put simply, respiratory failure is the _____ ."

2. What are the blood gas criteria for respiratory failure? _____

   A. PaO_2: _____

   B. $PaCO_2$: _____

3. What are the two general types of respiratory failure based on the type of physiologic impairment?

   A. Type I: _____

   B. Type II: _____

Chapter **41** Respiratory Failure and the Need for Ventilatory Support

Egan's lists seven causes of hypoxemia. Of these, decreased F_IO_2, diffusion defect, and perfusion/diffusion impairment are not commonly seen in the acute care setting. $\dot{V}/\dot{Q}$ mismatch, shunt, venous admixture, and hypoventilation are common.

- $\dot{V}/\dot{Q}$ mismatch is usually a result of poorly ventilated areas that still get blood flow. A typical example would be bronchospasm.
- Shunt occurs when there is no ventilation at all. A typical example would be pneumonia or ARDS.
- Hypoventilation occurs in an essentially normal lung when CO_2 displaces O_2. A typical example would be a drug overdose.
- Venous admixture is a low oxygen level in the blood returning to the vena cava/lungs. A typical example would be CHF with low cardiac output or low hemoglobin.

It's not too hard to tell these conditions apart.

- $\dot{V}/\dot{Q}$ mismatch responds to oxygen therapy.
- Shunt does not respond to oxygen therapy.
- Hypoventilation presents with a normal A-a gradient and responds to . . . ventilation!
- Venous admixture needs more cardiac output/more hemoglobin to deliver the Os.

4. What is the classic blood gas presentation of acute hypoxemic respiratory failure due to $\dot{V}/\dot{Q}$ mismatch or shunt? (Remember this one; it will show up to haunt you on the boards! Check out the Mini-Clini "Differentiating Causes of Hypoxemia" for some help.)

_____

5. What is the relationship between $PaCO_2$ and alveolar ventilation?

6. *Egan's* states that there are three major groups of disorders responsible for acute hypercapnic respiratory failure (Type II). Give two examples of specific disorders representative of each category. Table 41-2 provides a complete list.

A. Decreased ventilatory drive

1. _____

2. _____

B. Respiratory muscle fatigue/failure

1. _____

2. _____

C. Increased work of breathing

1. _____

2. _____

7. Give an example of a condition that could cause greatly increased CO_2 production.

_____

8. How does the body compensate for chronically elevated carbon dioxide levels associated with COPD or obesity

hypoventilation syndrome? _____

9. What happens to the normal blood gas classification of respiratory failure in patients with chronic respiratory failure?

10. Identify the five most common factors that lead to acute-on-chronic failure.

A. _____

B. _____

C. _____

D. _____

E. _____

11. Name four treatment goals for this group of patients.

A. _____

B. _____

C. _____

D. _____

12. The complications from treating acute respiratory failure are as life threatening as the failure itself! Identify the likely causes of these pulmonary complications.

A. Emboli _____

B. Barotrauma _____

C. Infection _____

13. Give one example of each of these nonpulmonary complications of life in the ICU.

A. Cardiac _____

B. Gastrointestinal _____

C. Renal _____

Chapter **41** **Respiratory Failure and the Need for Ventilatory Support**

14. Oh, go ahead; tell me three more complications associated with prolonged visits to the unit.

A. _____

B. _____

C. _____

TUBE 'EM

15. What is the primary goal of mechanical ventilation?

_____

16. Your board exams will expect you to identify these classic criteria for mechanical ventilation. Remember that no one criterion mandates ventilation (except apnea). See Table 41-3.

Mechanism	Normal and Critical Values
A. $PaCO_2$	_____
B. pH	_____
C. VC (ml/kg)	_____
D. MIP	_____
E. MVV	_____
F. V_E	_____
G. V_D/V_T	_____
H. $P(A - a)O_2$ on 100%	_____
I. P/F ratio	_____

You need to learn these values! Make flash cards. Make a memory matrix. Just do it.

17. Oxygenation indices like P/F ratio and A-a gradient are useful in determining the severity of failure. What P/F ratio is considered an indicator of profoundly impaired oxygenation? Hint: see Table 41-3 and consider checking other sections in *Egan's* on oxygenation.

18. Why is it useful to consider pH when evaluating carbon dioxide levels to determine the need to intubate and ventilate a patient?

_____

406

19. Define "MIP" and give the minimal value for most patients.

    A. _____

    B. _____

20. State the three types of muscle fatigue and give the cause.

    A. _____

    B. _____

    C. _____

21. Respiratory *muscle weakness* is most likely to occur in what patient group?

    _____

22. Name three conditions that frequently lead to respiratory *muscle fatigue.*

    A. _____

    B. _____

    C. _____

STRATEGIES

Noninvasive ventilation is our best new strategy for supporting patients in failure. Chapter 45 will cover this in-depth. Here's an overview.

23. Define *noninvasive ventilation.*

24. NIV can blow off the CO_2 and improve the Os via several mechanisms. List at least three.

    A. _____

    B. _____

    C. _____

25. NIV is useful for treating COPD with respiratory failure. State two benefits of this therapy.

    A. When is NIV useful for COPD?

B. When is it less effective?

C. Do COPD patients actually tolerate this procedure?

26. What cardiac condition is also treated by NIV?

27. Briefly discuss the use of NIV in respiratory failure with asthma.

28. Is NIV useful for treating ALI and ARDS? What does the evidence show? (Good and bad!)

29. Why is NIV unlikely to help with obesity hypoventilation syndrome?

30. What about NIV for patients who have progressive neuromuscular disorders like ALS? Please discuss.

Invasive ventilatory support is accomplished with an artificial airway and a mechanical ventilator. These methods are the traditional ways we manage respiratory failure and are quite effective. You must consider that noninvasive ventilation simply doesn't work well with patients who have upper airway problems, excess secretions, and poor mask fit. Others simply can't tolerate the mask. However, the most common time we need to be more aggressive is when the condition is expected to resolve slowly and the patient will need to be supported longer than a mask can be worn tightly strapped to the face.

31. Name the three variables you will set in volume ventilation.

    A. _____

    B. _____

    C. _____

32. Name the three set variables in pressure ventilation

    A. _____

    B. _____

    C. _____

33. What two variables are always set by the operator regardless of volume or pressure modes?

    A. _____

    B. _____

34. List the three unusual methods of ventilation listed in the book.

    A. _____

    B. _____

    C. _____

SPECIAL CASES

35. What is the main strategy for reducing lung injury in ARDS according to Chapter 41?

36. How does hyperventilation result in reduced ICP in head injury?

37. What is the target $PaCO_2$ in these cases?

_____

38. What is the chief concern regarding use of PEEP to increase oxygenation in patients with acute head injuries?

39. Air-trapping, or hyperinflation, as a result of obstructive lung disease (COPD, asthma) causes what two complications in mechanically ventilated patients?

A. _____

B. _____

40. How are tidal volume and flow rate manipulated to reduce complications in mechanically ventilated COPD patients?

A. Tidal volume _____

B. Flow rate _____

41. What surprising technique was found to reduce auto-PEEP?

_____

42. What is the specific goal in regard to CO_2 in respiratory failure in the chronic hypercapnic patient with COPD?

SUMMARY CHECKLIST

Complete the following sentences by writing in the correct term(s) in the blank(s) provided.

43. Acute respiratory failure is identified by a $PaCO_2$ > _____ mm Hg and/or a

PaO_2 < _____ mm Hg in an otherwise healthy individual (at sea level, of course).

44. _____ respiratory failure is usually due to $\dot{V}/\dot{Q}$ mismatch or intrapulmonary

_____, or _____.

45. _____ respiratory failure results from inadequate drive, respiratory

muscle _____, or excessive work of _____.

46. Chronic respiratory failure may be represented by ABGs demonstrating _____ with

evidence of metabolic compensation or _____ reflecting chronic hypoxemia.

47. The _____ status of the patient is the most important factor determining the need for ventilator support.

48. Excessive _____ is the most common cause of respiratory muscle fatigue.

49. Only patients with rapidly reversible conditions should undergo _____ ventilation in the acute setting.

50. The goal of therapy in acute hypercapnic respiratory failure is to guarantee a set _____ ventilation.

CASE STUDIES

Case 1

An alert, anxious 25-year-old woman presents in the emergency department complaining of chills, fever, and shortness of breath. An arterial blood gas is drawn on room air with these results:

pH	7.45
$PaCO_2$	32 mm Hg
PaO_2	50 mm Hg
HCO_3^-	23 mEq/L

51. Interpret this blood gas. _____

52. What is the A-a gradient? _____

53. What type of respiratory failure is present? _____

54. What do you recommend for initial respiratory treatment?

Case 2

A 27-year-old is brought to the emergency department by paramedics following a drug overdose. The patient is obtunded. Blood gases are drawn on room air:

pH	7.24
$PaCO_2$	60 mm Hg
PaO_2	65 mm Hg
HCO_3^-	26 mEq/L

55. Interpret this blood gas. _____

56. What is the A-a gradient? _____

57. What type of respiratory failure is present? _____

58. What is the appropriate initial respiratory treatment in this case?

Chapter **41** **Respiratory Failure and the Need for Ventilatory Support**

An alert 56-year-old man with a history of COPD presents in the emergency department complaining of dyspnea, which has worsened over the last few days. A blood gas is drawn on room air:

pH	7.26
$PaCO_2$	70 mm Hg
PaO_2	50 mm Hg
HCO_3^-	32 mEq/L

59. Interpret this blood gas. _____

60. What is the A-a gradient? _____

61. What type of respiratory failure is present? _____

62. What initial respiratory treatments are indicated? What are we trying to avoid?

WHAT DOES THE NBRC SAY?

The information presented in Chapter 41 forms a fundamental basis for our understanding of respiratory failure. It is highly complex, combining blood gases, pathophysiology, and more. The NBRC is passionate about your understanding of this material and will present you with many similar situations. Assess. Interpret. Recommend. Treat. Modify. When you are working on these problems, always start by interpreting the ABG. Do this in the context of the patient's history. COPD should raise a red flag that suggests you think hard before you interpret or act. Here are some examples. Circle the best answer.

63. An RT is asked to evaluate a lethargic 50-year-old woman who is in respiratory distress following abdominal surgery. She is breathing spontaneously, on a 50% air-entrainment mask, at 32 breaths per minute. ABG results show:

pH	7.28
$PaCO_2$	55 mm Hg
PaO_2	60 mm Hg
HCO_3^-	26 mEq/L

Based on this information, what would you recommend?
A. Provide intubation and mechanical ventilation.
B. Increase the F_IO_2 to 1.
C. Administer IPPB.
D. Administer bronchodilator therapy via SVN.

64. An alert, anxious 60-year-old man with a history of CHF presents in the ED with respiratory distress. Auscultation reveals bilateral inspiratory crackles. He has peripheral edema. ABG results drawn on a partial rebreathing mask show:

pH	7.45
$PaCO_2$	35 mm Hg
PaO_2	40 mm Hg
HCO_3^-	23 mEq/L

The most appropriate therapy for improving oxygenation would be
A. Provide intubation and mechanical ventilation.
B. Administer oxygen therapy via nonrebreathing mask.
C. Administer oxygen therapy via CPAP.
D. Administer bronchodilator therapy via SVN.

65. A man is being mechanically ventilated immediately after surgery for a closed head injury. Settings are:

Tidal volume	700 ml
Rate	10
Mode	AC
F_IO_2	0.40
PEEP	0

ABGs show:

pH	7.37
$PaCO_2$	44 mm Hg
PaO_2	86 mm Hg
HCO_3^-	24 mEq/L

Which of the following ventilator changes would you recommend at this time?
A. Increase the F_IO_2.
B. Decrease the volume.
C. Increase the rate.
D. Increase the PEEP.

66. An adult patient is being mechanically ventilated following respiratory failure. Settings are:

Tidal volume	800 ml
Rate	12
Mode	AC
F_IO_2	0.60
PEEP	3 cm H_2O

ABGs show

pH	7.37
$PaCO_2$	41 mm Hg
PaO_2	43 mm Hg
HCO_3^-	22 mEq/L

Which of the following ventilator changes would you recommend at this time?
A. Increase the F_IO_2.
B. Decrease the volume.
C. Increase the rate.
D. Increase the PEEP.

67. A patient with a history of hypercapnia and COPD is intubated and placed on the ventilator following respiratory failure. 24 hours later, the patient is alert and breathing spontaneously.

Settings are

Tidal volume	800 ml
Rate	12
Mode	CMV (AC)
F_IO_2	0.30
PEEP	0 cm H_2O

ABGs show:

pH	7.48
$PaCO_2$	41 mm Hg
PaO_2	60 mm Hg
HCO_3^-	30 mEq/L

413

Which of the following ventilator changes would you recommend at this time?
A. Decrease the F_IO_2.
B. Decrease the volume.
C. Change to pressure-controlled ventilation (PCV).
D. Change to synchronized intermittent mandatory ventilation (SIMV).

68. A 77-year-old man with COPD is admitted with acute bronchitis. Room air blood gas results show

pH	7.52
$PaCO_2$	45 mm Hg
PaO_2	50 mm Hg
HCO_3^-	36 mEq/L

What intervention would be appropriate at this time?
A. CPAP with 24% oxygen
B. 28% Air entrainment mask
C. nasal cannula at 5 L/min
D. simple mask at 8 L/min

69. CPAP is indicated for treatment of patients with _____.
A. respiratory failure secondary to shunting
B. apnea
C. ventilatory failure with hypercapnia
D. hypoxemia secondary to V/Q mismatch

Between the cases, the chapter, and these questions you should be getting the general idea!

FOOD FOR THOUGHT

Remember Table 41-3, the one about measurable indications for ventilatory support? Your boards expect you to know this information, as part of the decision to intubate and ventilate or as part of the decision to wean.

70. What clinical situations or condition suggests using ABGs to evaluate the need to intubate and ventilate? Compare this with situations better assessed by measures such as VC and MIP.

42 Mechanical Ventilators

Any sufficiently advanced technology is indistinguishable from magic.
Arthur C. Clarke

Once upon a time there were only three modes of ventilation: control, assist-control, and IMV. Ventilators were driven by pistons or bellows and an occasional lightbulb glowed or buzzer sounded when there was a problem. Volume cycled, pressure limited was, well—just exactly what it sounded like. Times have changed. Ventilators cost more than new cars. Whether or not the explosion of technology in ventilator design has improved health care has yet to be determined, but you will have to try to make sense of it anyway.

WORD WIZARD

Match these definitions to the key terms.

Definitions	Terms
1. _____ breath initiated by the ventilator	A. spontaneous breath
2. _____ causes a breath to end	B. control variable
3. _____ manipulated by machine to cause inspiration	C. limit variable
4. _____ controls the magnitude of inspiration	D. cycle variable
5. _____ combination of machine and spontaneous breaths	E. intermittent mandatory ventilation
6. _____ machine breaths only—no spontaneous	F. trigger variable
7. _____ spontaneous breaths only—no machine breaths	G. CMV
8. _____ causes a breath to begin	H. CSV
9. _____ breath initiated and ended by the patient	I. mandatory breath

HOW VENTILATORS WORK

10. What is a ventilator?

11. Describe the desired output of the ventilator in terms of the patient.

12. Identify two settings where ventilators use DC back-up power sources.

    A. _____

    B. _____

13. How are most modern intensive care ventilators powered?

_____

14. Identify one setting where electrical power is undesirable.

_____

15. Other than compressed gas, what mechanisms are used to drive a ventilator?

_____

I'M IN CONTROL

16. What does the output control valve do?

    A. Regulates: _____

    B. Shapes: _____

17. A. Setting an appropriate expiratory time is clinically important to avoid what dangerous condition?

    _____

    B. How many time constants is minimum for safe exhalation? _____

    C. What about pressure control: how many inspiratory time constants do you need to get a good volume?

    _____

18. What are the three variables that ventilators control or manipulate?

    A. _____

    B. _____

    C. _____

19. Identify the five types of control circuits used in ventilators.

    A. _____

    B. _____

    C. _____

    D. _____

    E. _____

20. State two advantages of fluidic control circuits.

    A. _____

    B. _____

416

21. Control variables are how a ventilator manipulates inspiration. Fill in the blanks below to show what is constant and what changes for each control variable.

	CONTROL VARIABLE	CONSTANT	VARIES WITH CHANGES IN LUNGS
A.		Pressure	
B.		Volume	
C.		Flow	

PHASE

22. Describe the basic purpose of the following phase variables in terms of the breathing cycle.

	PHASE VARIABLE	PORTION OF BREATHING CYCLE CONTROLLED
A.	Trigger variable	
B.	Target variable	
C.	Cycle variable	
D.	Baseline variable	

23. Name the three ways to trigger the ventilator.

A. _____

B. _____

C. _____

24. Time triggering divides each minute into segments allotted for each breath. This is the total cycle time. If the rate is 12 breaths per minute, what is the total cycle time? Hint: Divide the minute into 12 equal parts!

25. What is the normal setting range for pressure triggering? Flow triggering?

A. Pressure _____ to _____ cm H_2O

B. Flow _____ to _____ below the baseline flow

26. Which ventilator uses volume triggering?

_____

27. Pressure support ventilation (PSV) is an example of a mode that has a target (pressure) but is cycled off by another variable (flow). Define the term "target variable."

_____

28. Define the term "cycle variable."

_____

29. What is the most common application of pressure cycling?

_____

30. Give the basic idea behind volume cycling.

_____

31. Explain the concept of time cycling.

_____

32. What is the usual cycling parameter for pressure support ventilation?

_____

33. Define the term "baseline variable."

_____

34. What is the effect of PEEP on oxygenation? What about FRC?

_____

35. Explain what is meant by these acronyms. Which is the default value for ventilators?

A. ZEEP: _____

B. NEEP: _____

C. PEEP: _____

MODE

36. Define the phrase "mode of ventilation."

_____

37. You will need to decide on a control variable to end inspiration. What are the two primary ways to end inspiration?

A. _____

B. _____

38. What does "dual control" mean?

_____

39. Define spontaneous and mandatory breaths. Give another term for each.

A. Spontaneous: _____

B. Mandatory: _____

418

40. Explain the basic sequence of ventilation represented by each of these terms.

A. CMV _____

B. CSV _____

C. IMV _____

Recap

- All ventilators offer a mode that intermixes spontaneous breaths with ventilator breaths. This is called intermittent mandatory ventilation (IMV).
- All adult ventilators offer a mode that is machine breaths only. Common names are continuous mandatory ventilation (CMV) and assist-control.
- All adult ventilators offer the choice of volume-controlled ventilator breaths (VC) and pressure-controlled ventilator breaths (PC) for any mode that offers a machine breath.
- All adult ventilators have a mode that is spontaneous breathing without machine breaths. This is called spontaneous or continuous positive airway pressure (CPAP) mode, or continuous spontaneous ventilation (CSV).
- All adult ventilators offer a way to augment spontaneous breaths with a pressure boost. This is called pressure support (PS or PSV). If you want to overcome work caused by the artificial airway you use a special form of pressure support called "tube compensation."
- Some ventilators offer specialized modes like APRV, but this is really pressure-controlled (PC) IMV.

You may enjoy reading about the different controls. Ventilators actually have things like cruise control. Adaptive controls are truly exciting because the ventilator is capable of operating independently from the therapist.

WAVEFORMS

Ventilator waveforms have been around for a long time, but there was a time when you couldn't really see them in action. Most modern ventilators are capable of displaying waveforms graphically so you can apply them clinically. For example, if you see that expiratory flow does not return to baseline before the next breath starts, you know that the patient is not able to exhale completely. You can then adjust the ventilator to allow complete exhalation, or try to treat the problem (by giving a bronchodilator, for example).

There are two ways to help you learn waveforms:

- One method of learning this difficult subject is to practice drawing the waveforms.
- The other way is to go to a ventilator in the classroom or lab setting. Attach the ventilator to a test lung, turn on the graphics, adjust the ventilator to deliver different settings, and look at the waveforms that are produced. It will help you if an instructor is handy to guide you through this procedure!

Once you learn to identify the various waveforms, you can move on to the next step, which is to learn the problem pictures, what they mean clinically, and how to fix the problem.

41. Draw the following flow patterns. Look at Figure 42-11 for help.

A. Rectangular (square) _____

B. Decreasing ramp _____

C. Sinusoidal _____

Most ventilators allow the therapist to select the flow waveform from at least two of these three patterns. The pressure waveform will be determined by the mode you select.

Chapter **42** **Mechanical Ventilators**

What sounds like *Star Trek*™ and looks like an ATM on steroids? Welcome to the console, or interface for your new ventilator. The NBRC "hospital" is pretty accurate in their expectations of your abilities in this area. Just like the medical center, your boards think you should be able to set mode, trigger, targets, cycles, and alarms. Naturally, we'll go more in-depth in the next chapter, so this is your place to get started on the theory.

42. What are the two basic choices for patient triggering?

43. Do ventilators display the alarm events in terms of priorities?

44. What happens when there are a lot of false alarms?

45. What did the studies show in terms of what percentage of alarms are clinically significant?

TYPES OF VENTILATORS

46. Describe the volume and breath rate for conventional ventilation.

47. Give one example of an unconventional ventilator.

48. Describe some of the key features of the critical care ventilator.

49. Discuss high-frequency ventilation.

    A. Airway

    B. Example of a ventilator

    C. Typical rates

50. Discuss high-frequency oscillation

    A. Airway

    B. Example of a ventilator

    C. Typical rates

51. What are the two basic interfaces for the critical care ventilator and the patient?

    A. _____

    B. _____

52. Describe the typical subacute ventilator. Give an example. What's special about the oxygen system?

53. Discuss oxygen and battery issues for the ventilator in the home setting.

54. Give the two basic options for noninvasive ventilators.

A. _____

B. _____

55. Give four clinical reasons to use the noninvasive ventilator.

A. _____

B. _____

C. _____

D. _____

CASE STUDIES

Case 1

A 21-year-old patient is placed on a ventilator following a closed head injury. The physician desires to control this patient's ventilation to achieve a specific CO_2 level in the arterial blood.

56. Would you select volume or pressure ventilation to best achieve this goal?

_____

57. Would you recommend a convention ICU ventilator or high-frequency option?

_____

A 35-year-old woman with asthma is placed on a Puritan-Bennett 840 ventilator in IMV mode. The ventilator is set for volume control ventilation at a rate of 10, the total rate is 28, and alarms are sounding. The graphics and clinical signs show the patient and machine are not in sync.

58. Would you recommend switching to pressure control or maintaining volume control? Explain, please.

WHAT DOES THE NBRC SAY?

Your board exams will ask you some material from this chapter and much more from the applications in Chapter 43. *Here are a few practice questions. Circle the best answer.*

59. A patient with ARDS is being ventilated with the following settings.

    Mode   AC
    V_t 800
    Rate   14
    F_IO_2 80%
    PEEP   15 cm H_2O

    Peak pressures are unacceptably high while oxygenation remains poor. Which of the following changes may be beneficial in this situation?
    A. Change the PEEP to 20 cm H_2O.
    B. Increase the F_IO_2 to 100%.
    C. Initiate high-frequency oscillation ventilation.
    D. Place the patient on BiPAP by mask.

60. A resident asks you to identify which of the basic modes of ventilation on an ICU ventilator will permit spontaneous breathing for a patient with neuromuscular disease. You would select:
    1. CMV
    2. IMV
    3. CSV
        A. 1 and 3
        B. 1 and 2
        C. 2 and 3
        D. 1, 2, and 3

61. A patient in the early stages of ARDS is intubated. The physician states that he wishes to minimize the possibility of volutrauma or barotrauma. Which of the following modes would you recommend?
    A. volume-controlled ventilation
    B. manual ventilation
    C. CPAP
    D. pressure-controlled ventilation

62. An 80-kg (176-lb) patient is being ventilated in volume control mode. During a ventilator check, the therapist notes that the compliance has decreased from 40 ml/cm H_2O to 35 ml/cm H_2O. What effect will this change in compliance have on volume?
    A. no effect
    B. increased minute volume
    C. decreased minute volume
    D. decreased tidal volume

Not all modes are used in all parts of the country. What are your hospitals using? Does practice vary between community hospitals and the trauma center? A good starting point for the new therapist is to learn a lot about the modes that are most commonly used in current practice where you live and where you do your clinical training. For example, if you are being assigned to do clinical in a small hospital where CMV and AC are the main modes, don't go in with the idea that you will implement bilevel mode on the 840 or APRV. Instead, learn as much as you can about the art of using CMV. The best RTs can make the best of whatever mode is used in their institution while acting as resources for the nurses and physicians. They pull the other modes out of their bag of tricks when the opportunity arises, *but only after making themselves experts*. Introducing a new ventilator or new mode of ventilation is fraught with hazards if in-service training doesn't come along with the changes.

43 Physiology of Ventilatory Support

Life is like riding a bicycle. You don't fall off unless you stop pedalling.
Claude Pepper (attributed)

Mechanical ventilation can be a life-sustaining procedure, but it is not natural. There are physiologic consequences to applying positive pressure to the lungs and chest. For better or for worse, we're currently married to this technology and you will need to understand what happens when you connect the patient to the machine.

WORD WIZARD

There aren't too many new words to learn in Chapter 43. Look up the definitions in your glossary and write them out next to the words listed below.

1. barotrauma _____

2. time constant _____

3. biotrauma _____

4. transrespiratory pressure _____

5. patient–ventilator asynchrony _____

6. atelectrauma _____

7. mean airway pressure _____

8. transpulmonary pressure _____

LIFE UNDER PRESSURE

9. Which pressure is responsible for maintaining normal alveolar inflation?

_____

10. Which pressure gradient is required to expand the lungs and chest wall together?

_____

11. Which pressure causes airflow in the airways?

_____

12. What happens to transpulmonary pressure during normal inspiration? Exhalation?

A. Inspiration _____

B. Exhalation _____

13. What happens to transpulmonary pressure during inspiration with a negative pressure ventilator? Exhalation?

   A. Inspiration _____

   B. Exhalation _____

14. What is "tank shock"?

   _____

15. What happens to the airway and pleural pressures during inspiration with a positive pressure ventilator?

   _____

EFFECTS OF MECHANICAL VENTILATION

There are so many effects of mechanical ventilation that we need to break them down into little pieces to understand what happens when you attach that circuit to the ET tube!

16. What is the normal range of tidal volume during spontaneous breathing?

   _____

17. It's important to set a tidal volume on the ventilator based on pathophysiology. What volume would you set for a patient with:

   A. ARDS _____

   B. COPD _____

   C. Normal lungs _____

18. Besides increasing the volume, how can you increase minute ventilation with the ventilator?

   _____

19. What effect does minute ventilation have on $PaCO_2$?

   _____

20. Where is gas distributed by a normal spontaneous breath? What about a positive-pressure breath?

   A. Spontaneous _____

   B. PPV _____

21. How does perfusion, or blood flow, in the lung change during PPV?

   _____

22. What's the net effect of all this redistribution on the $\dot{V}/\dot{Q}$ ratio?

   _____

23. How would poor ventilator management result in respiratory acidosis?

   _____

24. There are several ways you could assess this problem. Explain the importance of each the following:

A. Draw arterial blood _____

B. Check electrolytes _____

C. Check ECG _____

25. How would poor ventilator management result in respiratory alkalosis?

_____

26. There are several ways you could assess this problem. Discuss each of the following:

A. Draw arterial blood _____

B. Check electrolytes _____

C. Check ECG _____

27. Discuss the two methods for treating metabolic acidosis in mechanically ventilated patients. Each can be a *lifesaving maneuver*, so think carefully on this one!

A. Bicarbonate administration

B. Minute ventilation

WHAT ABOUT OXYGENATION?

Remember type I failure? The mechanical ventilator can be used to improve oxygenation through a variety of methods.

28. Explain how mechanical ventilation improves oxygenation for each of the following causes of hypoxemia:

A. Hypoventilation _____

B. $\dot{V}/\dot{Q}$ mismatch _____

C. Shunt _____

29. What range of F_IO_2 can a modern ICU ventilator deliver?

_____

Chapter **43** **Physiology of Ventilatory Support**

30. State the formula for each of the following:

A. DO_2 _____

B. Alveolar air _____

C. Arterial oxygen content _____

D. Minute ventilation _____

31. How is optimal PEEP determined in terms of F_IO_2 and PaO_2?

_____

LUNG MECHANICS

32. How long does it take for 95% of the alveoli in a normal lung to fill with air?

A. Time constants _____

B. Real time _____

What about 98% of alveoli? _____ 99%? _____

33. What are the two major factors that affect alveolar time constants?

A. _____

B. _____

34. Compare a restrictive disorder like ARDS and an obstructive problem like COPD in terms of the time it takes for alveolar filling and emptying. Mark the blanks with an ↑ or ↓ to indicate how you would adjust the ventilator for these two groups of patients.

A. ARDS needs _____ inspiratory time and _____ expiratory time.

B. COPD needs _____ inspiratory time and _____ expiratory time.

C. Asthma needs _____ inspiratory time and _____ expiratory time.

35. You could help prolong the inspiratory phase for your restricted patient by making the following adjustments:

A. Inspiratory time setting should be _____.

B. Inspiratory flow setting should be _____.

36. You could help prolong the expiratory phase for your obstructed patient by making the following adjustments:

A. Inspiratory flow should be _____.

B. Mandatory ventilator rate should be _____.

C. Tidal volume should be _____.

37. What is meant by the term "peak inspiratory pressure"? What's the abbreviation?

_____

38. What is meant by the term "plateau pressure"? What's the symbol?

_____

39. We can protect patient lungs from damage caused by pressure by maintaining plateau pressures at less than

_____ cm H_2O.

40. See if you know how to adjust mean airway pressure. It's a little complicated! Circle "T" for "true" if the choice is one that would *raise the mean airway pressure*.
    A. Increase peak pressure   T   F
    B. Decrease inspiratory time   T   F
    C. Synchronized IMV   T   F
    D. Increase PEEP levels   T   F
    E. Constant pressure pattern (PC mode, $\downarrow$ ramp flow)   T   F

41. How does increasing airway pressure affect the FRC and oxygenation?

    A. FRC _____

    B. Oxygenation _____

42. Does inspiratory positive pressure ventilation by itself increase the FRC? What can you add to maintain this

    capacity? _____

43. What will happen to compliance when too much PEEP is applied? Could you adjust the PEEP based on the changes

    in compliance? _____

44. Your vent patient has atelectasis and needs lung recruitment. You'll want to apply up to _____ cm

    H_2O PEEP for up to _____ to _____ minutes.

45. The pressure-volume curve is useful for establishing the point where the lung begins to open up. Give three names for this "lower" point.

    A. _____

    B. _____

    C. _____

46. Why does dead space increase during mechanical ventilation?

_____

WORK OF BREATHING

Ventilators are intended to decrease the work of breathing. Many patients who are in respiratory failure are exhausted and their breathing muscles need a break to recover.

47. What happens to the diaphragm if the ventilator does the work for too long?

_____

48. What type of triggering reduces WOB in older ventilators? What about newer vents?

_____

49. What inspiratory maneuver can be added to IMV to reduce the work of breathing through the ET tube and ventilator

circuit? _____

50. Since you can't really measure WOB at the bedside, what three variables does the experienced therapist use to determine whether WOB is excessive?

A. _____

B. _____

C. _____

PHYSIOLOGIC EFFECTS OF VENTILATORY MODES

Mechanical ventilation is lifesaving. Unfortunately, it can also damage the lung. The RT is the advocate for the patient's lung tissue!

51. Look at Table 43-2 and give two negative pulmonary effects of too much PEEP.

A. _____

B. _____

52. Why is PEEP a problem with severe unilateral lung disease?

53. Identify two potential harmful effects of controlled CMV.

A. _____

B. _____

54. Name two advantages of IMV.

A. _____

B. _____

55. What is the most common application of VC-CMV?

_____

56. What is the primary reason for using PC-CMV?

_____

57. Compare how flow is set in PC versus VC mode.

_____

58. What are some of the possible benefits of APRV?

_____

59. PSV overcomes airway _____ and improves tidal _____.

60. *Egan's* says that PSV will result in four beneficial effects. Name them.

A. _____

B. _____

C. _____

D. _____

61. In BiPAP, IPAP is the same as _____ and EPAP is the same as _____.

62. Bilevel CPAP was originally developed for treatment of obstructive sleep apnea. It has also been shown to be useful in acute care settings. Explain.

A. COPD _____

B. ARDS _____

63. What is the effect of CPAP on ventilation?

_____

64. Identify the important physiologic effect of CPAP.

_____

65. Explain ASV in terms of

A. Therapist inputs _____

B. Microprocessor controlled _____

66. PAV is designed to improve what important relationship?

_____

67. Automatic tube compensation is not a mode of ventilation. What is it really?

_____

DOWN WITH THE GOOD LUNG!

68. Patients with unilateral lung disease greatly benefit from what type of positioning?

_____

69. What unique position improves oxygenation in ARDS?

_____

NOT JUST THE LUNGS

Amazingly enough, positive pressure ventilation affects almost every important organ system in the body including the heart, kidney, liver, brain, and the gut.

70. Briefly explain the negative effects of PPV on the heart.

_____

71. Why can patients with stiff lungs such as ARDS tolerate higher levels of PEEP in terms of the effect on heart and

blood vessels? _____

72. Normal patients can easily compensate for moderate increases in airway pressure. What patients are especially sensitive to the cardiovascular effects of PPV?

_____

73. Fluids can help a patient tolerate ventilation and so can drugs. Which drug would you use to treat

A. Low cardiac index _____

B. Low blood pressure _____

74. How can you use the ventilator to temporarily manage increased ICP?

_____

75. Explain the mechanism behind the drop in urine output in ventilated patients.

A. Direct _____

B. Indirect _____

76. There is a high incidence in GI bleeding in ventilator patients, usually due to stress ulceration of the gastric mucosa. Name the two pharmacologic agents used to protect the GI tract.

A. Cytoprotective _____

B. Acid suppression _____

432

77. ICP is not the only CNS problem associated with mechanical ventilation. The ICU experience results in fear, anxiety, and pain. Name one sedative and one analgesic that may help.

A. Acute sedation _____

B. Long-term management of anxiety _____

C. Analgesics

    1. Hemodynamically stable _____

    2. Unstable _____

We'd like to get the patient to level 2 or 3 on the Ramsay Scale.

VENTILATOR-INDUCED LUNG INJURY

78. Chest cuirass and poncho-type negative-pressure ventilators are still used in some settings. Hypoventilation can result from what two problems?

A. _____

B. _____

79. Positive pressure ventilation has long been associated with barotrauma. List three of the clinical signs of pneumo-thorax.

A. Chest motion _____

B. Percussion note _____

C. Breath sounds _____

80. Tension pneumothorax is life-threatening in a ventilated patient. How and where is this treated?

A. How?

B. Where in the chest?

81. What is volutrauma, and how is it prevented?

82. Air-trapping in ventilator patients can result in what condition?

_____

83. Oxygen toxicity may damage lung tissue. Every effort should be made to reduce the F_IO_2 to what value?

_____

84. List three ways to reduce the risk of ventilator-associated pneumonias.

A. Positioning _____

B. Nebulizers or MDIs _____

C. Reduce condensates _____

And, of course, the essential antiinfection procedure...

SUMMARY CHECKLIST

Fill in the blanks, thanks.

85. Positive physiologic effects of PPV include improved _____ and ventilation, and decreased

_____ of breathing.

86. No single _____ pattern has been demonstrated to be more physiologically effective than another.

87. Research indicates better ventilator synchrony and gas exchange with the _____ flow pattern than

the _____ flow pattern.

88. _____-triggering appears to be a better choice than _____-triggering when it is
available on the ventilator.

89. PEEP is applied to restore _____ in restrictive disease and _____ the airways in
obstructive disease.

90. PEEP allows the RCP to decrease the _____, thereby avoiding the complications of

_____ toxicity.

91. Positive pressure ventilation is detrimental to the $\dot{V}/\dot{Q}$ ratio primarily by shifting _____ to areas

that are less _____.

92. PPV may decrease venous _____ and cardiac _____.

93. PPV may cause hepatic and gastrointestinal malfunction primarily due to decreased _____ of

those _____ beds.

Case 1, Part 1

A trauma patient is stabilized after a motor vehicle accident. He is intubated and transported to the ICU, where you place him on a ventilator. As soon as you put him on the machine, his blood pressure falls dramatically.

94. What should you do (right away!)?

_____

95. What is the most likely cause of hypotension in a trauma patient who has been

placed on positive pressure ventilation?

_____

Part 2

Two days later, the patient has developed poor lung compliance and hypoxemia associated with noncardiogenic pulmonary edema (ARDS). He is being ventilated on VC-CMV, 12,900, +15 cm H_2O PEEP, and F_1O_2 70%. Blood gases show pH 7.37, $PaCO_2$ 38, and PaO_2 55. Peak inspiratory pressure is 60 cm H_2O, and plateau pressure is 50 cm H_2O.

96. There are two serious problems here. Identify them.

    A. Serious problem No. 1 _____

    B. Serious problem No. 2 _____

97. What change(s) in ventilator strategy would you suggest?

    A. Problem No. 1

    B. Problem No. 2

WHAT DOES THE NBRC SAY?

Not much, actually. Nothing new, that is. Of course you need to be able to recognize the harmful effects of PPV. If the patient develops a pneumothorax, you would assess, recognize, and recommend treatment. Chapter 40 reviews each of the common modes of ventilation, and the board exams are quite clear that you should be familiar with them.

FOOD FOR THOUGHT

98. If the newest modes of ventilation are not proven to alter patient outcomes, why should we use them?

99. Patients on ventilators have a really high incidence of GI bleeding. Why is GI bleeding such a big deal to RTs?

44 Initiating and Adjusting Invasive Ventilatory Support

Paralyze resistance with persistence.
Woody Hayes

A long time ago, in an ICU far, far away, there was a one-size-fits-all approach to mechanical ventilation. It was easier that way, but we did not realize how this could harm the patient. Chapter 44 is one of the best and most important chapters in *Egan's* because it details a clear-cut plan for initiating and managing the ventilator in terms of what's wrong with the patient (i.e., custom-made ventilation). The concept of pathophysiology-based mechanical ventilation is so important that the NBRC included an article on the concept in their newsletter. So, whether you are talking about board exams or clinical practice, this is an important chapter.

FIRST THINGS FIRST

Here is a step-by-step approach. See if it works for you. First, read the chapter and highlight key points. Next, map out a plan. For example:
- **Step One.** Decide whether to use positive or negative pressure. Easy because negative pressure is pretty much used for long-term neuromuscular problems and chest wall disorders. It's used in the hospital only if the patient brings it in.
- **Step Two.** Full ventilator support, or partial support? Pick full support if the patient is apneic or paralyzed by drugs, or exhausted from struggling to breathe. Remember to use this for a short period of time to avoid muscle atrophy. Partial support is good for patients with a drive to breathe, those being weaned, or to minimize adverse effects of positive pressure.
- **Step Three.** Select volume or pressure control. Volume control works pretty well and is especially good when you want to control minute ventilation and $PaCO_2$. Pressure control is great when you need to keep the pressures low to prevent lung injury with ARDS or ALI. PC is also good when you want to let the patient control the flow and volumes. It's more comfortable and flexible.
- **Step Four.** Pick a mode. Assist-control (CMV) and IMV are the most common and best understood of all the modes. Pressure support is almost always added to IMV to help reduce work of breathing.
- **Step Five.** Select settings for ventilation. Rate, volume, F_IO_2, and PEEP should be set according to pathophysiology. Alarm settings are pretty standardized.
- **Step Six.** Assess the patient after you initiate your choices. Make changes to meet your goals for the patient. Comfort and synchrony, gas exchange and hemodynamics—that's what you want to look at.

CASE STUDIES

Let's go right to the cases and find out if you understand how to initiate and adjust ventilatory support. Five basic types of lungs and ten specific disorders make up almost every case of mechanical ventilation.

Table 44-4 is dynamite! It covers most of the bases. Your five basic types of lungs are:
- Normal lungs—like a young OD patient: 8 to 10 ml/kg for tidal volume
- Normal lungs—like a neuromuscular patient: 10 to 12 ml/kg for tidal volume
- Obstructed lungs—like acute exacerbation of COPD or asthma: 8 to 10 ml/kg for tidal volume
- Stiff lungs—like ARDS/ALI: 6 to 8 ml/kg for tidal volume. Can go lower to keep pressures down.
- Kids get 8 to 10 for tidal volume depending on age; on boards, usually 10.

Let's get to work! You will need Tables 44-3, 44-4, and 44-5 to help with the cases. Boxes 44-4, 44-7, 44-10, and 44-12 are good, too. You will also need information from other chapters like airway management, acid-base, and monitoring and management!

A 5 foot 5 inch, 60-kg (132-lb) young woman attempted suicide by drug overdose. She is unconscious and breathing slowly and shallowly. The emergency physician elects to intubate this patient.

1. What size ET tube would be appropriate for an adult female?
   A. 6.0-mm inside diameter
   B. 7.0-mm outside diameter
   C. 7.5-mm inside diameter
   D. 8.0-mm inside diameter

2. In the emergency setting, how will you assess proper tube placement?
   1. Auscultate the chest.
   2. Auscultate the epigastrium.
   3. Attach an exhaled O_2 monitor.
   4. Observe chest wall motion.
      A. 1 and 2
      B. 1 and 3
      C. 2, 3, and 4
      D. 1, 2, and 4

After the intubation is completed, a small amount of white secretions are suctioned from the airway. The physician requests a room air ABG at this point. Results show:

pH	7.25
$PaCO_2$	60 mm Hg
PaO_2	55 mm Hg
HCO_3^-	26 mEq/L

Vital signs are:

HR	115
BP	125/75
RR	26
Temp	37

A chest film is taken, which reveals the tip of the endotracheal tube to be 4 cm above the carina with no sign of a pneumothorax.

3. What action would you recommend in regard to the ET tube placement?
   A. Advance the tube 2 to 3 cm.
   B. Withdraw the tube 2 to 3 cm.
   C. Maintain current placement.
   D. Remove the tube and insert a laryngeal mask airway.

4. The ABG results are interpreted as _____.
   A. metabolic acidosis with severe hypoxemia
   B. respiratory acidosis with moderate hypoxemia
   C. partially compensated respiratory alkalosis with mild hypoxemia
   D. partially compensated metabolic alkalosis with moderate hypoxemia

The patient is transported to the ICU. The physician requests that you initiate mechanical ventilation.

5. Calculate ideal body weight. One formula for women is 105 + 5 (height − 60). The answer will be in pounds, and you need to divide by 2.2 to convert to kilograms. Box 44-8 uses 45.5 + 2.3 (height in inches − 60) to get the answer in kilograms. The answers will be slightly different but this won't change outcomes.
   A. 45 kg
   B. 59 kg
   C. 65 kg
   D. 130 kg

6. Which of the following volumes would you recommend?
   A. 400 ml
   B. 600 ml
   C. 720 ml
   D. 1000 ml

7. What mode and rate would you select?
   A. VC-IMV, 18
   B. VC-CMV, 12
   C. VC-IMV, 6
   D. VC-CMV, 8

8. ·What type of humidification system would you recommend for this patient?
   A. heated wick humidifier set at 35° C
   B. HME
   C. heated passover humidifier
   D. bubble humidifier

One week later, the patient is alert and weaning is initiated. When the rate is decreased to 5, however, the patient's spontaneous respiratory rate rises to 30 and tidal volumes drop to 200 ml.

9. To help resolve this problem you might recommend initiation of _____.
   A. CMV
   B. AC
   C. PSV
   D. APRV

Case 2

Paramedics bring a 5 foot 2 inch, 50-kg (110-lb) 65-year-old woman with a history of COPD to the emergency department for treatment of dyspnea. She is wearing a nasal cannula set at 2 L/min. ABGs are drawn. Results show:

pH	7.30
$PaCO_2$	70 mm Hg
PaO_2	45 mm Hg
HCO_3^-	34 mEq/L

Vital signs are	
HR	100
BP	100/70
RR	34
Temp	39

Noninvasive positive pressure breathing is attempted with bilevel ventilation, but the patient is unable to tolerate the mask and fights the system. A decision is made to intubate and initiate mechanical ventilation. The patient is given a small amount of sedation and intubated nasally with a 6.5-mm ID tube. Settings are:

Mode	VC-SIMV
Rate	10
V_T	400 ml
F_IO_2	28%
PEEP	0
Peak flow	20 LPM
Flow pattern	Decelerating ramp
Sensitivity	1.5 cm H_2O below baseline

439

10. How long should you wait before drawing an ABG to assess the results of these settings?
    A. 5 minutes
    B. 20 minutes
    C. 40 minutes
    D. 60 minutes

11. What is the maximum desirable plateau pressure during mechanical ventilation?
    A. 15 cm H_2O
    B. 25 cm H_2O
    C. 30 cm H_2O
    D. 40 cm H_2O

During your first ventilator check the following observations are made.

PIP	40 cm H_2O
Plateau	35 cm H_2O
Set rate	10
Total rate	30
Exhaled V_T	425 ml
Spontaneous V_T	100 ml
I:E ratio	1:1.5

12. What high pressure alarm limit should you set?
    A. 35 cm H_2O
    B. 45 cm H_2O
    C. 50 cm H_2O
    D. 65 cm H_2O

13. What value should you set for the low minute ventilation alarm?
    A. 3.5 L
    B. 6.0 L
    C. 7.2 L
    D. 8.0 L

14. Which of the following would result in a lower work of breathing for this patient?
    1. addition of 100 ml mechanical deadspace
    2. initiation of PSV at 5 cm H_2O
    3. changing to flow-triggering 2 L/min
    4. addition of 10 cm H_2O PEEP
       A. 1 and 2 only
       B. 2 and 3 only
       C. 1 and 3 only
       D. 2, 3, and 4

15. What action should you take to increase the I:E ratio?
    A. Increase the peak flow.
    B. Increase the tidal volume.
    C. Increase the set rate.
    D. Increase the F_IO_2.

16. What I:E ratio would provide sufficient time for exhalation and prevent auto-PEEP in this COPD patient?
    A. 1:1
    B. 1:2
    C. 1:4
    D. 1:10

A 5 foot 6 inch woman who weighs 100 kg (220 lb) is in the ICU following surgery for multiple injuries sustained in a motor vehicle accident. She has an arterial line and a pulmonary artery catheter in place. Her chest radiograph shows bilateral infiltrates consistent with ARDS. The ET tube is in good position.

Current ventilator settings are:

Mode	Volume-controlled CMV
V_T	1000
Rate	12
F_iO_2	0.70
PEEP	5 cm H_2O
Peak flow	60 L/min, decelerating ramp
Sensitivity	1.0 cm H_2O below baseline

17. What is this patient's approximate ideal body weight?
    A. 50 kg
    B. 60 kg
    C. 80 kg
    D. 100 kg

18. What initial tidal volume would you recommend to prevent further lung injury?
    A. 480 ml
    B. 600 ml
    C. 720 ml
    D. Maintain current setting

The following data are obtained:

HR	110, NSR with occasional PVCs
BP	110/75 mm Hg
SpO_2	88%
PA	38/8 mm Hg
PCWP	12 mm Hg
CO	5.8 L/min
SvO_2	59%

19. With regard to the patient's oxygenation, what action would you recommend?
    A. Increase the F_iO_2.
    B. Increase the PEEP.
    C. Add mechanical dead space.
    D. Maintain current settings.

A PEEP trial is conducted with the following results.

PEEP	Cstat	PaO₂	CO
5	22	57	5.8
10	25	66	5.7
15	30	72	5.9
20	25	77	5.2
25	22	85	4.8

20. What PEEP level would you recommend?
    A. 5
    B. 10
    C. 15
    D. 20
    E. 25

441

The patient continues to deteriorate over the next 2 days. Her compliance and PaO_2 have decreased, while PIP has increased to 60 cm H_2O to maintain a normal $PaCO_2$.

21. Which of the following ventilator modes could be considered as alternatives?
    1. pressure-control CMV
    2. SIMV volume control
    3. APRV
    4. CSV-CPAP
        A. 1 and 3 only
        B. 2 and 3 only
        C. 2 and 4 only
        D. 1 and 4 only

22. Which of these techniques are used with ARDS to reduce lung injury or improve oxygenation?
    1. expiratory retard
    2. prone positioning
    3. permissive hypercapnia
    4. unilateral lung ventilation
        A. 1 and 2
        B. 2 and 3
        C. 1 and 4
        D. 3 and 4

Case 4

A respiratory student who fell down the stairs while reading *Egan's* suffered a closed-head injury. The student is 5 feet 5 inches tall and weighs 60 kg. ICP and blood pressure are elevated. She is being ventilated with these settings.

Mode	VC-CMV
Rate	12
V_T	600
F_IO_2	.30
PEEP	0

Blood gases on these settings are:

pH	7.40
$PaCO_2$	40
PaO_2	55
HCO_3^-	24

23. This blood gas should be interpreted as _____.
    A. normal with moderate hypoxemia
    B. respiratory alkalosis with mild hypoxemia
    C. compensated respiratory acidosis with severe hypoxemia
    D. compensated metabolic alkalosis with moderate hypoxemia

24. With regard to the oxygenation, what change would you suggest?
    A. Increase the PEEP.
    B. Increase the rate.
    C. Change to APRV.
    D. Increase the F_IO_2.

25. With regard to the ventilation, what change would you suggest?
    A. Increase the rate.
    B. Increase the tidal volume.
    C. Change to SIMV.
    D. Add mechanical dead space.

26. What is the formula for calculating the rate needed to produce a desired change in $PaCO_2$?
    A. $PaCO_2$ measured × set rate ÷ $PaCO_2$ desired
    B. $PaCO_2$ desired × set rate ÷ $PaCO_2$ measured
    C. $PaCO_2$ measured × $PaCO_2$ desired ÷ set rate
    D. $PaCO_2$ measured × PaO_2 measured ÷ set rate

27. What rate would you suggest for this patient if the desired $PaCO_2$ is 30 mm Hg?
    A. 8
    B. 10
    C. 14
    D. 16

28. How long should you maintain a head injury patient in a hyperventilated state? Hint: See Chapter 43.
    A. 2 to 4 hours
    B. 6 to 8 hours
    C. 12 to 24 hours
    D. 24 to 48 hours

Case 5

A 5 foot 7 inch 27-year-old woman who weighs 140 lb with a long history of asthma including previous intubation and mechanical ventilation presents in the emergency department with high-pitched, diffuse wheezing. She is barely able to talk due to her dsypnea. She has not responded to two consecutive SVN treatments with 5 mg of albuterol and 0.5 mg of Atrovent. Peak flows are not measurable, and SpO_2 is 92% on 2 L via nasal cannula. She is using her accessory muscles to breathe and has some intercostal retractions on inspiration. She is started on IV SoluMedrol, continuous bronchodilator therapy, and ECG monitoring. One hour later, she is lethargic and breath sounds are virtually absent. You draw an ABG with the following results:

pH	7.29
$PaCO_2$	55 mm Hg
PaO_2	64 mm Hg
HCO_3^-	24 mmol
SaO_2	90%

29. What action would you recommend at this time?
    A. continuation of present therapy
    B. oral intubation with 7.5 ET tube and mechanical ventilation
    C. trial of NIPPV via bilevel mask ventilation
    D. tracheostomy and mechanical ventilation

30. The emergency physician elects to move the patient to the MICU as soon as she is stabilized. You assist in the transport. In the ICU, you are asked to set up the ventilator. You would select:
    A. VC-SIMV 14, 400, 0.40 F_IO_2, +3 PEEP, +5 PSV
    B. VC-CMV 12, 750, +5 PEEP, 0.40 F_IO_2
    C. APRV high PEEP 30, low PEEP 20, 0.60 F_IO_2, 1 second release time
    D. CPAP (CSV) +10 PEEP, 0.30 F_IO_2

31. What pharmacologic agent is recommended at this time?
    A. inhaled corticosteroids
    B. sedation with midazolam
    C. paralysis with tubocurarine
    D. respiratory stimulus with doxapram

Chapter **44** Initiating and Adjusting Invasive Ventilatory Support

32. Bronchodilator therapy is also indicated. How will you need to adjust the dosage for administration to a ventilated patient?
    A. Give the standard dose.
    B. Increase the dose to 2 to 4 times normal amount.
    C. Decrease the dose by half the normal amount.
    D. Give the standard dose intravenously.

33. Which of the following are major concerns when ventilating severe asthmatics?
    1. pulmonary barotrauma
    2. development of auto-PEEP
    3. ventilator asynchrony
    4. high airway pressures
       A. 1 and 2
       B. 1, 3, and 4
       C. 2, 3, and 4
       D. 1, 2, 3, and 4

34. An appropriate peak flow and flow pattern for this patient would include
    A. 40 L/min with a decelerating flow waveform.
    B. 20 L/min with a square flow waveform.
    C. 100 L/min with a sinewave flow pattern.
    D. 50 L/min with an accelerating flow waveform.

35. What alteration to the mode of ventilation might be useful to prevent barotrauma and improve comfort?
    A. addition of mechanical dead space
    B. using a heated humidifier
    C. switching to pressure control
    D. utilizing inverse ratio ventilation

Case 6

A 6 foot, 176-lb 66-year-old man has been brought to the SICU following coronary artery bypass graft surgery. He has no history of lung disease. He is intubated with a No. 8 oral ET tube. The anesthesiologist asks you to select ventilator settings.

36. What tidal volume is appropriate for this postoperative patient?
    A. 500 ml
    B. 650 ml
    C. 800 ml
    D. 950 ml

37. Why should you add a small amount of PEEP to the system?
    A. to prevent auto-PEEP
    B. to prevent atelectasis
    C. to prevent cardiogenic pulmonary edema
    D. to prevent barotrauma

38. What is your primary goal for this patient?
    A. Prevent ventilator-associated barotrauma.
    B. Prevent ventilator-associated pneumonia.
    C. Control air-trapping.
    D. Wean and extubate as quickly as possible.

Those are six of the common situations you need to be able to manage. The other three are:

Unilateral Lung Disease

39. What position is useful in this type of patient? What special form of ventilation can be used?
    A. Position

    B. Special form of ventilation

Neuromuscular Disorders

40. What adjustment to tidal volume might be made?

CHF

41. When your patient is in CHF, he or she has pulmonary edema. What adjustment may help improve oxygenation and work of breathing? What are the choices besides intubation?

WHAT DOES THE NBRC SAY?

The Examination Matrix is quite clear on this subject. You should be able to:
- Initiate and adjust ventilators when settings are specified (and when they're not)
- Initiate and adjust all the primary modes like CMV and IMV
- Select appropriate tidal volume, minute volume, and respiratory rate

You should also know when to modify
- Mode
- Tidal volume
- F_IO_2
- Inspiratory plateau
- PEEP and CPAP levels
- Pressure support and pressure control
- Alarm settings
- Mechanical dead space
- Mean airway pressure
- Inverse ratio ventilation

If you can understand and apply the material in this chapter, you are well on your way to passing your boards and becoming a great therapist!

42. A patient with CHF is placed on the ventilator. The respiratory therapist should
    A. obtain a sputum sample for culture.
    B. assess changes in intracranial pressure.
    C. assess changes in blood pressure.
    D. obtain a chest x-ray.

Chapter **44** **Initiating and Adjusting Invasive Ventilatory Support**

43. A patient is receiving mechanical ventilation via volume-controlled CMV (or assist control if you like) with a mandatory rate of 14. Peak inspiratory pressures are in the low 50s. The physician wants to maintain the mean airway pressure but lower the peak pressure. What would the RCP recommend?
   A. Increase the mandatory rate.
   B. Increase the inspiratory flow.
   C. Initiate pressure-controlled ventilation.
   D. Initiate IMV with pressure support.

44. What is an appropriate range for respiratory rate (f) when using high-frequency oscillation ventilation with newborns?
   A. 1-2 Hz
   B. 3-5 Hz
   C. 10-15 Hz
   D. 20-30 Hz

45. A patient with ALI due to trauma from a motor vehicle accident is placed on mechanical ventilation. The man is 182 cm (6 feet) tall and weights 100 kg (220 lb). With respect to ventilator settings, what tidal volume would you recommend?
   A. 480 ml
   B. 800 ml
   C. 960 ml
   D. 1200 ml

46. An apneic patient is placed on mechanical ventilation following surgery. What range of rate is typical for initiating mechanical ventilation on an adult patient?
   A. 4-8
   B. 8-12
   C. 12-20
   D. 20-30

47. A patient is being mechanically ventilated in CMV mode. When the patient begins to inhale, airway pressure drops to –4 cm H_2O below baseline before a breath is started. What control needs to be adjusted?
   A. frequency
   B. PEEP
   C. pressure support
   D. sensitivity

48. A patient with ARDS is being mechanically ventilated with a PEEP of 10 cm H_2O and an F_IO_2 of 0.80. When the patient is removed from the ventilator for suctioning, he experiences decreased oxygen saturation and increased heart rate. What should the respiratory therapist recommend?
   A. Decreasing the PEEP to 5 cm H_2O
   B. Changing to a closed suction system
   C. Giving SVN with albuterol 2.5 mg
   D. Increasing the F_IO_2 on the ventilator

49. A 70 kg patient is ventilated on IMV mode with a rate of 8, tidal volume of 700, F_IO_2 of 0.40, PEEP of 4 cm H_2O, pressure support of 4 cm H_2O and an inspiratory flowrate of 45 L/min. The patient is breathing 22 times per minute in between the machine breaths with a tidal volume of 150 ml. What change should the respiratory therapist recommend?
   A. Increasing the peak inspiratory flow rate
   B. Increasing the respiratory rate
   C. Increasing the set tidal volume
   D. Increasing the pressure support

50. A 50-kg adult female is mechanically ventilated following a cardiac arrest. What tidal volume setting is recommended for this patient?
    A. 200 ml
    B. 300 ml
    C. 400 ml
    D. 500 ml

   There are literally hundreds more questions like this on the subject of initiating and managing mechanical ventilation. Whole books have been written on this subject alone!

FOOD FOR THOUGHT

51. What are the two most common ventilator strategies currently in use in the United States?

52. What are the common ventilator modes (and adjuncts like PEEP, PSV, etc.) where you are training or working?

53. How can you determine correct pressure and inspiratory time when you switch from volume-controlled to pressure-controlled ventilation?

Chapter **44** **Initiating and Adjusting Invasive Ventilatory Support**

45 Noninvasive Ventilation

Thou knows't the mask of night is on my face.
William Shakespeare

Noninvasive positive-pressure ventilation (NIV) by mask has been used in home care for many years, especially in the treatment of sleep-disordered breathing. Other forms of noninvasive ventilation like rocking beds and pneumobelts have been around since the 1930s. In the 1970s and 1980s, patients were ventilated with IPPB and mask to try to avoid intubation. But it was not until 1989 that serious efforts were made to use NIV as a means of treating acute respiratory failure. Increased technology in NIV ventilators and advances in mask designs have enabled the modern respiratory therapist to put noninvasive ventilation on the front lines of acute respiratory care in the management of COPD, asthma, and cardiogenic pulmonary edema. NIV is even used in the chronic care setting to relieve symptoms of hypoventilation and improve quality of life.

WORD WIZARD

We've been looking for less invasive ways to help people breathe since the first invasive airway management with

tracheostomy tubes was performed 350 years ago. In the 1930s a rubber inflatable device called a _____

was strapped to the abdomen to help patients with _____ disease to help move the diaphragm. Later, a

_____ bed was designed to help with weaning. Motion _____ was a hazard of the bed. Negative

pressure ventilators like the _____ lung were used to treat polio patients but were large and bulky. A chest

_____ covers only the chest and looks like a turtle shell. New positive pressure devices became popular in

the 1980s. _____, or inspiratory positive airway pressure, helps to inflate the lung during inspiration. Positive

pressure devices can be used at home to treat nocturnal _____, or they can be used in place of more invasive
methods in the ED or the ICU.

GOALS AND INDICATIONS

1. Four important goals of NIV in the acute care setting are to

   A. Avoid _____

   B. Improve _____

   C. Decrease _____

   D. Relieve _____

2. In the acute care setting, NIV is indicated for more than a dozen conditions. Name at least five.

   A. _____

   B. _____

   C. _____

   D. _____

   E. _____

3. NIV is also indicated for the chronic care setting. List five conditions:

A. _____

B. _____

C. _____

D. _____

E. _____

4. What is the standard of care for acute COPD exacerbation?

_____

5. Patients with status asthmaticus suffer a high degree of complications when intubated and mechanically ventilated. What were the results of Meduri's study on NIV in treating status asthmaticus?

_____

6. In what specifc group of COPD patients is NIV recommended when weaning from mechanical ventilation is difficult?

7. Compare mask CPAP to mask ventilation in the treatment of acute cardiogenic pulmonary edema. When does NIV outperform CPAP? Which one is first-line therapy?

_____

8. NIV should be used for what group of patients with community-acquired pneumonia?

_____

9. Should NIV be used to treat hypoxemic respiratory failure?

10. List four other indications for noninvasive ventilation in the acute care setting.

A. _____

B. _____

C. _____

D. _____

11. Briefly discuss the use of NIV to prevent post-extubation failure of high-risk patients.

12. What three criteria does the Rule of Thumb on page 1137 say should be met before implementing NIV in acute respiratory failure?

    A. _____

    B. _____

    C. _____

NIV AND CHRONIC CARE

13. NIV is used in the chronic care setting to treat some of the many causes of nocturnal hypoventilation. Describe the pathophysiologic "vicious cycle" that takes place in nocturnal hypoventilation.

14. How long does it take for NIV to reverse this process?

    _____

15. When should you try NIV in restrictive thoracic disorders like kyphoscoliosis?

    _____

16. Describe the ideal treatment of ALS with NIV. What are some benefits? What gas exchange indicator is useful for knowing when to start?

17. What does the Academy of Neurology have to say about ALS and NIV?

18. How would you use NIV for the long-term care of COPD rather than an acute exacerbation?

SELECTION AND EXCLUSION CRITERIA

19. How is the need for ventilatory assistance established? See Box 45-3.

    A. Respiratory rate   _____

    B. Dyspnea   _____

    C. $PaCO_2$ _____

    D. pH   _____

    E. P/F ratio   _____

20. Many patients might benefit from NIV but are excluded because we know it won't work for them. Name at least four of these criteria. Check Box 45-4.

    A. _____

    B. _____

    C. _____

    D. _____

Bottom line: The acute respiratory failure must be reversible within a few days! NIV is a short-term therapy for the acutely ill patient.

21. Once you put the patient on the noninvasive ventilator there are some predictors of success that can be measured. Look at Box 45-5 to find the values for:

A.	Respiratory acidosis	
B.	pH	
C.	Improvement in gas exchange	
D.	RR and HR	

22. Describe the two basic parts of the decision-making process for the patient with chronic restrictive thoracic disease.

A.

B.

23. Discuss some of the contraindications or exclusion criteria for chronic patients who might otherwise need NIV.

TOOLS OF THE TRADE

Masks (Interfaces)
You get to play with a lot of masks in noninvasive ventilation: nasal, full-face, and total face.

24. Which type of mask is most commonly used for NIV?

_____

25. How can you pick the right mask size—besides plain ol' trial and error?

_____

26. The oral mask has a lot of potential problems. List at least four.

A. _____

B. _____

C. _____

D. _____

27. Describe the total face mask. Where is it used? What are the advantages and disadvantages?

28. Why can't you use a standard resuscitation mask for this task?

29. What type of mask do studies show to be most effective in the acute care setting?

Ventilators

Positive-pressure ventilators to ventilate critically ill patients via ET usually need a sealed system to operate. Noninvasive ventilators are made to work with leaks. It will help if you understand the following terms:

- CPAP—breathing at an elevated baseline pressure during inspiration and exhalation
- EPAP—elevated pressure at exhalation
- IPAP—elevated pressure during inspiration

Figure 45-12 reproduced here shows a picture of these three concepts.

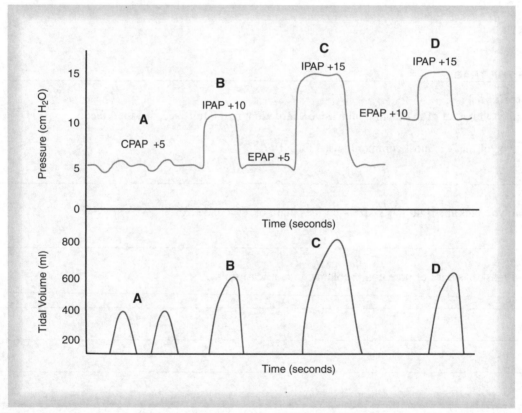

Figure 45-12 (from text). Changes in noninvasive ventilator settings (IPAP and EPAP) and corresponding effects on V_T. **A,** Spontaneous breathing on CPAP of 5 cm H_2O. **B,** Patient-triggered breath with the addition of 5 cm H_2O of pressure support (noninvasive ventilator settings are IPAP 10 cm H_2O and EPAP 5 cm H_2O). **C,** Pressure support was increased to 10 cm H_2O (NIV settings are IPAP 15 cm H_2O and EPAP 5 cm H_2O). Higher V_T occurs as pressure support is increased in **A** and **B. D,** IPAP 15 cm H_2O and EPAP 10 cm H_2O. Increasing EPAP setting. Results in lower V_T because pressure support was decreased to 5 cm H_2O.

30. What happens to tidal volume when you increase the EPAP without increasing the IPAP?

---

31. What are some of the problems with using standard critical care ventilators to deliver mask ventilation? What new mode may help?

START ME UP

Once you've chosen a ventilator and a mask that fits, you have to select mode and settings just like you did for invasive mechanical ventilation.

32. How should you position the patient?

_____

33. How should you prepare the patient for the experience?

34. Give initial settings for use with a noninvasive ventilator

    A. IPAP/ventilatory pressure: _____

    B. EPAP/PEEP: _____

35. What pressure could open the esophagus?

    A. Esophagus opens at _____

    B. Put in an NG tube and _____

36. You won't be setting a tidal volume, but you still want a good one. What volume would you like to achieve? Which control do you increase if the volume is too low?

    A. Goal: _____

    B. Adjust: _____

37. What two adjustments can be made to improve oxygenation?

Table 45-1 gives a clear overview of what controls to manipulate to get the results you need. You have to do a little fine-tuning to make this work. Don't forget to encourage and reassure the patient.

38. See if you have the basic idea:

   A. Increase _____ to increase tidal volume.

   B. Increase _____ to improve oxygenation and FRC.

   C. Set the rate at _____ and increase the rate to decrease _____.

39. While you can initiate NIV anywhere, what unit should the patient be in while they are on NIV?

WHAT COULD GO WRONG?

40. Use Table 45-2 to help you find out what could go wrong and how to fix it!

SIDE EFFECT	OCCURRENCE	REMEDY
Masks		
A. Discomfort		
B. Claustrophobia		
C. Skin breakdown		
Flow		
D. Congestion		
E. Sinus pain		
F. Dryness		
G. Air leaks		
Bad stuff		
H. Aspiration		
I. Low blood pressure		
J. Pneumothorax		

WHAT DOES THE NBRC SAY?

This subject is not a big part of the exams because it is relatively new; however, you can expect several questions. Here's what the matrix says you should know:
- CPAP devices—mask, nasal, or bi-level
- Patient breathing circuits—noninvasive ventilation
- Noninvasive ventilators (equipment))
- Mechanical ventilation—adjust noninvasive positive pressure ventilation

They don't tell you much, do they? So, for the exams, it's really three things:
- Do you know when to recommend a trial of NIV?
- Which ventilator would you pick for acute? Chronic?
- Can you state the initial vent settings?
- What should you change if O_2 is low? If CO_2 is high?

Questions 41-44 refer to the following scenario. Circle the best answer.

A 60-kg, 70-year-old patient with COPD does not wish to be intubated and has an advanced directive supporting his wishes. The patient is admitted to the medical ICU in respiratory failure. ABGs reveal: pH 7.25, $PaCO_2$ 66, PaO_2 50.

41. What mode of therapy would the respiratory therapist recommend in this situation?
    A. nasal cannula at 6 L/min
    B. nonrebreathing mask at 10 L/min
    C. continuous positive airway pressure
    D. noninvasive positive pressure ventilation

42. NIV is initiated on spontaneous mode with F_IO_2 0.40, IPAP of 8 cm H_2O and EPAP of 2 cm H_2O. ABGs reveal: pH 7.29, $PaCO_2$ 54, PaO_2 52, HCO_3 30. The respiratory therapist should recommend what change in regard to the carbon dioxide levels?
    A. Increase the respiratory rate setting.
    B. Increase the tidal volume setting.
    C. Increase the IPAP.
    D. Increase the EPAP.

43. What should the RT recommend to improve oxygenation?
    A. Increase the respiratory rate setting.
    B. Increase the tidal volume setting.
    C. Increase the IPAP.
    D. Increase the EPAP.

44. What exhaled tidal volume would you target for this patient?
    A. 200 ml
    B. 350 ml
    C. 475 ml
    D. 600 ml

46 Monitoring the Patient in the Intensive Care Unit

The best monitor is a knowledgeable, observant and dedicated healthcare professional.

Donald F. Egan, MD

Truer words were never spoken. ICU monitoring has reached a level of complexity that is as dazzling as it is expensive. The amount of data available to the critical care clinician is staggering. The key to success in this endeavor is to combine appropriate information gathering with sound clinical assessment. You can't learn that from a book! What you can do is learn the basics: normal values, waveforms, terms, and most common problems and situations you will encounter. When you go out into the clinical setting you can learn to apply this new information.

WORD WIZARD

Match these key terms to the definitions that follow.

Terms	Definitions
1. _____ afterload	A. pressure the ventricle has to contract against
2. _____ Swan-Ganz catheter	B. pressure stretching the ventricle at the onset of contraction
3. _____ Q_S/Q_T	C. unreal events seen on monitors often caused by movement
4. _____ Apache score	D. popular system for measuring neurologic impairment
5. _____ V_D/V_T	E. hemodynamic monitoring device placed in the pulmonary artery
6. _____ PaO_2/F_IO_2 ratio	F. amount of wasted ventilation per breath
7. _____ preload	G. noninvasive measurement oxygenation
8. _____ maximal inspiratory pressure	H. popular acute illness index
9. _____ Glasgow Coma Scale score	I. bedside test for respiratory muscle strength
10. _____ artifacts	J. physiologic shunt

RESPIRATORY MONITORING

Quick, memorize Table 46-1! Just kidding, you probably already know this stuff. Right?

11. Gas exchange at the lung is best monitored by what test? What test is best for immediate continuous assessment of oxygenation?

A. Gas exchange _____

B. Continuous _____

12. Tissue oxygenation depends on seven factors. That's a lot more complicated than just measuring one number like blood oxygen saturation. List four of these factors, and give the correct abbreviation.

A. _____

B. _____

C. _____

D. _____

459

13. What is the most serious clinical limitation of using pulse oximetry to assess the respiratory status?

_____

14. Pulse oximetry is affected by many factors. Name four. (See Box 46-2.)

A. _____

B. _____

C. _____

D. _____

15. What is the value for normal oxygen consumption?

_____

16. What does the Fick equation measure?

_____

17. PaO_2/F_IO_2 ratio is the most reliable index of gas exchange. What is the normal ratio? What ratio suggests ARDS?

A. Normal _____

B. ARDS _____

18. The most accurate and reliable measure of pulmonary oxygenation efficiency is direct calculation of shunt. State the classic shunt equation.

Qs/Qt = _____

19. What two blood gas samples are needed to calculate shunt?

A. _____

B. _____

Be sure to check out the Murray Lung Score in Box 46-3. It is a simple, inexpensive way to quantify lung dysfunction.

MONITORING VENTILATION

20. What is the gold standard for assessing the adequacy of ventilation?

_____

21. Efficiency of ventilation is assessed by measuring physiologic dead space.
State the modified Bohr equation. (Another testing favorite!)

V_D/V_T = _____

22. List the normal and critical values for dead space–to–tidal volume ratio.

A. Normal _____   _____

B. Critical is > _____ and predicts failure to wean.

460

23. What is the formula for measuring minute ventilation?

_____

24. What is the difference between arterial and end-tidal CO_2 in normal subjects?

_____

25. Capnometry is extremely useful in two emergency situations. Name them.

A. _____

B. _____

26. What test has to be done to validate the CO_2 value of the capnometer?

_____

27. Name the parts of the normal capnograph tracing seen here.

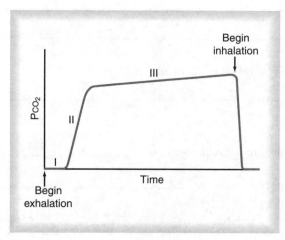

Time-based capnograph.

A. I _____

B. II _____

C. III _____

MONITORING CHEST WALL MECHANICS

28. The pressure–volume curve is a ventilator graphic that can show compliance and lower inflection points. The lower inflection point may help you set what ventilator parameter?

_____

29. The upper "inflection" (or deflection if you like) point may point out what problem?

_____

Compliance

30. Compliance shows stiffness of the lungs. What is the formula for calculating compliance? (Be sure to subtract PEEP.)

      C = Change in _____ /change in _____ or $(V_T/P_{plat} - PEEP)$

31. What is normal compliance?

_____

32. Low compliance on a patient with ARDS may drop to what values?

_____

Resistance

33. What is the formula for calculating airway resistance?

      R_{aw} = _____

34. What is normal airway resistance? What's normal for a ventilated patient?

    A. Normal _____

    B. Ventilated patients _____

35. Effects of what therapy can be measured by resistance changes?

_____

Peak and Plateau Pressures

36. What is the safe maximum value for peak pressure? _____

37. What are the maximum safe plateau pressures? _____

When peak pressures rise, it is due to either increased resistance or decreased compliance. Take a look at the peak and plateau pressures. When they move up together, the problem is compliance. When the peak pressure goes up and the plateau stays the same, the problem is airway resistance. Box 46-7 gives common clinical conditions that alter compliance and resistance.

Auto-PEEP

Auto-PEEP occurs when lungs don't empty well (obstructive disease) or when there is a high minute ventilation (ARDS). It causes all kinds of problems from difficulty in triggering the ventilator to hemodynamic compromise.

38. What ventilator maneuver unmasks auto-PEEP?

_____

39. Explain how adjustment of extrinsic (ventilator) PEEP is related to the level of intrinsic (auto) PEEP.

40. Explain what happens to oxygenation, arterial blood pressure, and venous return when you increase MAP.

41. What is the primary goal of manipulating MAP?

_____

Work of Breathing

Research hospitals have several methods of measuring the work of breathing including the use of esophageal balloons.

42. The simplest way to monitor work of breathing is to monitor the patient's _____ breathing rate,

_____ , and the f/V_T ratio.

43. What score for the rapid shallow breathing index is a good predictor of weaning success?

_____

Please note that higher values are used in older patients.

MONITORING MUSCLE STRENGTH

44. What two values are measured at the bedside?

    A. _____

    B. _____

45. What is a normal VC? What VC indicates poor muscle strength?

    A. Normal _____

    B. Poor _____

46. What are the benefits of measuring MIP compared to VC?

    A. _____

    B. _____

47. How long should you measure MIP? _____

48. Why should you use one-way valves when you measure MIP?

Chapter **46** **Monitoring the Patient in the Intensive Care Unit**

Most hospitals require ventilator checks every 2 hours. You need to record a number of values, assess the patient, and evaluate the information gathered so you can make any necessary changes.

49. Briefly discuss the five areas you need to check.

   A. Airway _____

   B. Vent settings _____

   C. Gas exchange _____

   D. Respiratory mechanics _____

   E. Alarms _____

50. Ventilator graphics allow rapid determination of a number of variables. Look at Box 46-8, and list five of the parameters you can check.

   A. _____

   B. _____

   C. _____

   D. _____

   E. _____

51. Table 46-2 explains how to do a patient–ventilator system check. The check is one of the most frequent and common activities that RTs perform. Explain the key steps listed below.
   A. Before entering the room

   B. Explain

   C. Observe

   D. Drain

E. Airway

F. Inspect

G. Auscultate

H. Note pressures (at least three)

I. IMV

J. Graphic artistry

MATHEMATICS

A lot of important math problems were presented in the last section of Chapter 46. Before you go on to the dreaded *hemodynamics* section, make sure you understand the math. You can look back at the text or just read along. Practice will help you gain understanding.

Shunt

You will at least have to recognize the classic shunt equation. At best, you should be able to calculate it (even though computers are used in the clinical setting). Let's see if you can estimate shunt using the formula from *Egan's*.

Let's do it together first.

A patient is breathing 100% oxygen. The PaO$_2$ is 200. What is the estimated shunt?

- PAO$_2$ = (760 − 47) × 1.0 − PaCO$_2$ (assume 40). Say 673 for PAO$_2$.
- Now plug the numbers into the formula: 673 − 200 = a 473–mm Hg difference between A and a!
- If there is a 5% shunt for each 100-mm Hg difference, the estimated shunt is 473/100 × 5 or 24%.

Your turn.

Chapter **46** **Monitoring the Patient in the Intensive Care Unit**

52. A patient is breathing 100% oxygen. P_B is 747 (conveniently), $PaCO_2$ is 47 (goodie), and PaO_2 is 300. Estimate the shunt.

A. PAO_2 =

B. A − a =

C. Shunt =

Fick

Fick was *the* physiologist. You can use his equation to calculate cardiac output or oxygen consumption. This isn't used much in the clinical setting, but it can be on your boards.

Let's do one together.

What is cardiac output for a patient who has a $\dot{V}O_2$ of 250, a CaO_2 of 19, and a CvO_2 of 14?

Plug the numbers into the formula:

- QT (total perfusion or cardiac output) = $\dot{V}O_2/CaO_2 − CvO_2 \times 10$ or…
- QT = 250/19 − 14 × 10 = 250/5 × 10 = 250/50 = 5 L/min

Your turn.

53. What is cardiac output for a patient who has an oxygen consumption of 200 ml/min, an arterial content of 20 vol%, and a venous content of 16 vol%?

A. Formula _____

B. Calculation _____

C. Answer _____

You could rearrange this to calculate oxygen consumption if you knew the cardiac output. For example, what is the oxygen consumption for a patient who has a cardiac output of 4 L/min, CaO_2 of 17, and CvO_2 of 13?

$$\dot{V}O_2 = 4 \times 17 − 13 \text{ or } 160 \text{ ml/min. You can keep on rearranging all you like.}$$

Minute Ventilation

That was fun; now try an easy one. Exhaled minute ventilation is respiratory rate × tidal volume. $V_E = f \times V_T$. For example, a patient has a respiratory rate of 12 and a tidal volume of 500, so the exhaled minute ventilation is 6000 ml, or 6 L.

54. What is the V_E for a patient who has a respiratory rate of 8 and a tidal volume of 400?

A. Formula _____

B. Calculation _____

C. Answer _____

What about a patient who has ventilator breaths and spontaneous breaths (SIMV)?

55. A patient has a set rate of 6 and a machine volume of 700. The patient has 10 spontaneous breaths at 300 ml. What is the total V_E?

Bohr

$V_D/V_T = (PaCO_2 - PECO_2)/PaCO_2$. First we'll calculate the physiologic dead space–to–tidal volume ratio, and then we'll use it in combination with minute volume.

For example: W

What is the dead space–to–tidal volume ratio for a patient who has an arterial CO_2 of 40 and an exhaled CO_2 of 30?

$$40 - 30/40 = 10/40 \text{ or } 25\% \text{ Normal}$$

Your turn.

56. Calculate V_D/V_T for a patient who has an arterial CO_2 of 40 and an exhaled CO_2 of 20.

    A. Formula _____

    B. Calculation _____

    C. Analysis _____

Now combine this with the minute volume equation to calculate *alveolar* minute ventilation. Use respiratory rate of 12, tidal volume of 500, $PaCO_2$ of 40, and $PECO_2$ of 30.
- The new formula says: $V_A = f(V_T - V_D)$.
- Dead space is 25%. So multiply the tidal volume by 0.25 to get the dead space volume. $500 \times 0.25 = 125$ ml.
- Now plug in the numbers. $V_A = 12(500 - 125)$ or $12 \times 375 = 4500$ ml.

57. Calculate alveolar minute ventilation for a patient who has a rate of 10, tidal volume of 500, arterial CO_2 of 40, and end-tidal CO_2 of 28.

    A. Formula _____

    B. Calculation _____

    C. Answer _____

Expect some combination of this material on your board exams!

Compliance

Like dead space, compliance calculations are simplified on the board exams. We'll do it both ways here.

First, static effective compliance the simple way.

A patient has an exhaled volume of 600 ml. The plateau pressure is 35 and the PEEP is 5.

$$\text{Compliance is } 600/35 - 5 \text{ or } 600/30 = 20 \text{ ml/cm } H_2O$$

Your turn.

58. Calculate static effective compliance for a patient who has an exhaled volume of 1000, plateau pressure of 35, and PEEP of 10.

    A. Formula _____

    B. Calculation _____

    C. Compliance_____

In clinical practice it may be important to subtract the compressed volume with some ventilators. A comparison will make this clear. The patient in the example had a volume of 600 and compliance of 20. But, if the PIP was 40 cm H_2O and the circuit expansion factor is 5 ml/cm H_2O, then the volume lost to expansion is 200 ml (factor × PIP)! The new compliance calculation is

$$(600 - 200)/(35 - 5) \text{ or } 400/30 = 13 \text{ ml/cm } H_2O$$

You try:

59. Calculate compliance for a patient who has a tidal volume of 800, PIP of 50, plateau of 35, and PEEP of 5. The circuit factor is 4 ml/cm H_2O.

A. Formula _____

B. Calculation _____

C. Compliance_____

Some ventilators compensate for tubing compliance so you don't need to do this step!

Resistance

A look at the difference between PIP and plateau is useful for clinical estimates of airway resistance as well. First, you need to use a square or constant flow pattern on most modern ventilators. Next, you need to determine the flow rate in liters per second, not liters per minute.
   Here is an example:
   Calculate resistance for a patient who has a PIP of 50 cm H_2O, plateau of 40 cm H_2O, and flow rate of 60 L/min.

60 L/min converts to L/sec this way: 60 L/min ÷ 60 sec/min = 1 L/sec. Now calculate:

PIP – plateau ÷ flow = 50 – 40 ÷ 1 = 10 cm H_2O/L /sec

Now your turn.

60. Calculate airway resistance for a patient who has a peak pressure of 50 cm H_2O, plateau pressure of 40 cm H_2O, and flow rate of 30 L/min.

A. Convert flow to liters per second _____

B. Resistance formula _____

C. Calculation _____

D. Airway resistance is _____

If you are doing patient care, you may not have to calculate to see that resistance or compliance has changed. Look at the difference between peak pressure and plateau pressure. If the difference has increased and all else is stable, then the resistance has also increased. Some ventilators will perform compliance and resistance calculations for you. The manual calculations will give slightly different answers than the ventilator. Policy will determine the way you do the numbers at any particular hospital.
   Remember, if the patient is actively breathing spontaneously, it will be very difficult to make accurate calculations. These are really intended for full ventilatory support.

ASSESSMENT OF HEMODYNAMICS

Here at last. The dreaded hemodynamics strikes terror into the hearts of residents, nurses, and respiratory care students everywhere . . . but it will be okay. Break it down into small pieces: indications, complications, normal values, equipment, waveforms. You can do it! Let's start with invasive arterial monitoring.

Arterial lines

61. Identify the two main sites for arterial cannulation in adults.

A. _____

B. _____

62. What are the two indications for an indwelling arterial line?

A. _____

B. _____

468

63. List the normal values for these systemic arterial parameters. Check Table 46-3.

A. Systolic _____

B. Diastolic _____

C. Mean _____

When the arterial line doesn't agree with manual measurements, the manual method is safer. One problem may be that the pressure transducer is not the level of the heart. A transducer that is above the heart results in *lower* pressures on the monitor.

Another problem may be a "dampened" tracing. This means the waveform is flattened out. Clots and air bubbles in the system are common causes of a dampened tracing.

Equipment

One more area you need to become familiar with is the basic parts of the system. Take a look at this picture.

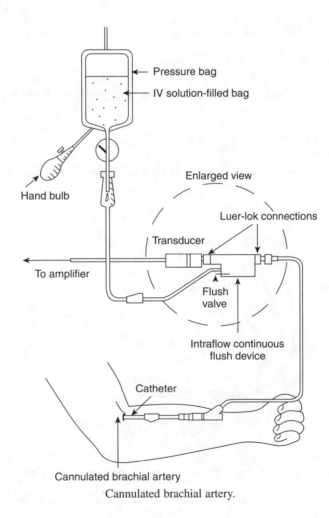

Cannulated brachial artery.

Starting at the top, you see a **pressurized IV bag** that may also contain heparin to help reduce the chance of clotting. The main thing is the pressure. Without it, blood from the patient could back up into the system, and we wouldn't be able to **flush,** or wash out blood, back into the artery. The **transducer** converts the arterial pressure waveform to an electronic signal that can be sent to the amplifier and displayed on the monitor.

Special **stiff,** or **noncompliant, IV tubing** connects from the transducer and continuous flush device to the catheter that is in the artery. This tubing prevents the arterial pressure wave from being damped as it passes up to the transducer (just like when ventilator tubing expands as a breath passes through it and we lose some in the expansion).

There now, that wasn't too bad.

Chapter **46 Monitoring the Patient in the Intensive Care Unit**

Flow-directed, balloon-tipped, pulmonary artery catheter…oh, let's just call it a "Swan."

Dr. Swan and Dr. Ganz are credited with developing this nifty tube for looking at the pressures inside the heart and lungs. So, many people still call it a "Swan" or "Swan-Ganz" catheter. Pulmonary artery catheter (PAC) is more generic. Pulmonary artery monitoring **is** a complex subject, but you can make it much simpler if you start by learning certain basic pieces of information. (You can also pass your boards.)

64. Name six conditions that suggest insertion of a PAC.

A. _____

B. _____

C. _____

D. _____

E. _____

F. _____

65. Measurement of PCWP is especially helpful in separating noncardiogenic (ARDS) and cardiogenic pulmonary edemas (CHF). What value for PCWP suggests ARDS?

_____

66. Look at the catheter itself. Identify the labeled parts. (Check Figure 46-15 for clues.)

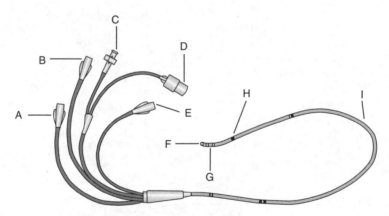

Quadruple-channel pulmonary artery catheter.

A. _____

B. _____

C. _____

D. _____

E. _____

F. _____

G. _____

470

H. _____

I. _____

Pneumopnugget

67. Label the following four waveforms. (Look at Figure 46-16 if you get lost).

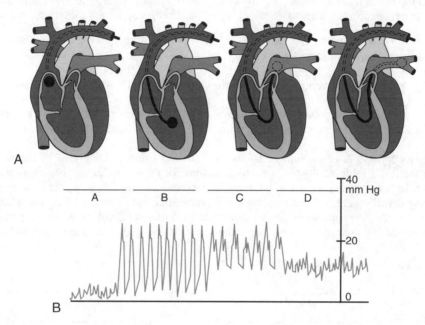

A, Position of pulmonary arterial catheter in heart. *B*, As monitored by pressure tracings.

Pneumopnugget

These are the four patterns seen on insertion and during normal monitoring. Just like in ECGs, there are abnormal patterns, too, but don't worry about them yet. Each of the normal waveforms corresponds to an anatomic location. So if, for example, the catheter is supposed to be in the pulmonary artery but you see a right ventricular waveform, you know something is wrong (maybe it is pulled back too far). Or, if the waveform appears wedged when it isn't supposed to be, perhaps the catheter has migrated too far forward.

68. List the normal values for these parameters. (See Table 46-3.)

A. Central venous pressure (CVP) _____

B. Right atrial pressure (RA) _____

C. Pulmonary artery

  1. Systolic _____

  2. Diastolic _____

D. Pulmonary artery wedge pressure (PWP, PCWP, PAWP) _____

WHAT DOES IT ALL MEAN?

Interpretation of PAC readings is a pretty complex subject. Right atrial pressure (RAP) and CVP are often used interchangeably. CVP represents preload to the right side of the heart. It can be a good indicator of the fluid volume status of the patient. It could also tell us if there is a backup in the system between the right atrium and the left atrium, like pulmonary hypertension, a blood clot, heart failure, or a defect in the tricuspid valve. The wedge pressure does much the same for the left side. Under normal circumstances it shows us the left ventricular preload. Considered along with CVP, it helps decide about the fluid balance. If both CVP and PWP are low, you should consider hypovolemia.

Here is where the RT must really think. Because both values are measured inside the chest, and positive pressure ventilation increases intrathoracic pressure, it is possible for the ventilator to affect the readings. The pressure tracings will move up and down with positive pressure breaths, so you may be able to detect this by watching the tracing increase and decrease as the ventilator cycles. But PEEP makes a constant increase in pressure, and PEEP levels above 10 cm H_2O, especially in hypovolemic patients, can artificially elevate the values, especially the wedge pressure. A high value usually means the patient has too much fluid, so someone might conclude the patient needs to lose some fluid when really he or she is dry! A complete explanation of what to do about this would keep you here a long time, but here are some ideas:

1. Measure pressure values from the PAC at end exhalation. You will need to run off a printed strip to do this, since the digital values on the monitor are averaged.

2. Do not take the patient off the ventilator to measure values, especially if the patient is on a high level of PEEP.

3. Correct the PAC values if the patient is on a high level of PEEP. This is not simple—remember that the degree of pressure transmitted also depends on lung compliance, so learn more about this before you try it.

You can use the catheter to look at other things besides overall fluid balance. Diagnosis of certain conditions is aided by information from the PAC. Table 46-4 provides a look at some of these conditions. For example, compare ARDS to left ventricular failure. In both conditions, the pulmonary artery pressure may increase, the radiograph shows infiltrates, and breath sounds may reveal crackles. Both patients have hypoxemia and decreased lung compliance. But, the failing left ventricle causes the wedge pressure to go up, whereas ARDS does not. Combine this with patient history and other assessments, and you get the big picture. Certain other values can be measured besides pressure, so let's look at those next.

69. List the normal values for these parameters.

A. Cardiac output (CO) _____

B. Cardiac index (CI) _____

C. Systemic vascular resistance (SVR) _____

D. Pulmonary vascular resistance (PVR) _____

With the Swan, cardiac output is measured via thermodilution. This is very helpful information, especially in the administration of drugs that support cardiac function, or if you want to know if changes in the ventilator are affecting the heart. The problem is that cardiac output is not personal enough. For example, you would expect a sumo wrestler to have a bigger cardiac output than an elderly woman, but both would be technically within the normal range at 5 L/min of output. If you divide the output by the body surface area, you derive cardiac index, and this is more useful, because everyone should have the same range for cardiac index. Anyone who drops below 2.5 is in trouble!

Another useful calculation is vascular resistance. It's just like airway resistance (PIP − plateau/flow), only now we want to know how much pressure drop occurs when we push the blood through the vessels. Let's look at the pulmonary vascular resistance formula, because you might have to calculate this on your boards.

$$PVR = MPAP - PAWP/CO$$

If you have a patient with a mean pulmonary artery pressure of 12 mm Hg, CVP of 4 mm Hg, and cardiac output of 4 L/min, you get 12 − (4/4) = 2 mm Hg/L/min for the resistance. Sometimes this number is multiplied by 80 to convert it to dynes. Either way, PVR is normally quite low.

70. What common respiratory vessel problem results in vasoconstriction, or elevated vascular resistance in the pulmonary vessels? Hint: PVR, Table 46-3.

_____

71. Calculate PVR for a patient who has a mean pulmonary artery pressure of 15 mm Hg, CVP of 3 mm Hg, and CO of 5 L/min.

Sometimes you need to be able to calculate mean arterial pressure so you can work the resistance problem. Remember that MAP = systolic pressure + (2 × diastolic)/3.

72. Calculate mean pulmonary artery pressure if systolic pulmonary artery pressure is 25 mm Hg and diastolic pulmonary artery pressure is 10 mm Hg.

Remember to learn the basics and normal values. When you are looking at the data, think about where in the heart or lungs the pressure is being measured. That will help give you a clue about what part of the system has become abnormal. To increase your expertise you will have to go to the clinical setting and look at the patient data from the PAC and learn interpretation at the bedside.

NEUROLOGIC MONITORING

73. Why are the pupils of interest in assessing neurologic status?

74. Why shouldn't you check a patient's gag reflex?

75. Name one of the breathing patterns that suggests a neurologic deficit.

76. Describe what happens to the brain for each of the ICP values below.

    A. 10 to 15 mm Hg

    B. 15 to 20 mm Hg

    C. 30 to 35 mm Hg

77. The Glasgow Coma Scale is a popular tool used to assess acute neurologic deficits. What do the following scores mean?

    A. 9 to 13

    B. <8

78. What two tests are commonly used together to monitor renal function?

79. Define polyuria and oliguria in terms of actual daily output.

80. How is liver function usually evaluated?

TROUBLESHOOTING THE PATIENT–VENTILATOR SYSTEM

81. Troubleshooting revolves around what two general problem areas? (See Box 46-12.)

A. _____

B. _____

82. Use Table 46-7 to help you identify common problems.

		CLUE	POSSIBLE PROBLEM	CORRECTIVE ACTION
A.		Sudden increase in PIP	1.	
			2.	
B.		Gradual increase in PIP	1.	
C.		Sudden decrease in PIP	1.	
			2.	
D.		Decreased minute/tidal volume	1.	
			2.	
E.		Increased minute or tidal volume	1.	
			2.	

83. Use Box 46-12 to help you identify four patient-related causes of sudden respiratory distress.

A. _____

B. _____

C. _____

D. _____

84. List four ventilator-related causes of sudden respiratory distress.

A. _____

B. _____

C. _____

D. _____

85. Regardless of the source of the problem, what is always the first priority?

_____

86. If there is any doubt as to the cause or solution of a problem, what action should you take?

87. How can you check the patency of the artificial airway?

88. Sedation and paralysis may be needed outside of the normal sedation humanely given in the ICU. Some patients cannot tolerate the ventilator without medication. The key is to avoid oversedation and troubleshoot all the physiologic stuff like hypoxia first. Give examples of drugs in the following classes:

A. Tranquilizing agents

1. _____

2. _____

3. _____

B. Narcotic analgesics

1. _____

2. _____

C. Neuromuscular blocking agents

1. Long-term (nondepolarizing) _____

2. Short-acting (depolarizing) _____

D. Sedative/hypnotics and miscellaneous _____

The flavor of the month for this one is propofol (Diprivan). Rapid acting with a short half-life, it's easy to get out of the system when the nurses turn off the IV! Amidate, or etomidate, is a great drug for managing the airway that has some advantages over the paralyzing agent Anectine.

WHAT DOES THE NBRC SAY?

The issue of hemodynamics in the board exams is a bit tricky. Hemodynamics used to be a heavy hitter, with 10 or more questions on the Written Registry. The last revision of the exams removed most of this material. Now you see only a few questions, and they are less technical in regard to equipment and focus more on identifying clinically important material that all ICU staff needs to understand. Because whole textbooks are devoted to hemodynamic monitoring or ventilator management, *Egan's* cannot possibly give you everything you need. It is a great place to start, and it clearly summarizes the main points. Chapter 46 will make an excellent reference when you go to prepare for the tests. Here are some sample questions. Circle the best answer.

89. A 42-year-old patient with a cervical spine injury is being mechanically ventilated in control mode. As you enter the room, the low pressure alarm is sounding. The patient is connected to the ventilator, but you do not see his chest moving. Your first action would be to _____.
A. manually ventilate the patient with the resuscitation bag
B. check the alarm settings
C. observe the exhaled volumes
D. manually ventilate the patient with the mechanical ventilator

90. After insertion of a Swan-Ganz catheter via the left subclavian vein, a patient's compliance quickly drops. The high pressure alarm on the ventilator is activated. Breath sounds are absent over the left chest, and the trachea is deviated to the right side. The patient appears extremely anxious. What action should the RCP take?
A. Use a capnometer to assess ventilation noninvasively.
B. Recommend administration of Versed.
C. Call for a portable chest radiograph.
D. Recommend chest tube insertion.

91. A 38-year-old woman with a diagnosis of myasthenia gravis is being mechanically ventilated. As you enter the room, the high pressure alarm is sounding. The patient appears anxious. Auscultation reveals coarse bilateral rhonchi. What action should you take at this time?
A. Manually ventilate the patient.
B. Check the alarm setting.
C. Recommend sedation.
D. Suction the patient.

92. An 89-year-old woman with emphysema is being mechanically ventilated. The high pressure and high rate alarms are being activated. Breath sounds are clear. Pulse oximetry and vital sign values are within normal limits. Hemodynamics are normal. ABGs are stable. The patient is very agitated, and her respiratory rate is 32. What are your recommendations?
A. Administer Versed.
B. Increase the alarm limit.
C. Suction the patient.
D. Call for a portable chest radiograph.

93. The data below are reported for a patient:
PCWP   25 mm Hg
PAP   40/24 mm Hg
CI   1.9 L/min/m²

These data suggest which of the following?
A. noncardiogenic pulmonary edema
B. cardiogenic pulmonary edema
C. pulsus paradoxus
D. hypovolemia

94. When properly placed, the distal tip of the Swan-Ganz catheter will be located in the _____.
A. left atrium
B. right atrium
C. right ventricle
D. pulmonary artery

Questions 95 through 97 refer to the following situation:
A patient is intubated and placed on the ventilator after she develops respiratory failure following hip replacement surgery. The following values are recorded:

$PaCO_2$	50 mm Hg
PaO_2	60 mm Hg
F_IO_2	0.40
$PECO_2$	10 mm Hg
Tidal volume	800 ml
Respiratory rate	20

95. These data indicate a dead space–to–tidal volume ratio of _____.
    A. 20%
    B. 40%
    C. 60%
    D. 80%

96. What is the exhaled minute volume?
    A. 8.0 L
    B. 12.0 L
    C. 16.0 L
    D. 20.0 L

97. What is the alveolar minute volume?
    A. 3.2 L
    B. 11.2 L
    C. 12.8 L
    D. 16.0 L

98. The following information is recorded for a patient:
    $\dot{V}O_2$ 200 ml/min
    CaO_2 16 vol %
    CvO_2 12 vol %

    What is the cardiac output?
    A. 2.0 L/min
    B. 3.0 L/min
    C. 4.0 L/min
    D. 5.0 L/min

99. The hemodynamic data below are recorded for a patient who is being mechanically ventilated.
    Cardiac output   3.5 L/min
    PAP   16/8 mm Hg
    PWP   4 mm Hg
    CVP   2 mm Hg
    HR   125/min

    These data probably indicate _____.
    A. hypovolemia
    B. pulmonary hypertension
    C. fluid overload
    D. pulmonary embolism

FOOD FOR THOUGHT

There was an editorial in the journal *Respiratory Care* a few years ago entitled something like this: "The pulmonary artery catheter—it goes in through your arm and you pay through the nose." Think about three questions in relationship to this idea. First, do you think it is important to use top-of-the-line technology in every setting? Second, if your loved one were ill, what would you want for them? Third, do you think the average person understands the complexity of "the high cost of medicine"?

Discontinuing Ventilatory Support

> *I'm losing.*
> Reported as the last words of Frank Sinatra

It's relatively easy to initiate mechanical ventilation, and some patients are equally easy to get back off. Unfortunately, there is still no magic number that tells you a patient will be successfully weaned or removed from support. You will have to customize the job for each patient. Sometimes this task takes all our skills and resources to accomplish. Sometimes it can't be done!

WORD WIZARD

Please write the meaning of these terms. This simple task will help you talk the talk when you're in the ICU. Most of these little letters are on your board exams as well.

ASV _____

ATC _____

CPAP _____

MMV _____

PSV _____

PMV _____

RSBI _____

SBT _____

SAT _____

SIMV _____

FIRST THINGS FIRST

1. What is the purpose of mechanical ventilation? (Don't explain, just look at the first sentence in Chapter 47 in *Egan's!*)

2. What is the basic idea about removing the ventilator?

3. How often should the ventilated patient be evaluated for the ability to discontinue ventilatory support?

_____

4. What's the difference between weaning from and discontinuing ventilator support?

A. Wean _____

B. Discontinue _____

5. What are the three basic methods for discontinuing?

A. _____

B. _____

C. _____

6. Regardless of the reason for initiating mechanical ventilation, what has to happen before you can get the patient off the ventilator?

_____

REASONS FOR VENTILATOR DEPENDENCE

7. Patients may need mechanical ventilation for apnea, ventilatory failure, or hypoxemia. They may remain dependent because of what four general factors?

A. _____

B. _____

C. _____

D. _____

8. State the four factors that determine total ventilatory workload.

A. _____

B. _____

C. _____

D. _____

9. What do fever, shivering, agitation, trauma, and sepsis have in common?

_____

10. List two causes of increased dead space ventilation.

A. _____

B. _____

11. Name four common causes of decreased lung compliance.

A. _____

B. _____

C. _____

D. _____

12. Name three causes of decreased thoracic compliance.

A. _____

B. _____

C. _____

13. State three causes of increased airway resistance.

A. _____

B. _____

C. _____

14. Why are artificial airways implicated in increased airway resistance?

_____

15. Give examples of conditions that adversely affect ventilatory capacity. Check out Box 47-2 for clues.

A. CNS drive

1. _____

2. _____

3. _____

4. _____

B. Muscle strength

1. _____

2. _____

3. _____

4. _____

Ok, so now you have this giant shopping list of things that could make removal from the ventilator difficult. Sometimes one thing, like reduced drive to breathe from drugs, is the problem. That's easy to solve. You can give an antidote (like Narcan for heroin or morphine), cleanse the blood (dialysis, for example), or just wait for the effects to wear off (anesthesia, for instance). Or, you might run into something a little more complicated. Like a depressed COPD patient with congestive heart failure (CHF) who has a small ET tube, bronchospasm, malnutrition, CO_2 retention, and electrolyte disorders along with the lung infection that put him on the ventilator in the first place! That's a plate full of issues to be resolved prior to weaning. See Box 47-3: *Factors that Contribute to Ventilator Dependence* if you need this to get more complicated.

481

Careful, systematic assessment is an especially important part of your approach to ventilator discontinuance.

16. What is the first thing you should evaluate whether you are considering weaning or taking the patient off the ventilator? *The single most important thing.*

    _____

17. What are the four questions you should ask?

    A. _____

    B. _____

    C. _____

    D. _____

    Once the patient is stable and things are looking up, you can take a look at the weaning indexes. Do they work? Like everything else, they sometimes work. Even though indexes have limitations, we still need to gather the information because it helps quantify the patient's overall status.

18. Your board exams will expect you to identify these classic criteria for weaning from mechanical ventilation. Remember that no one criterion mandates that you wean or don't wean! Use Table 47-1 to help out with this question. Again, YOU MUST KNOW THIS FOR THE BOARD EXAMS!

Measurement	Critical Value
A. $PaCO_2$	_____
B. pH	_____
C. VC (ml/kg)	_____
D. Spontaneous V_T	_____
E. Spontaneous rate	_____
F. V_E	_____
G. MVV	_____
H. MIF (NIF, MIP)	_____
I. V_D/V_T	_____
J. $P(A - a)O_2$ on 100%	_____
K. P/F ratio	_____
L. PaO_2	_____
M. Qs/Qt	_____
N. F_IO_2	_____
O. f/V_T	_____
P. Compliance	_____

Another giant menu to memorize and then apply to clinical care. (If it seems overwhelming, break it down into small pieces; learn a few at a time.)

19. Describe the breathing patterns that may cause problems with weaning or discontinuance.

20. Physical assessment of respiratory muscles may be useful. Describe what you are looking for in this area.

21. Rapid shallow breathing index may be the best overall predictor of weaning outcomes. Calculate the index for a patient who has a spontaneous rate of 25 with a spontaneous volume of 350 ml. What are the criteria for success?

    A. Formula _____

    B. Calculation _____

    C. Criteria _____

22. How could you modify the criteria to be a better predictor with elderly patients?

    _____

23. What do you have to do with the ventilator patient to get the RSBI?

24. Give the PaO_2, F_IO_2, and PEEP values that should be met prior to weaning.

    A. PaO_2 _____

    B. F_IO_2 _____

    C. PEEP _____

25. Explain why both low and high pH values are problematic in weaning.

26. Identify the critical values for confirming cardiovascular stability? (Refer to Table 47-2.)

Measurement	Values Inconsistent with Weaning
A. Heart rate	
B. Systolic pressure	
C. Diastolic pressure	
D. Hemoglobin	
E. Cardiac index (CI)	

27. Describe the ways that renal function may affect weaning.

A. Electrolytes _____

B. Fluid balance and urine output _____

C. Metabolic acidosis _____

28. Describe the ideal CNS status you'd like to see.

29. What two classes of drugs tend to interfere with weaning?

30. Because many factors are associated with success, weaning indexes are becoming more popular. What is a weaning index? Which one is the most useful?

31. What turns out to be the best approach after all?

_____

PREPARING THE PATIENT

A quick glance at Box 47-6 should amuse you or scare you—more than 60 factors to improve before attempting to discontinue the ventilator! The RT should start by optimizing those parts of the patient's medical condition over which they have direct control, and focus on psychological and environmental factors they can influence.

32. Name two drug therapies the RT can utilize to reduce airway resistance.

   A. _____

   B. _____

33. How else can the RT improve conditions in the airway?

   _____

34. What time of day should weaning activities be conducted?

   _____

35. What percentage of patients may develop "ICU psychosis" or other psychological disturbances after a few days in the unit?

   _____

36. How can the RT help the patient get adequate sleep?

   _____

37. Describe the environmental considerations that may improve patient well-being.

   _____

38. What three methods does *Egan's* identify for helping patients communicate?

   A. _____

   B. _____

   C. _____

WEANING METHODS

When the original problem is resolving, the indexes look good, and you've optimized as many factors as possible, you must get down to the business of discontinuing the ventilator. Rapidly or slowly, you have several methods to choose from.

39. List the three basic methods of discontinuing support.

   A. _____

   B. _____

   C. _____

40. Instead of putting the patient on a T-piece with an aerosol, you could use one of the spontaneous (CSV) ventilator modes. Name these two modes and suggest appropriate levels of support.

A. _____

B. _____

41. Describe the specific advantage of using the ventilator instead of the T-tube.

_____

42. What is the typical minimum length of time for a spontaneous trial when you are going for rapid discontinuance?

_____

43. How should you position the patient prior to the trial breathing period?

_____

Rapid discontinuance works really well on patients who have been on the ventilator for a short period of time (e.g., a postoperative patient, an OD who is now awake, that sort of thing). Wouldn't it be nice if more patients fell into this category? For the more difficult customer, you basically have three choices: T-piece, SIMV, or SBT.

44. Describe the T-piece (T-tube) trial for gradual weaning.

_____

45. What F_IO_2 is ideal for T-piece weaning?

_____

46. What happens at night?

_____

47. Describe the variation of this method where the patient is kept on the ventilator.

48. What are the biggest drawbacks to T-piece weaning?

49. Compare T-piece to IMV weaning.

Chapter **47** **Discontinuing Ventilatory Support**

50. Why do you think IMV (SIMV) is such a popular weaning method in the United States?

51. What does research show about SIMV?

_____

52. Describe pressure support ventilation (PSV).

_____

53. Pressure is normally set to achieve what initial range of tidal volume?

_____

54. From what level of PSV may a patient be extubated?

_____

55. What is an SAT? Why do we do it?

56. *Egan's* gives a formula for estimating the level of pressure support needed to overcome work of breathing. Calculate the level needed for a patient who has a PIP of 50 cm H_2O, plateau pressure of 30 cm H_2O, a ventilator flow rate of 60 L/min, and a spontaneous inspiratory flow rate of 30 L/min. (You can look at Mini-Clini, *Setting Pressure Support Levels,* for help.)

A. Formula _____

B. Calculation _____

C. Answer _____

If you're just trying to overcome work of breathing through the ET tube, it's a lot easier to use the "tube compensation" modes found on newer ventilators. The machine does the calculating for you. Other times you want to set PSV to achieve a desired tidal volume, either in units of ml or ml/kg. Another way to set PSV is to increase the pressure until the spontaneous rate drops to a desirable level.

SPONTANEOUS BREATHING TRIALS

Spontaneous breathing trial (SBT) is the hottest of the hot for ventilator discontinuance! Remember, this should be done formally and systematically by the therapist. The first SBT is a brief screening trial. Box 47-8 gives a step-by-step procedure for you.

57. How long is the first SBT?

_____

58. The formal SBT is at least _____ minutes and no longer than _____ minutes.

59. The SBT is sometimes performed with a T-piece or, if the patient stays on the vent, with PSV of _____ cm

H$_2$O or CPAP of ≤ _____ cm H$_2$O.

60. Monitor the patient during the trial. You should stop the SBT if distress occurs.

Assessment	Signs of Serious Distress
A. Mental status	
B. Respiratory rate	
C. Heart rate	
D. Blood pressure	
E. SpO$_2$	

61. When should you repeat the SBT if the patient fails the first trial?

_____

62. Describe mandatory minute ventilation (MMV).

_____

63. Describe adaptive support ventilation (ASV).

64. Describe the three basic ways NIV is used to assist weaning. Comment on each.

A.

B.

C.

65. Discontinuance is a relatively simple process of using SBTs along with protocols. Weaning is another story. What does the summary for this section say about "the best approach"?

Table 47-4 of *Egan's* summarizes the pros and cons of the various weaning methods.

MONITORING THE PATIENT

66. What are the two easily monitored and reliable indicators of patient progress during weaning?

A. _____

B. _____

67. What is the single best index of ventilation? How do you integrate this information with the clinical picture?

_____

68. What is the simplest way to monitor oxygenation during weaning?

69. Give the expected and excessive changes for each of the following parameters. Check out Table 47-6 if you get lost.

Parameter	Expected	Deleterious
A. Respiratory rate	_____	_____
B. PaO_2	_____	_____
C. $PaCO_2$	_____	_____
D. Heart rate	_____	_____
E. Blood pressure	_____	_____

The NBRC will expect you to know these changes well. So do your instructors. (So does the patient!)

EXTUBATION

Weaning and extubation are separate issues. We know this, but other clinicians may not be as clear, so the RT has to be a strong advocate in the decision to remove or maintain the artificial airway. Failed extubation may be hazardous to your patient's health. A study published in *Respiratory Care* indicated that a failure rate (patient requiring reintubation) of 10% to 20% was acceptable in the medical ICU population. In the surgical ICU (uncomplicated postoperative patients), a failure rate of less than 5% is OK. Failure rates above 20% probably mean you are not assessing the patients carefully enough. Failure rates below 10% probably mean you are keeping the patient on the ventilator too long!

70. What is the important thing to remember about the presence of the artificial airway in terms of weaning? What can be done about it?

_____

71. What is the minimum ability required for personnel performing routine extubation?

_____

72. What is the minimum ability required for personnel performing high-risk extubation?

_____

73. What are common patient complaints following extubation?

74. Describe the cuff leak test.

75. Identify the appropriate treatment for postextubation stridor.

A. Mild _____

B. Moderate _____

C. Severe _____

76. What patients are at risk for aspiration following extubation? How can you minimize the risk?

_____

FAILURE TO WEAN

As much as we all want to get the patient off the vent, it doesn't always work.

77. Identify five common causes of weaning failure from Box 47-13.

A. _____

B. _____

C. _____

D. _____

E. _____

78. The ICU is no place for the long-term ventilator patient. It's too expensive, and the staff is not usually trained to deal with the issues. What are the alternative care sites?

_____

490

79. Table 47-7 is a monster! Identify strategies for each of the following problems.

Problem	Management Strategy
A. Anemia	_____
B. Tube-related WOB	_____
C. Bronchospasm	_____ _____
D. Secretions	_____ _____
E. Dyspnea	_____ _____
F. Muscle fatigue	_____ _____
G. Hemodynamics	_____ _____
H. Infection	_____
I. Metabolic	_____ _____
J. Nutrition	_____ _____
K. Exercise	_____ _____
L. Psychological	_____ _____ _____
M. Sleep	_____ _____ _____
N. Pain	_____ _____

Many of these techniques are useful once the patient is removed from the ICU and placed in an alternate site. A skilled, multidisciplinary approach is needed for the chronic ventilator patient. In the end, some patients will remain on the machine for life.

80. Who should be involved in the decision to terminate life support?

_____

81. Discuss the three factors mentioned in your text used to help make the decision.

CASE STUDIES

Case 1

A 61-year-old woman is placed on the ventilator for respiratory failure for CHF and COPD. Twenty-four hours later, the physician asks for your recommendation regarding weaning. Breath sounds reveal coarse crackles in both bases. Pedal edema is present as well. The following information is obtained.

Spontaneous RR	28
Spontaneous V_t	0.2 L
MIF	−18 cm H_2O
VC	0.6 L
HR	116
BP	90/60
pH	7.33
$PaCO_2$	35 mm Hg
PaO_2	65 (on F_IO_2 0.5)
Cardiac index	2.3

82. What is your assessment of her respiratory status?

83. Has the primary problem been resolved?

84. What is the rapid shallow breathing index?

85. Explain your recommendation regarding initiating weaning. If you recommend weaning, also recommend the method.

A 61-year-old man is placed on the ventilator following open-heart surgery. Twelve hours later, the patient is awake and the physician asks for your recommendation regarding weaning. The following information is obtained:

Spontaneous RR	14
Spontaneous V_T	0.2 L
MIF	−35 cm H_2O
VC	1.2 L
HR	116
BP	90/60
pH	7.37
$PaCO_2$	35 mm Hg
PaO_2	85 (on F_IO_2 0.35)

86. What is your assessment of his respiratory status?

87. Has the primary problem been resolved?

_____

88. What is the rapid shallow breathing index?

_____

89. Explain your recommendation regarding initiating weaning. If you recommend weaning, also recommend a technique.

A 61-year-old is placed on the ventilator following an acute episode of Guillain-Barré syndrome. At 21 days later, the patient is regaining strength and movement in his limbs. The physician asks for your recommendation regarding weaning. The following information is obtained:

Spontaneous RR	22
Spontaneous V_T	0.22 L
MIF	−20 cm H_2O
VC	1.0 L
HR	116
BP	90/60
pH	7.38
$PaCO_2$	37 mm Hg
PaO_2	70 (on F_IO_2 0.40)

90. What is your assessment of his respiratory status?

_____

91. Has the primary problem been resolved?

_____

92. What is the rapid shallow breathing index?

_____

93. Explain your recommendation regarding initiating weaning. If you recommend weaning, also recommend a technique.

A 5 foot 2 inch, 50-kg, 80-year-old woman has been on the ventilator for 2 days following open-heart surgery due to hemodynamic instability. The vitals are now stable. The physician wants you to conduct a spontaneous breathing trial. You suction the patient and sit her up for trial. Pretrial respiratory rate is 22, MIP is −45 mm Hg, and spontaneous volume is 400 ml. She is placed on a T-piece for 3 minutes with 40% oxygen. After 3 minutes, the f is 25, MIP is −40, and V_T is 420.

94. What would you recommend at this time?

_____

95. What is the RSBI? _____

96. How long does she need to succeed on the trial before you would consider extubation?

_____

It's clear that weaning and discontinuance are important topics. But is weaning really specified in the exam matrices? The Examination Matrix states that you should "Initiate and modify weaning procedures" and "wean or change weaning procedures and extubation." The key to understanding this subject is in the ways mechanical ventilation is applied. Modes like PSV, SIMV, IMV, CPAP, and PEEP are frequently cited in different areas of these test preparation tools. This makes it difficult to know exactly how many questions on weaning will be on an individual test. It could vary from a few (two or three) to many (five to seven)!

Here are some examples for your thinking pleasure. Circle the best answer.

97. Which of the following would you evaluate prior to initiating T-piece weaning?
    1. PaO_2
    2. Gag reflex
    3. Spontaneous respiratory rate
    4. Urine output
       A. 1 and 2 only
       B. 1 and 3 only
       C. 2 and 4 only
       D. 3 and 4 only

98. A patient being assessed for readiness to wean has the following values:

pH	7.36
$PaCO_2$	42 mm Hg
PaO_2	67 mm Hg (F_iO_2 40%)
MIP	−25 cm H_2O
Pulse	105
Respirations	20
VC	12 ml/kg

    What action should the RT recommend at this time?
    A. Initiate a T-piece trial.
    B. Continue with mechanical ventilation.
    C. Initiate breathing exercises to strengthen ventilatory muscles.
    D. Repeat the vital capacity maneuver.

99. Which of the following indicates a readiness to wean?
    A. spontaneous rate of 28
    B. spontaneous tidal volume of 200 ml
    C. negative inspiratory force of 18 cm H_2O
    D. minute volume of 8 L/min

100. An alert patient is being mechanically ventilated. Settings are:

Mode	SIMV
Rate	2
Tidal volume (set)	800
F_iO_2	0.30
PEEP	5 cm H_2O

    ABG results 30 minutes after initiating these settings are:

pH	7.37
$PaCO_2$	38 mm Hg
PaO_2	75 mm Hg

    What should the RT recommend at this time?
    A. Increase the set rate to 4.
    B. Discontinue mechanical ventilation.
    C. Decrease the PEEP to 0 cm H_2O.
    D. Decrease the F_iO_2 to 0.21.

101. A 70-year-old, 70-kg (154-lb) patient with a history of COPD is being mechanically ventilated. The patient is alert, but making no spontaneous efforts.

Mode	AC
Rate	12
Tidal volume (set)	800
F_IO_2	0.40
PEEP	3 cm H_2O
pH	7.51
$PaCO_2$	38 mm Hg
PaO_2	95 mm Hg
HCO_3^-	36 mEq/L

Which of the following should the RT recommend?
1. Change to SIMV mode.
2. Decrease the F_IO_2.
3. Decrease the set rate.
4. Decrease the PEEP.
   A. 1 and 2 only
   B. 1 and 3 only
   C. 1, 2, and 3 only
   D. 1, 3, and 4 only

102. A patient is being ventilated in the SIMV mode with a rate of 8, volume of 800, and F_IO_2 of 0.40. ABG results show:

pH	7.47
$PaCO_2$	33 mm Hg
PaO_2	88 mm Hg
HCO_3^-	23 mEq/L

What action should the RT recommend in response to these findings?
A. Increase the tidal volume.
B. Increase the F_IO_2.
C. Change to AC mode.
D. Reduce the rate.

103. A patient on SIMV experiences difficulty each time you try to reduce the rate below 6. The patient becomes tachypneic with a rate of 28 and a spontaneous volume of 200. Which of the following modifications would be *least* useful in this situation?
A. adding pressure support ventilation
B. T-piece weaning
C. trial of extubation
D. changing to flow-by or flow triggering

It's not too difficult to wean patients on paper if you know your *values!* Watch out for COPD patients who are being overventilated or overoxygenated by the machine.

FOOD FOR THOUGHT

104. What is the single best approach to weaning?

_____

48 Neonatal and Pediatric Respiratory Care

The only creatures that are evolved enough to convey pure love are dogs and infants.
Johnny Depp

Whether you dream of working with this special population, in a community hospital where you will need the skills and knowledge periodically, or just want to do well on your boards, you will find Chapter 48 is just what the doctor ordered for mastering neonatal and pediatric care. It's a comprehensive and comprehensible overview of the care and feeding of little ones who can't breathe. This is a very long chapter, packed with a huge amount of information, so make an extra large pot of coffee for this one. (If you need a refresher on fetal lung development and anatomic differences between kids and adults, you'll find it in Chapter 8.)

WORD WIZARD

You have probably noticed that medical terminology is important and medicine likes acronyms. Here's a final set to help you build up your baby talk. Write out the words to these letters.

A. AGA _____

B. CPAP _____

C. ECMO _____

D. HFV _____

E. INO _____

F. PEFV _____

G. PPHN _____

H. ELBW _____

I. VLBW _____

J. PDA _____

K. ROP _____

FETAL ASSESSMENT

1. Assessment of the newborn begins with maternal history. Identify three conditions that are likely to result in a baby that is small for its gestational age. (Refer to Table 48-1.)

   A. _____

   B. _____

   C. _____

2. Identify five maternal factors likely to lead to premature delivery.

A. _____

B. _____

C. _____

D. _____

E. _____

3. What maternal metabolic condition is likely to result in an infant who is large for its gestational age?

_____

4. The fetus can be assessed by a variety of methods. Briefly describe each of the following tests. Think "When would I recommend this test?" and you'll be thinking like an RT (One who passes the Registry Exams…!
   A. Ultrasonography

   B. Amniocentesis (Be sure to include LS ratio and PG. Also, include normal and abnormal values and what the terms mean.)

   C. Fetal heart rate monitoring (Be sure to discuss accelerations and deaccels and heart rate values and what they mean.)

   D. Fetal blood gas analysis (Include normals and describe the relationship between fetal scalp gases and arterial blood gases.)

5. When are Apgar scores taken? _____

6. You *simply must* learn the Apgar scoring system. (Refer to Table 48-2.)

	SIGN	**0**	**1**	**2**
A.	Heart rate			
B.	Respiration			
C.	Muscle tone			
D.	Reflex			
E.	Color			

Hint: You could make up some kind of mnemonic to help you remember the five signs like "Heart Rate Must Really Count."

7. What term is used to describe the following weeks of gestation?

   A. Before 38 weeks _____

   B. 38 to 42 weeks _____

   C. After 42 weeks _____

8. Name the two common systems used for assessing gestational age based on physical characteristics and neurologic signs.

   A. _____

   B. _____

9. Explain the abbreviations and identify the weights that correspond to the following terms.

	ABBREVIATION	**FULL NAME**	**WEIGHTS/PERCENTS**
A.	VLBW		
B.	LBW		
C.	AGA		
D.	LGA		
E.	SGA		

10. Why does anyone care about birth weight and gestational age?

11. State the normal range for a full-term infant's vital signs.

    A. Heart rate _____

    B. Respiratory rate _____

    C. Blood pressure _____

12. Describe the usual way to take an infant's heart rate. Where do you place the stethoscope?

    A. Method _____

    B. Stethoscope placement _____

13. Why is it important to check the pulses in different areas of the baby's body?

14. Infants in respiratory distress typically exhibit one or more of these five signs. Explain the significance of each sign.

    A. Nasal flaring _____

    B. Cyanosis _____

    C. Expiratory grunting _____

    D. Retractions _____

    E. Paradoxical breathing _____

One therapy can often be effectively applied when you see several of these signs. What is it?

15. What scoring system is used to grade the severity of underlying lung disease?

    _____

16. Once the decision is made to administer surfactant to a premature infant you will need to adjust both of these (list how you will adjust each):
    A. Ventilating pressure

    B. F_IO_2

Preterm

Post-term

17. What are the two usual sites for obtaining blood gas samples in infants according to Chapter 48?

A. _____

B. _____

18. The pulse oximeter can be a useful tool if you know the rules for babies. Discuss right and left placements and two defects that commonly cause hypoxemia. Where does that probe go?

A. Right _____

B. Left _____

C. Defects _____

D. Probe _____

19. List the ABG values for preterm and term infants at birth. (Refer to Table 48-4.)

	PARAMETER	PRETERM (1 TO 5 HOURS)	NORMAL TERM (5 HOURS)	NORMAL PRETERM INFANTS (5 DAYS)
A.	pH			
B.	$PaCO_2$			
C.	PaO_2			

20. Newborns have meaningful breath sounds.
    A. List four causes of stridor.

    B. Explain how wheezing is treated in kids.

Oxygen Therapy

21. Considering the hazards, we need to agree on the safe limits for oxygen therapy. Give the accepted ranges for these parameters.

    A. F_IO_2 < _____ %

    B. Preemie SpO_2 _____ to _____

22. Hyperoxia is associated with ROP and BPD in some infants. What do these acronyms stand for?

    A. ROP: _____

    B. BPD: _____

23. Which babies are most likely to get ROP?

24. How could oxygen cause heart problems to worsen in some newborns?

25. Compare the use of the following oxygen delivery devices. (Refer to Table 48-6.)

	DEVICE	AGE	ADVANTAGE	DISADVANTAGE
A.	AEM			
B.	Cannula			
C.	Incubator			
D.	Hood			
E.	Tent			

Bronchial Hygiene

26. Name four conditions in which secretion retention is common in children.

    A. _____

    B. _____

    C. _____

    D. _____

27. Identify one other situation where bronchial hygiene therapy may be useful.

28. Because infants cannot cough on command, how will you get the mucus out once it is mobilized?

29. Why is it so important to monitor ALL aspects of infants who need bronchial hygiene therapy?

30. How can you monitor hypoxemia during head-down positioning?

Humidity and Aerosol Therapy

31. What type of device is used for patients who are intubated?

_____

32. What's important about volume and water level for babies on ventilators in terms of humidification?

33. What factors could affect the delivery of humidity from a servo-controlled heated humidifier to an infant who is mechanically ventilated?

There are three reasons why continuous nebulization is usually avoided in infants and toddlers. First, you can get problems with fluid balance in really little ones. All these nebs increase the risk of infection. Finally, these aerosol generators make so much noise they can harm babies!

SAY "YES" TO AEROSOL DRUG THERAPY

34. State the three methods you can use to give aerosol medications to children.

    A. _____

    B. _____

    C. _____

35. What would you add to the MDI or SVN to deliver an MDI to an infant?

36. What is the dosage range for albuterol delivered by SVN? See Table 48-7.

    _____

37. What is the dosage range and frequency for racemic epinephrine?

    A. Dose _____

    B. Frequency _____

38. What is the dosage and treatment schedule for nebulized budesonide?

    A. Dose _____

    B. Treatment schedule _____

39. Which kids should not get Atrovent for their asthma?

40. When should you avoid Serevent or Advair?

41. Cromolyn is an asthma medication that is not ever given as a _____ drug.

42. Before you use Mucomyst as a mucolytic you should pretreat with what drug?

AIRWAY MANAGEMENT

43. Identify the correct ET size and suction catheter size for these children. (Refer to Table 48-8.)

	AGE/WEIGHT	ET INTERNAL DIAMETER (ID)	LENGTH (ORAL)	SUCTION
A.	<1000 g			
B.	1000 to 2000 g			
C.	2000 to 3000 g			
D.	>3000 g			
E.	2 years			
F.	6 years			

44. State the two formulas for calculating tube diameter and length.

A. Tube ID No. 1 _____ Tube ID No. 2 _____.

B. Tube length oral No. 1 _____ Tube length nasal No. 2 _____.

45. What is the consequence of placing an ET tube that is too small in an infant?

46. Estimate the correct tube size for a 4-year-old using the first formula in question 44.

47. Estimate the correct tube size for a child who is 122 cm (48 inches) tall.

_____

48. Which laryngoscope blade is usually used for infant intubation?

_____

49. What is the main difference between infant or pediatric ET tubes and adult ET tubes?

_____

50. What airway can be used as an alternative to intubation in children?

51. What are the recommended vacuum pressures for suctioning infants and children?

  A. Infants _____

  B. Children _____

52. Identify the criteria for initiating chest compressions after delivery.

_____

ADVANCED FUN AND GAMES

53. Play with baby's FRC by applying CPAP. What is the specific indication for CPAP? Give the blood gas values.

  A. Indication _____

  B. Blood gas values _____

54. Name four signs of respiratory distress that suggest using CPAP. (Refer to Box 48-4.)

  A. _____

  B. _____

  C. _____

  D. _____

55. Discuss adjustment of CPAP in infants.
  A. Start at

  B. Adjust in increments of

56. CPAP is usually administered to an infant via what old and what new type of interface? What about kids?

A. Babies (2 types) _____

B. Kids _____

HIGH-FLOW NASAL CANNULA

Most cannulas work, but only at low flows due to humidification issues. New humidifiers allow you to go higher.

57. What is the range of flow given for the new cannulas?

_____

58. What problem may occur if the prongs on a high-flow system fit tightly in the nares?

MECHANICAL VENTILATION

59. You know you have respiratory failure and the need to ventilate when:

A. $PaCO_2 <$ _____

B. $PaO_2 >$ _____

60. You suspect you need to ventilate with what pulmonary diseases? Check out Box 48-5.

A. _____

B. _____

C. _____

D. _____

61. Give the range of PIP for infants for initiating time-cycled pressure limited ventilation.

_____

62. Identify the inspiratory time ranges that should be set for these age groups.

A. Neonates _____

B. Older children _____

63. Ventilator rates should be adjusted to maintain a normal range of what ABG value?

_____

64. What PEEP levels are usually used in neonates for initiating ventilation?

_____

65. What range of volumes is normally used when volume ventilation is selected?

_____

66. Why would it be common to observe lower exhaled than inhaled volumes in pediatric patients? Hint: Think about the type of airway used.

_____

67. List at least five things you should consider prior to extubating a baby.

A. _____

B. _____

C. _____

D. _____

E. _____

HIGH FREQUENCY VENTILATION

68. HFV is often initiated as "rescue therapy." Explain.

69. Identify the two common characteristics of HFV.

A. V_T _____

B. Rate _____

70. What are the three types of HFV? Which is more common?

A. _____

B. _____

C. _____

Most common? _____

71. How would you wean a patient from HFV?

Nitric oxide (NO) is an FDA-approved drug. When you inhale this gas, it's called iNO. NO selectively vasodilates pulmonary vessels surrounding the functional alveoli.

72. What effect does NO have on oxygenation? ECMO?

_____

73. Two big problems exist with NO inhalation. Explain.
    A. Rebound pulmonary hypertension

    B. Altered hemoglobin

You can read more about this gas in Chapter 38: Medical Gas Therapy.

EXTRACORPOREAL MEMBRANE OXYGENATION

Hours of Boredom, Moments of Terror

An RT who performs extracorporeal membrane oxygenation (ECMO) describes her job as pretty routine until something goes wrong. ECMO is a fascinating and vital form of therapy where RTs play a leading role. Over 16,000 neonates have been treated with ECMO with a 78% survival rate.

74. What does ECMO do?

75. Describe the two basic forms of ECMO.
    A. VA

    B. VV

76. Give three examples of neonatal conditions where ECMO is being used after conventional medical therapies fail.

A. _____

B. _____

C. _____

WHAT DOES THE NBRC SAY?

The exam matrices make detailed references to the material in Chapter 48. Here's a partial list:
- Perinatal data
  - Maternal history
  - Perinatal history
  - Apgar scores
  - Gestational age
  - L/S ratio
  - Preductal and postductal oxygenation studies
- Equipment
  - Oxygen hoods and tents
  - Specialized ventilators: high frequency

The Clinical Simulation Examination Matrix makes it clear that you will have one pediatric and one neonatal problem. That material is covered in Chapter 34.

While Chapter 48 covers some of this information, you would be wise to consider taking a neonatal resuscitation program (NRP) and pediatric advanced life support (PALS) course before you take the boards. Those two courses are specifically mentioned in the matrix.

Here are some sample multiple-choice questions. Circle the best answer.

77. Which of the following tests would be useful in determining lung maturity?
    A. sweat chloride
    B. L/S ratio
    C. fetal hemoglobin
    D. pneumogram

78. Calculate the Apgar score for a crying infant who has a heart rate of 120, actively moves, sneezes when a catheter is put in the nose, but has blue extremities.
    A. 5
    B. 6
    C. 7
    D. 9

79. The simplest way to apply CPAP to treat hypoxemia in an infant is to use _____.
    A. nasal prongs
    B. nasal mask
    C. full-face mask
    D. oxygen hood

80. Excessive oxygen delivery to newborns may raise the risk of
    A. pneumonia
    B. retinopathy
    C. cystic fibrosis
    D. PPHN

81. What vacuum pressure would you set for suctioning a newborn?
    A. 40-60 mm Hg
    B. 60-80 mm Hg
    C. 80-100 mm Hg
    D. 80-120 mm Hg

82. What laryngoscope blade would you select for intubation of a newborn?
    A. Miller
    B. Macintosh
    C. LMA
    D. Fiberoptic

83. What size endotracheal tube would you recommend for a 1500-g preemie?
    A. 2.5
    B. 3.0
    C. 3.5
    D. 4.0

FOOD FOR THOUGHT

If you choose to work in this field, it would be a good idea to take the Neonatal/Pediatric Specialist Examination to test your knowledge and demonstrate your competence in this specialty area.

49 Patient Education and Health Promotion

Quit worrying about your health. It will go away.
Robert Orben

Teaching can be very satisfying—when learning is taking place! It's equally frustrating to try to learn when teaching is disorganized or the objectives are unclear. Client and community education really go to the far ends of the spectrum. It is tremendously rewarding to help someone quit smoking, learn to be more independent, or to teach children how to manage their asthma. These are REAL victories in the battle for better health! On the other hand, you can go nuts trying to get your message across to some people. Chapter 49 provides you with valuable ideas on how to develop, conduct, and measure the outcomes of a health education program. You can use this information in school, with patients, in the community, and in teaching co-workers. Let's go do some educating!

WORD WIZARD

Make sure you have a good grasp of the key terms in this chapter before you apply them. Write out the definition for each of these terms. You can use the chapter or the glossary.

1. Affective domain _____

2. Cognitive domain _____

3. Health education _____

4. Health promotion _____

5. Psychomotor domain _____

PATIENT EDUCATION

Respiratory care practitioners have always been on-the-spot instructors at the bedside, but the role of RT as formal educator has increased dramatically in the past few years as health care delivery methods and settings have changed.

Overview

6. What are the top five causes of death in the United States?

1. _____

2. _____

3. _____

4. _____

5. _____

7. Why is educating the public about these illnesses so important?

_____

What's in a Domain?

8. Why should you consider developing written objectives for patient teaching?

_____

9. How can you state an objective in measurable terms?

   A. Begin with a _____

   B. Write an action _____

   C. Add a condition _____

   D. Write a standard _____

10. Give an example of an objective for each of the following learning domains. (Oh, go ahead, take one out of *Egan's*.)

	DOMAIN	OBJECTIVE
A.	Cognitive	
B.	Affective	
C.	Psychomotor	

11. Which of the learning domains should be evaluated before you proceed with patient education?

_____

12. Maslow's hierarchy of needs (pretty useful if you apply it) explains why a dyspneic patient will not be very receptive to learning a new skill. How can you assess readiness to learn?

_____

13. What is the key to motivating patients to learn?

_____

14. What is the key to teaching psychomotor skills? How can you confirm that a patient or family member has learned a new skill? (This is a board exam question, by the way!)

_____

15. Give an example from the text of how to relate psychomotor skills a patient uses every day to help make the transition from everyday life to therapy.

_____

F.A.T. T.I.P.S.*

Now that you've reviewed some important ideas about teaching, let's take a look at:

CRYSTAL CLEAR CLASSROOM COMMANDMENTS
- I. Meet immediate patient needs *first*.
- II. Create an educational setting.
- III. Include hearing, seeing, touching, writing, speaking.
- IV. Keep sessions short.
- V. Repeat, repeat, repeat!
- VI. Allow plenty of time to practice skills.
- VII. Spend time preparing for the session.
- VIII. Organize your materials and presentation.
- IX. Personalize and customize the learning experience.
- X. Be enthusiastic!!!

If you think about your own learning experiences, you will have no difficulty believing in these powerful ideas for improving your teaching abilities. (Make a copy and mail them to someone!)

Teaching Children

Respiratory therapists teach children more than any other group. Cystic fibrosis and asthma are common conditions you will encounter in the NBRC hospital and the clinical setting.

16. How is teaching children different from teaching adults? How is it the same? (Refer to Boxes 49-1 and 49-2.)

17. Where could you find resource materials to help in teaching children with asthma? (Check out the Mini-Clini on page 1273.)

_____

18. What suggestions are given for rewarding performance?

Evaluation

19. What process answers the question "Has the patient learned?" When should you begin to develop this process?

20. Describe some of the formal and informal ways you can tell if a patient has met affective domain objectives.

HEALTH EDUCATION

Naturally, RTs are expected to be role models (see the AARC guideline) who demonstrate healthy behaviors in public. Imagine giving a patient information about nicotine intervention when you smell like cigarettes yourself! Role models aren't enough, however, to achieve large-scale improvements in public health.

21. The primary goal of health education is to _____ people's _____.

22. Learning activities must incorporate values and beliefs of the learner. What four factors need to be considered in this area?

    A. _____

    B. _____

    C. _____

    D. _____

23. How do the personal characteristics of the educator impact on learning?

AN OUNCE OF PREVENTION IS WORTH...

24. State the four major preventable causes of death in the United States and explain the cause of each one.

    A. _____

    B. _____

    C. _____

    D. _____

25. Compare the standard medical approach to health in the United States with the public health model.

516

26. What are two broad goals of the Healthy People 2010 initiative?

27. Discuss how RTs might participate in the management of COPD through education?

28. Besides the hospital, name four other settings where RTs would be likely to function as individual counselors or public health advocates.

A. _____

B. _____

C. _____

D. _____

CASE STUDIES

Your text has several perfectly good cases in the form of "Mini-Clinis," so let's do something else. Suppose you had to teach your classmates how to use a peak flow meter. Write three objectives for this topic for each domain using behavioral terms.

29. Cognitive domain
A.

B.

C.

30. Affective domain
    A.

    B.

    C.

31. Psychomotor domain
    A.

    B.

    C.

32. How long would your teaching session last?

    _____

33. Give examples of how you would involve the following senses in your session.

    A. Hearing _____

    B. Seeing _____

    C. Touching _____

    D. Writing _____

    E. Speaking _____

34. Give an example of how you would measure learning for each domain.

A. Cognitive _____

B. Affective _____

C. Psychomotor _____

WHAT DOES THE NBRC SAY?

Well, you should be able to educate a patient. Here's an example.

35. The best way to ensure that a patient learned to properly administer a bronchodilator via MDI is to _____.
A. ask the patient to answer questions regarding inhaler use
B. give the patient appropriate literature regarding MDI use
C. ask the patient to demonstrate how to use the inhaler
D. have the patient explain when he is to use the MDI

FOOD FOR THOUGHT

36. Why do you think the public should be educated about the risk factors for the top five causes of death? After all, a lot of RTs are employed in taking care of patients who have ignored these risk factors.

37. How is teaching other caregivers different from teaching patients or family members?

50 Cardiopulmonary Rehabilitation

No one is useless in this world who lightens the burden of another.
Charles Dickens

Alvan Barach first recommended reconditioning programs for COPD patients over 60 years ago. Unfortunately, it was not until recently that these programs began in earnest around the nation. In the 1980s, it was often up to the individual therapist to try to provide and encourage these concepts for individual patients. Now there are many well-established inpatient and outpatient programs to meet the physical and psychosocial needs of patients with chronic lung disease.

While there are many good textbooks and patient teaching aids available, you will find that Chapter 50 provides an excellent overview of the subject. Even if you don't work in rehabilitation, you will be in a position to identify patients who can benefit from these services, and can play a key role in improving the quality of your patients' lives. You may also wish to participate in one of the Better Breather's Clubs founded by the American Lung Association, local health care organizations, or the closest chapter of the American Association for Respiratory Care.

WORD WIZARD

You can build impressive mental muscles by adding these words to your vocabulary. Match the following terms and acronyms to their definitions.

Terms and Acronyms	Definitions
1. _____ ADL	A. physical activities designed to strengthen muscles and improve O_2 utilization
2. _____ Borg scale	B. measure of an individual's ability to perform common tasks
3. _____ CORF	C. point where there is insufficient O_2 to meet the demands of energy metabolism
4. _____ Karvonen's formula	D. measure of an individual's perception of breathing difficulty
5. _____ progressive resistance	E. cardiac goal for aerobic conditioning based on 65% of maximum O_2 consumption
6. _____ OBLA	F. ratio of CO_2 production to O_2 consumption
7. _____ reconditioning	G. Medicare-approved facility that provides ambulatory rehab services
8. _____ respiratory quotient	H. common method used to calculate target heart rate for exercise
9. _____ target heart rate	I. training method that gradually increases muscle workloads

DEFINITIONS AND GOALS

Pulmonary rehabilitation is not the same animal as other types of rehab, although it can contain some of the same elements.

10. What is meant by the general term "rehabilitation"?

11. The definition of pulmonary rehabilitation is really long. Please put it into your own words.

12. What are the three general goals of pulmonary rehabilitation?

    A. _____

    B. _____

    C. _____

SCIENTIFIC BASIS FOR PULMONARY REHABILITATION

Exercise physiology plays an important role in our understanding of the benefits of reconditioning, but physiology alone is not sufficient to achieve desired outcomes in patients with COPD.

13. How do social sciences play a role in establishing ways to improve the patient's quality of life?

14. Why is MVV a useful pulmonary function test in regard to assessing physical activity?

15. How can you estimate MVV using simple spirometry?

    _____

16. Identify the three general ways that reconditioning will increase exercise tolerance.

    A. _____

    B. _____

    C. _____

17. Compare the roles of psychosocial and physical methods in terms of outcomes of rehabilitation.

18. Describe the two-way relationship of physical reconditioning and psychosocial support.

Program designs may vary, but the desired outcomes and basic components are similar.

19. Why is it so important to have specific objectives for the program goals? How should these objectives be stated?

    A.

    B.

20. State five accepted benefits of exercise reconditioning. (Refer to Box 50-1.)

    A. _____

    B. _____

    C. _____

    D. _____

    E. _____

21. Research literature clearly shows that rehabilitation has proven benefits. What is the effect of rehabilitation on the progression of the disease?

22. Name three common goals (*not objectives*) for rehab programs (Box 50-2).

    A. _____

    B. _____

    C. _____

23. Who manages the overall care in a program and screens the prospective patients?

    _____

24. What is the first step in patient evaluation for a pulmonary rehab program?

    _____

25. Name four tests that should be included with the physical examination.

A. _____

B. _____

C. _____

D. _____

26. Two tests are usually conducted to assess cardiopulmonary status. State two purposes for these tests.

A. Exercise evaluation

1. _____

2. _____

B. Pulmonary function testing

1. _____

2. _____

27. List two contraindications to exercise testing.

28. Identify four physiologic parameters that should be monitored during exercise testing.

A. _____

B. _____

C. _____

D. _____

29. Name two types of patients that are usually excluded from selection for rehab.

A. _____

B. _____

30. State the four general groups of patients included in pulmonary rehab programs.

A. _____

B. _____

C. _____

D. _____

524

31. What are the benefits of grouping patients together on the basis of severity and overall ability?

32. Give one benefit and one drawback of the open-ended program model.

   A. Benefit: _____

   B. Drawback: _____

33. Give one benefit and one drawback to the traditional closed design.

   A. Benefit: _____

   B. Drawback: _____

34. Describe the new Medicare coverage for pulmonary rehabilitation.

35. Describe two ways to set target heart rate for patient exercise.

   A. Formula _____

   B. Estimate _____

36. Describe a typical walking exercise program. What is our minimum walk time?

37. What is the basic concept behind ventilatory muscle training?

38. Briefly discuss the following high-priority program educational components.

   A. Breathing control

B. Stress management

C. Medications

D. Diet

39. What is the ideal class size for a rehab program? What external factor affects this ideal?

40. Give specific examples for each of the following sources of program reimbursement. (Check out Box 50-6.)

   A. Nongovernment health insurance _____

   B. Federal and state health insurance _____

   C. Ancillary insurance _____

   D. Other options _____

41. What is/are the most likely cause(s) of lack of measurable improvement within a pulmonary rehab program?

42. Potential hazards do exist. Give one from each category:

   A. Cardio _____

   B. Blood gas _____

   C. Muscular _____

   D. Miscellaneous _____

Case 1

An alert 55-year-old man with long-standing asthma and COPD is admitted for acute exacerbation of his illness following a "chest cold." This is the fourth admission for this patient in the past 3 months. He tells you that he has had to quit his job and take early retirement because of his lung problems.

43. What concerns does this situation raise?

44. Explain the benefits of entering a rehab program to this patient.

Case 2

A 57-year-old woman with chronic bronchitis is enrolled in your pulmonary rehab program. During walking exercises, she complains of dyspnea and will not continue with the walk.

45. What assessments would be useful in this situation?

46. Give several possible methods for modifying the exercise program to improve this patient's compliance.

WHAT DOES THE NBRC SAY?

In the case of pulmonary rehabilitation, the Examination Matrix is very specific:
1. Explain planned therapy and goals to patient in understandable terms to achieve optimal therapeutic outcome.
2. Educate patient and family in disease management.
3. Counsel patient and family concerning smoking cessation.
4. Instruct patient and family to assure safety and infection control.

You will only see about two multiple-choice questions per examination (CRT and WRE). The Clinical Simulation Matrix includes identical items but also specifically mentions that you may encounter a case of a patient with COPD who needs pulmonary rehabilitation. This means that rehab is a small but very important part of the credentialing process. Here are a few representative questions. Circle the answers.

47. A COPD patient has enrolled in a pulmonary rehabilitation program. The patient should be informed that the program will help provide all of the benefits *except* _____.
   A. increased physical endurance
   B. improved PFT results
   C. increased activity levels
   D. improved cardiovascular function

48. During an exercise test a patient is able to reach a maximum heart rate of 120. His resting heart rate is 70. What target heart rate would you recommend for this patient during aerobic conditioning?
   A. 70 beats per minute
   B. 85 beats per minute
   C. 100 beats per minute
   D. 115 beats per minute

49. Which of the following tests would be useful in assessing ventilatory reserve during exercise testing?
   A. forced vital capacity
   B. maximum voluntary ventilation
   C. body plethysmography
   D. single breath nitrogen washout

FOOD FOR THOUGHT

All through *Egan's* we find references to the Borg scale. This scale is a valuable tool that can be easily used at the bedside or in the rehab setting.

50. Describe the Borg scale.

51. What are the units of measurement on the scale?

_____

52. What is the value of this instrument?

Respiratory Care in Alternative Settings

Problems are only opportunities in work clothes.
Henry J. Kaiser

Egan's had to end with a beginning, and Chapter 51 introduces you to a fast-growing segment of the respiratory industry. As health care is being redefined on many levels, the work setting for our profession is moving outside the boundaries of the traditional medical center concept. Alternative care settings provide special challenges for the respiratory therapist, particularly the new graduate.

WORD WIZARD

No matter what else you got out of this book, you're bound to have a brain full of odd letter combinations. Don't worry, this is the last of the acronyms. Write out the meanings.

1. CMS _____

2. DME _____

3. PPS _____

4. NIV _____

5. SAHS _____

6. AARC _____

7. SNF _____

8. TTOT _____

RECENT TRENDS

9. What is the most common alternative site for health care?

_____

10. What was the overall effect of the PPS system? How has the BBA impacted RTs?

A. PPS

B. BBA

11. What were the results of the Muse study?

DEFINITIONS AND GOALS

12. Name the five areas of nonacute or alternative care.

    A. _____

    B. _____

    C. _____

    D. _____

    E. _____

13. Describe the LTACH and its relationship to respiratory care.

14. What is "subacute" care?

15. Name some of the most common respiratory care services provided in alternative settings.

    A. _____

    B. _____

    C. _____

    D. _____

16. What is the most common age group receiving subacute care?

    _____

17. State at least three of the benefits of respiratory home care.

    A. _____

    B. _____

    C. _____

Now give three typical disease states that need our help.

D. _____

E. _____

F. _____

STANDARDS

18. Why does government play a major role in setting standards for the regulation of postacute care?

_____

19. What is the purpose of the Medicare Provider Certification Program?

20. Who is responsible for accreditation of companies that provide home care services?

_____

21. What are the two types of accreditation for respiratory home care?

_____

TRADITIONAL ACUTE CARE

22. What do RTs like about working in the postacute care setting?

23. Compare traditional and alternative settings in terms of the following areas (Table 51-1).

AREA	TRADITIONAL	ALTERNATIVE
A. Diagnostic tests		
B. Equipment		
C. Supervision		
D. Patient assessment		
E. Work schedule		
F. Time constraints		

24. Explain the role of the following practitioners in the postacute care team. (Refer to Table 51-2.)

    A. Utilization and review _____

    B. Social services _____

    C. Physical therapy _____

    D. Physiatrist _____

    E. DME supplier _____

25. How can you confirm that a nonprofessional caregiver is able to perform care?

    _____

26. Discuss items in the home environment that must be assessed prior to discharge. Check out Box 51-1 if you get stuck.

    A. Accessibility

    B. Equipment

    C. Environment

OXYGEN THERAPY

Oxygen is the most common mode of respiratory therapy used outside the hospital and the one that is tested the most, too!

27. Why do so many people use oxygen in alternative care settings in the United States?

    _____

28. State two of the documented benefits of long-term oxygen therapy.

    A. _____

    B. _____

29. Describe the six elements that must be included in a home oxygen prescription.

A. _____

B. _____

C. _____

D. _____

E. _____

F. _____

30. The AARC Clinical Practice Guidelines for Oxygen in the Home clearly states the indications for oxygen outside the acute care hospital. You MUST know this, so cough it up!

A. Adults, etc., >28 days $PaO_2 \leq$ _____ mm Hg, or $SaO_2 \leq$ _____

B. Cor pulmonale, CHF, or critical >56% $PaO_2 \leq$ _____ or

$SaO_2 \leq$ _____.

C. Ambulation, sleep, or exercise if SaO_2 falls below _____%.

Seriously, only these patients will qualify for O_2 outside the hospital in most cases. You are expected to know these criteria for your boards, so you can discharge patients and advise the staff. Remember, the home care folks cannot qualify the patients because it is a conflict of interest.

31. What are the two primary uses of compressed oxygen cylinders in the alternative setting?

A. E cylinder _____

B. H cylinder (or M) _____

32. How do flowmeters used in alternative settings differ from those used in the hospital?

_____

33. Let's compare the advantages and disadvantages of the oxygen supply systems available for use in alternative settings (see Table 51-3). If you can get this down, you will be a really useful RT who can participate in discharge planning and actually help your patients and your organization.

SYSTEM	ADVANTAGE	DISADVANTAGE
A. Cylinders		
1.		
2.		
B. Liquid		
1.		
2.		
C. Concentrator		
1.		
2.		

Chapter **51** **Respiratory Care in Alternative Settings**

34. Liquid oxygen is weighed to determine the amount available. If a patient was using 3 L/min with a 100-lb system that was one-fourth full, how many hours would the gas last? (See Table 51-4.)

35. Explain how an oxygen concentrator works. KISS.

36. What is the typical range of oxygen percentage a concentrator will supply?

   A. 1 to 2 L/min _____

   B. >5 L/min _____

37. What effect will the concentrator have on a patient's electrical bill? (Remember that money is a BIG issue for fixed-income elderly who are ill.)

   _____

38. Describe some of the methods for avoiding communication problems with patients receiving home oxygen therapy.

   _____

39. In addition to providing a backup supply, what other precautions should be taken in terms of concentrator power supply?

40. List at least four areas that should be evaluated when checking a home patient's oxygen concentrator.

   A. _____

   B. _____

   C. _____

   D. _____

41. When a patient is placed on an oxygen-conserving device, how would you determine the correct liter flow to use?

42. What actions should a patient who is wearing transtracheal oxygen take if he believes the catheter isn't working properly?

43. In theory, how would a demand flow oxygen-conserving system benefit the patient?

44. What are the two main drawbacks to demand flow systems?

45. In what situations should a patient or caregiver be instructed to alter the prescribed flow setting?

46. State the three main problems associated with insertion of the transtracheal catheter (see Box 51-4).

    A. _____

    B. _____

    C. _____

47. Describe the basic methods for avoiding complications of transtracheal catheters.

VENTILATORY SUPPORT

48. Give examples for each of the three main groups of patients who are placed on ventilators in the alternative care setting (see Table 51-5).

    A. Nocturnal ventilation

        1. _____

        2. _____

        3. _____

B. Continuous mechanical ventilation

    1. _____

    2. _____

    3. _____

C. Terminally ill

    1. _____

    2. _____

49. Identify the three common settings where ventilatory support is delivered outside the hospital.

    A. _____

    B. _____

    C. _____

50. Invasive long-term ventilation is always provided via what type of airway?

    _____

51. Describe the emergency situations a family must be able to deal with in caring for a home ventilator patient.

52. Identify at least three situations where NIV is partly contraindicated.

    A. _____

    B. _____

    C. _____

53. Identify at least three situations where NIV is absolutely contraindicated.

    A. _____

    B. _____

    C. _____

54. What options exist for patients who do not want invasive ventilation and cannot use NIV?

55. What options are available on invasive positive pressure ventilator systems during power failures, or if a patient wishes to be mobile?

_____

56. What is the biggest challenge associated with NIV?

_____

57. Identify the three basic types of negative pressure ventilators.

A. _____

B. _____

C. _____

OTHER MODES OF POSTACUTE RESPIRATORY CARE

58. What is the primary use of bland aerosols in the postacute setting?

59. What is the major problem with delivery of bland aerosols?

_____

60. What are the two limits on Medicare reimbursement for compressor-driven SVNs in the alternative setting?

A. _____

B. _____

61. How can you prevent bacterial growth on suction catheters that are used repeatedly?

_____

62. State three common clinical problems or patient complaints associated with SAHS.

A. _____

B. _____

C. _____

63. What is the primary treatment for this condition?

_____

64. What is the most common clinical problem with the CPAP apparatus?

_____

65. Discuss solutions to the common complaint of nasal dryness.

66. Apnea monitors alert parents or caregivers of what three serious signs? How long do they need the monitor?

   A. Condition _____

   B. Duration of monitoring _____

PATIENT ASSESSMENT AND DOCUMENTATION

67. Describe the main areas you would check during initial screening of a patient following admission to a postacute care facility.

68. What areas would be important to assess **besides** the usual vital signs and evaluation of the respiratory system?

69. How often should a member of the home care team perform a follow-up evaluation for patients receiving respiratory care treatments? What factors should be considered in determining the frequency of visits?

EQUIPMENT DISINFECTION AND MAINTENANCE

70. Describe the process for cleaning a home nebulizer (for example):

   A. _____

   B. _____

   C. _____

   D. _____

71. Describe the guidelines for using water in humidifiers and nebulizers.

72. What is the most important principle of infection control in the home setting?

PALLIATIVE CARE

73. According to the World Health Organization, palliative care involves control of what two debilitating symptoms?

    A. _____

    B. _____

74. What is hospice?

CASE STUDIES

Case 1

A 70-year-old with COPD is discharged with an order for home oxygen. The room air blood gas prior to discharge is:

pH	7.47
$PaCO_2$	33 mm Hg
PaO_2	62 mm Hg
SaO_2	92%

Medicare returns the CMN as disapproved on the basis that this patient does not meet the criteria for saturation of PO_2 for home oxygen.

75. Make an argument for keeping the patient on oxygen based on your knowledge of respiratory physiology. You won't find a clear answer in the text. (This is a real case and we did get reimbursement! Hint: What does the low $PaCO_2$ and high pH indicate?)

Case 2

A home care patient whom you are seeing uses an oxygen concentrator. He calls you to say that he doesn't think he is getting an adequate amount of flow from his cannula.

76. What are some possible causes of this problem?

77. What would you suggest the patient do to quickly check the cannula?

An active 49-year-old with α_1-antitrypsin deficiency is to be discharged with home oxygen. The prescription is for 2 L/min continuous oxygen.

78. What system would you recommend for this patient to use at home?

79. What about a portable system?

WHAT DOES THE NBRC SAY?

Home care is included in the rehabilitation section of the examination matrix. You can expect only a few questions. Usually these relate to cleaning or home oxygen. Here are some representative questions. Circle the answer.

80. A patient with a tracheostomy is to receive humidification via a nebulizer in his home. With regard to water for the nebulizer, which of the following would be the most appropriate choice for the home setting?
   1. Sterile distilled water should be obtained from the DME provider.
   2. Tap water is sufficient for the home setting if the nebulizer is cleaned properly.
   3. Bottled water can be used as long as it is distilled.
   4. Tap water that is boiled may be used for up to 24 hours.
      A. 1 and 3
      B. 1 and 4
      C. 2 and 3
      D. 2 and 4

81. Which of the following actions would an RT perform during the monthly check of a home oxygen concentrator system?
   1. replacement of the silica pellets in the sieve bed
   2. analysis of the F_iO_2 delivered by the concentrator
   3. filter replacement
   4. evaluation of the concentrator's electrical system
      A. 1 and 2
      B. 2 and 3
      C. 1 and 4
      D. 3 and 4

82. A patient who is wearing a transtracheal oxygen catheter suddenly becomes dyspneic. The first action the patient should take would be to _____.
   A. call the physician
   B. clean the catheter
   C. increase the oxygen flow to the catheter
   D. remove the catheter and proceed to the emergency department

83. A patient who is using oxygen at home occasionally needs to go out for health care appointments. What type of portable system would you recommend for this patient?
   A. E cylinder with standard flowmeter
   B. E cylinder with conserving device
   C. small liquid oxygen reservoir
   D. Patients can go out for short periods without supplemental oxygen.

84. A respiratory care practitioner determines that a cuirass-type negative pressure ventilator is now reading a pressure of −20 cm H_2O, when it should be cycling at −35 cm H_2O. The patient is in no distress, but the measured tidal volume is 200 ml lower than the desired volume. The practitioner should _____.
   A. begin manual ventilation of the patient
   B. check for leaks in the system
   C. increase the vacuum setting
   D. increase the amount of air in the cuff

FOOD FOR THOUGHT

Concentrators have changed dramatically in the last few years.

85. Discuss the special features of these two high-tech sieves.
   A. Respironics Millenium M10

   B. Inogen One